# HEALTH SYSTEMS RESEARCH

Edited by W. van Eimeren

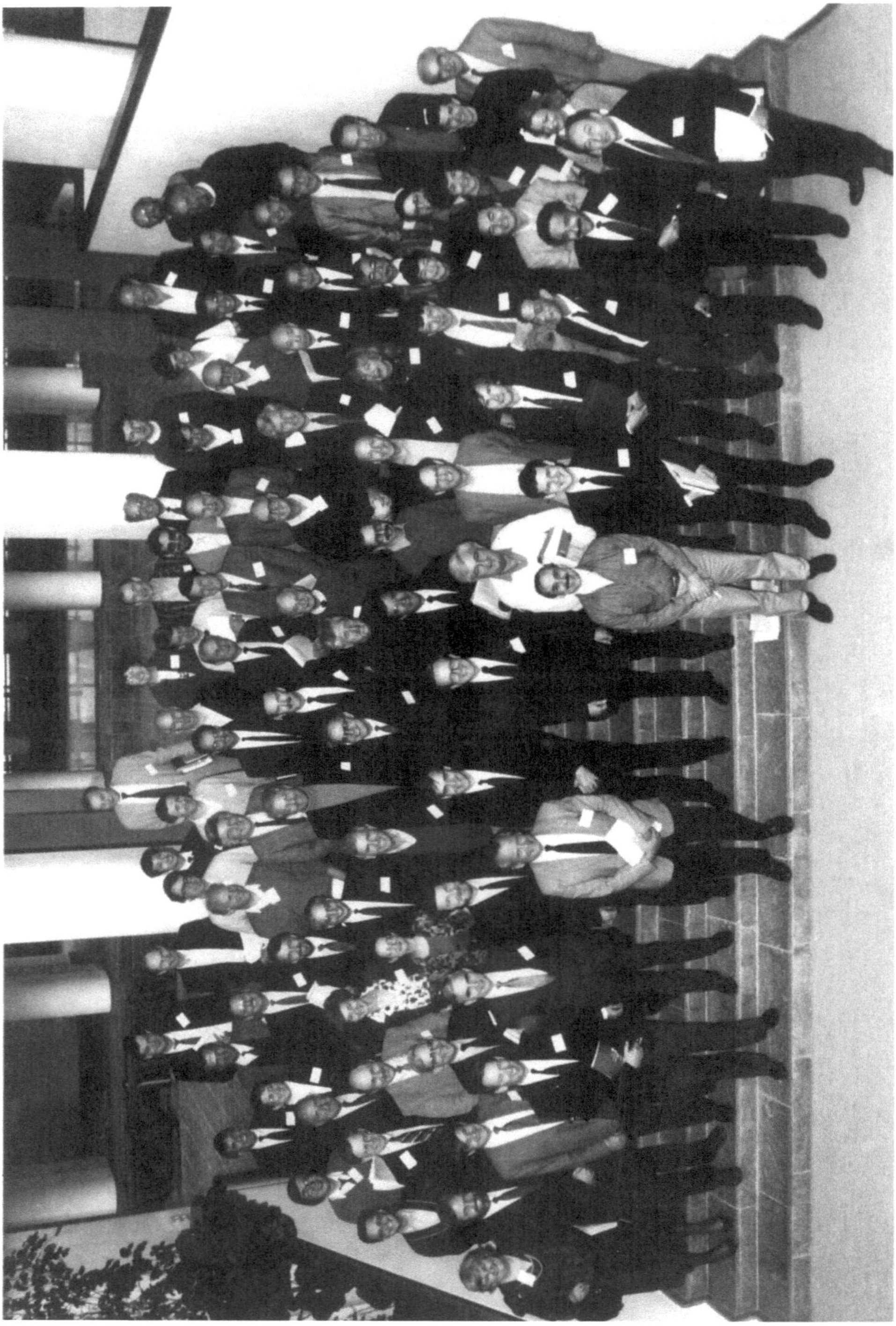

R. Dinkel B. Horisberger K. Tolo (Eds.)

# Improving Drug Safety – A Joint Responsibility

With 35 Figures and 21 Tables

Springer-Verlag
Berlin Heidelberg New York London
Paris Tokyo Hong Kong Barcelona

Dr. Rolf Dinkel
HealthEcon Ltd.
Steinentorstr. 19
CH-4051 Basel

Dr. Bruno Horisberger
Interdisciplinary Research Centre
for Public Health
Rorschacher Strasse 103c
CH-9007 St. Gallen

Prof. Kenneth W. Tolo
The University of Texas at Austin
Main Building 201
USA-Austin, Texas 78702

ISBN-13: 978-3-642-64762-8 e-ISBN-13: 978-3-642-61250-3
DOI: 10.1007/978-3-642-61250-3



Softcover reprint of the hardcover 1st edition 1991



2119/3140/543210 – Printed on acid-free paper

# Preface

As the focus on pharmaceuticals has broadened from concern for their cost and effectiveness to their real and potential risks and benefits, a critical question has been raised: whose responsibility is it to improve drug safety? In April 1990, this question became the theme for a conference at Wolfsberg, Switzerland, near the shores of Lake Constance. Called an "international dialogue conference" by its organizers, the meeting brought together leaders from the pharmaceutical industry, regulatory authorities, academia, medicine, consumer organizations and the media. Opening addresses were given by representatives of the Council for International Organizations of Medical Sciences (CIOMS), the International Federation of Pharmaceutical Manufacturers Associations (IFPMA), the Swiss International Pharmaceutical Agency, and the RAD-AR Consortium.

This book documents the papers presented and discussions held at this conference, which took the topic of risks and benefits of drug therapy one step further to responsibility. It includes a rich menu of issues for those who care about the evaluation of drug therapy, the ethics behind it, the expectations of the patient, and the role of traditional and nontraditional drug safety communications. The ideas expressed here come from different parts of the world but relate to common drug safety problems, observations, and scientific assessments; they provide insights into innovative approaches, cautious changes, and desired actions.

The papers in this volume are broadly divided into conceptual perspectives (ethics, how the knowledge about drug risks and benefits is generated and appraised, the expectations in drug safety) and operational perspectives (communication, discussion, and action).

The ethical perspectives in Parts III and XII come not only from academia and the World Health Organization but also from the pharmaceutical industry. Parts IV and V look at the generation of knowledge on drug risks and benefits from the view of national regulators, medical researchers, and an epidemiologist.

The complexities of assessment of the risk/benefit relationship are discussed in Part VI and the challenges are pointed out time and again. There are distortions, differing scientific evaluations, and personal judgments to be taken into consideration, as well as cultural influences.

Expectations in drug safety communication, of the media, the patient, the pharmacologist and the regulator, are all mentioned in Part VII. Some traditional channels of drug safety communications are discussed in Part VIII, while more innovative channels are described in Part IX. A special section (Part X) is devoted to the program for Risk/Benefit Assessment of Drugs – Analysis and Response (RAD-AR) in the USA, Europe, and Japan.

It became clear through the conference and the papers presented that an agenda for action is needed. One set of future directions is described in Part XIII. It is followed by the Wolfsberg Think Pieces, which were set out at the conclusion of the 1990 conference and which show how the leaders from various countries and fields of work viewed specific drug safety issues and how they thought responsibility for improving the situation could be shared.

The editors drew from about 50 manuscripts and countless pages of transcripted discussions from plenary sessions and workshops to compile a representative picture of the conference proceedings. They attempted to convey specific problems in an interdisciplinary dialogue without becoming mired in jargon and technicalities of the experts' knowledge. There was no space for a full-scale report on all the discussions that followed the presentation of the individual keynote addresses, the papers, and the working group reports. Nevertheless, we hope those who were present will find we have preserved the essence of the 1990 Wolfsberg meeting in this publication. What participants carried home with them in the way of contacts and insights has perhaps preserved and conveyed this even better.

Drug safety has become an area which decision makers realize must be open to complete and knowledgeable evaluation. More than that, some industry leaders at Wolfsberg maintained that good drugs mean good business. That comes close to what consumers are hoping for. Physicians and other health practitioners should be able to offer nothing less than good drugs, knowledge of their full capacity, and instruction on how to use them wisely.

# Contents

## *Part III: Ethical Perspectives*



## *Part IV: Generating Knowledge About Drug Risks*



## *Part V: Generating Knowledge About Drug Benefits*

## *Part VI: Assessing the Risk/Benefit Relationship*



## *Part VII: Expections in Drug Safety Communication*

## *Part XIII: An Agenda for Action*



## *Appendix*

# Participants

Frank Amon
Schering AG, Berlin, FRG

Dr. Richard B. Arnold
International Federation of Pharmaceutical Manufacturers Associations (IFPMA), Geneva, Switzerland

Prof. Paul Arntson
Northwestern University, Evanston, ILL, USA

Robert M. Bachmann
National Council on Patient Information and Education, Washington, DC, USA

Prof. Zbigniew Bankowski
Council for International Organizations of Medical Sciences (CIOMS), Geneva, Switzerland

Malcolm Barlow
SmithKline Beecham, Philadelphia, PA, USA

Dr. John F. Beary
Pharmaceutical Manufacturers Association (PMA), Washington, DC, USA

Dr. Bernard Bégaud
Centre de Pharmacovigilance Hôpital Pellegrin, Bordeaux, France

Dr. Christine Bergmann
Institut für Arzneimittelwesen, Berlin, GDR

Dr. Kamel Besseghir
Ares Serono, Geneva, Switzerland

Annette Bopp
Freelance Journalist, Hamburg, FRG

Dr. Dieter Bothe
Hoffmann-La Roche & Co. AG, Basle, Switzerland

Prof. Chris J. van Boxtel
University of Amsterdam, Amsterdam, Netherlands

Prof. Hans Harald Bräutigam
Die Zeit, Hamburg, FRG

Andreas Breitsprecher
Ciba-Geigy, Basle, Switzerland

Prof. Rudolf Bruppacher
Ciba-Geigy, Basle, Switzerland

Dr. Urs M. Bucher
Interpharma, Basle, Switzerland

Karin Buechner
HealthEcon AG, Basle, Switzerland

Dr. Dennis Burley
Centre for Pharmaceutical Medicine, Woking, Surrey, England

Dr. Erol Caglarcan
Action Policy Group, Duxbury, MA, USA

Peter Carpenter
Consultant in Public Communication, Atherton, CA, USA

Dr. Win Castle
Glaxo Group Research Ltd., Greenford, Middlesex, England

Dr. Diane Chen-Koch-Weser
F. Hoffmann-La Roche & Co. AG, Basle, Switzerland

Dr. Jill Dawson
Financial Times, London, England

Dr. Rolf Dinkel
HealthEcon AG, Basle, Switzerland

Jack Domeischel
G.D. Searle & Co., Chicago, ILL, USA

Dr. Jens Drolshammer
Lawyer, Zurich, Switzerland

Dr. Stanley A. Edlavitch
McGill University, Montreal, Canada

Prof. I. Ralph Edwards
Otago Medical School, Dunedin, New Zealand

Dr. Arthur Emmett
Ciba-Geigy, Summit, NJ, USA

Dr. G.A. Faich
Food and Drug Administration, Rockville, MD, USA

David Finer
Freelance Journalist, Stockholm, Sweden

MICHAEL FOLEY
Michael Foley Associates, Geneva, Switzerland

Prof. FERENC FOLLATH
Kantonsspital Basel, Basle, Switzerland

Prof. GEORGES M. FÜLGRAFF
Scientific Counselor and member of several committees in the European Community and FRG, Berlin, FRG

Prof. J.P. GIROUD
University Hospital Port Royal, Paris, France

Dr. ARNOLD J. GORDON
Pfizer, New York, NY, USA

Prof. SAMUEL GOROVITZ
Syracuse University, Syracuse, NY, USA

Dr. ETZEL GYSLING
Journalist, Wil, St. Gallen, Switzerland

Dr. J. HAAS
Boehringer Ingelheim GmbH, Ingelheim/Rhein, FRG

Dr. GILLIAN HALL
VAMP Health Ltd., London, England

Dr. T.B. HART
ICI Pharmaceuticals, Macclesfield, Cheshire, England

Dr. DAVID A. HENRY
Royal Newcastle Hospital, Newcastle, NSW, Australia

Dr. BRUNO HORISBERGER
Interdisciplinary Research Centre for Public Health, St. Gallen, Switzerland

G.W. VAN DEN HURK
Swiss Re-Insurance, Zurich, Switzerland

MICHAEL JEFFRIES
Journalist, Radnage, Bucks, England

Prof. JUDITH JONES
Degge Group, Arlington, VA, USA

KANYI KANEYUKI
Sankyo Co. Ltd., Tokyo, Japan

Dr. K.H. KIMBEL
Arzneimittelkommission der Deutschen Ärzteschaft, Cologne, FRG

STEPHEN KLAIDMANN
Georgetown University, Washington, DC, USA

Goro Koide
Nippon Broadcasting Corp., Tokyo, Japan

Dr. Juergen Krause
Goedecke AG, Freiburg, FRG

Prof. Gottfried Kreutz
Institut für Arzneimittel des Bundesgesundheitsamtes, Berlin, FRG

Dr. Peter Lauper
Ciba-Geigy, Basle, Switzerland

Prof. Klaus M. Leisinger
Ciba-Geigy, Basle, Switzerland

Guenter Lewandowski
Ciba-Geigy, Basle, Switzerland

Prof. William Lowrance
Rockefeller University, New York, NY, USA

Dr. Bryan R. Luce
Battelle, Washington, DC, USA

Prof. Nathan Maccoby
Stanford University, Palo Alto, CA, USA

Dr. Ronald D. Mann
The Royal Society of Medicine, London, England

Dr. R.H.B. Meyboom
Staatstoezicht op de Volksgezondheid, Rijswijk, Netherlands

Dr. Louis A. Morris
Food and Drug Administration, Rockville, MD, USA

Thomas Mueller
Basler Zeitung, Basle, Switzerland

Hisao Nakagawa
Ministry of Health and Welfare, Tokyo, Japan

Dr. Hassan Nour-Eldin
Hoechst AG, Frankfurt, FRG

Dr. Yasuo Ohashi
University of Tokyo, Tokyo, Japan

Akio Ohsawa
Ciba-Geigy, Takarazuka, Japan

Dr. Marisa Papaluca
Ministero della Sanità, Rome, Italy

Dr. Gwen Parr
Ciba-Geigy, Horsham, West Sussex, England

Dr. J.G. TEN PAS
Ciby-Geigy, Arnhem, Netherlands

Dr. JEAN PFANNER
Interkantonale Kontrollstelle für Heilmittel (IKS), Bern, Switzerland

Dr. ROBBERT A. PIEKE
AKZO / Organon International B.V., Oss, Netherlands

Dr. ERWIN RAHNER
Boehringer Ingelheim GmbH, Ingelheim/Rhein, FRG

Dr. BRUCE ROWSELL
Bureau of Pharmaceutical Surveillance, Ottawa, Canada

Dr. H. SCHULTE-SASSE
Kliniken der Freien Hansestadt Bremen, Bremen, FRG

PETER SIMON
F. Hoffmann-La Roche & Co. AG, Basle, Switzerland

MICHAEL SONNENREICH
Sonnenreich & Roccograndi P.C., Washington, DC, USA

Prof. WALTER O. SPITZER
McGill University, Montreal, Canada

Prof. KJELL STRANDBERG
National Board of Health and Welfare Department of Drugs, Uppsala, Sweden

TETSUO TAKEUCHI
Yamanouchi Pharmaceutical Co. Ltd., Tokyo, Japan

Prof. YASUMASA TANAKA
Gakushuin University, Tokyo, Japan

Dr. DAVID TAYLOR
Ciba-Geigy, Takarazuka, Japan

Prof. KENNETH TOLO
The Lyndon B. Johnson School of public affairs the University of Texas at Austin

Prof. DIONISIOS VARONOS
National Drug Organization (EOF), Athens, Greece

Dr. ROBERT VANDER STICHELE
State University of Gent, Gent, Belgium

Dr. JAN WILLEM VAN DER VELDEN
Duphar B.V., Weesp, Netherlands

Dr. ROBERT VERMEULEN
Janssen Pharmaceuticals N.V., Beerse, Belgium

Dr. Ursula Versteegen
Ciba-Geigy, Basle, Switzerland

Hans R. van der Voort
AKZO/Organon International B.V., Oss, Netherlands

Prof. Stuart R. Walker
Centre for Medicines Research, Carshalton, Surrey, England

Prof. Yongming Wang
Shanghai Medical University, Shanghai, People's Republic of China

Prof. Walter P. von Wartburg
Ciba-Geigy, Basle, Switzerland

Katharine Whitehorn
The Patients' Association, London, England

Dr. B.E. Wiholm
National Board of Health and Welfare, Uppsala, Sweden

Richard Williams
Ciba-Geigy, Basle, Switzerland

Prof. Ernlé W.D. Young
Stanford University Centre for Biomedical Ethics, Palo Alto, CA, USA

Susan Youngren
International Life Sciences Institute (ILSI), Washington, DC, USA

# Affiliations of Participants

## Academic Institutions and Hospitals

| | |
|---|---|
| Gakushuin University | Tokyo, Japan |
| Georgetown University | Washington DC, USA |
| Hôpital Pellegrin | Bordeaux, France |
| Kantonsspital Basel | Basle, Switzerland |
| Kliniken der Freien Hansestadt Bremen | Bremen, FRG |
| McGill University | Montreal, Canada |
| Northwestern University | Evanston, ILL, USA |
| Otago Medical School | Dunedin, New Zealand |
| Rockefeller University | New York, NY, USA |
| Royal Newcastle Hospital | Newcastle, NSW, Australia |
| Shanghai Medical University | Shanghai, China |
| Stanford University | Palo Alto, CA, USA |
| State University of Gent | Gent, Belgium |
| Syracuse University | Syracuse NY, USA |
| The Royal Society of Medicine | London, England |
| University Hospital Port Royal | Paris, France |
| University of Amsterdam | Amsterdam, Netherlands |
| University of Texas | Austin, TX, USA |
| University of Tokyo | Tokyo, Japan |

## Regulatory Authorities

| | |
|---|---|
| Arzneimittelkommission der Deutschen Ärzteschaft | Cologne, FRG |
| Bureau of Pharmaceutical Surveillance | Ottawa, Canada |
| National Drug Organization (EOF) | Athens, Greece |
| Food and Drug Administration | Rockville, MD, USA |
| Institut für Arzneimittelwesen | Berlin, GDR |
| Institut für Arzneimittel des Bundesgesundheitsamtes | Berlin, FRG |

| | |
|---|---|
| Interkantonale Kontrollstelle für Heilmittel (IKS) | Bern, Switzerland |
| Ministero della Sanità | Rome, Italy |
| Ministry of Health and Welfare | Tokyo, Japan |
| National Board of Health and Welfare | Uppsala, Sweden |
| Staatstoezicht op de Volksgezondheid | Rijkswijk, Netherlands |

**Pharmaceutical Manufacturers**

| | |
|---|---|
| AKZO/Organon International B.V. | Oss, Netherlands |
| Ares Serono | Geneva, Switzerland |
| Boehringer Ingelheim GmbH | Ingelheim/Rhein, FRG |
| Ciba-Geigy | Arnhem, Netherlands<br>Basle, Switzerland<br>Horsham, West Sussex, England<br>Summit, NJ, USA<br>Takarazuka, Japan |
| Duphar B.V. | Weesp, Netherlands |
| Glaxo Group Research Ltd. | Greenford, Middlesex, England |
| Goedecke AG | Freiburg, FRG |
| Hoechst AG | Frankfurt, FRG |
| F.Hoffmann-La Roche & Co. AG | Basle, Switzerland |
| ICI Pharmaceuticals | Maccelesfield, Cheshire, England |
| Interpharma | Basle, Switzerland |
| Janssen Pharmaceuticals N.V. | Beerse, Belgium |
| Pfizer | New York, NY, USA |
| Pharmaceutical Manufacturers Association (PMA) | Washington, DC, USA |
| Sankyo Co. Ltd. | Tokyo, Japan |
| Schering AG | Berlin, FRG |
| G.D. Searle & Co. | Chicago, ILL, USA |
| SmithKline Beecham | Philadelphia, PA, USA |
| Yamanouchi Pharmaceutical Co. Ltd. | Tokyo, Japan |

**International Organizations**

| | |
|---|---|
| Council for International Organizations of Medical Sciences (CIOMS) | Geneva, Switzerland |
| International Federation of Pharmaceutical Manufacturers Associations (IFPMA) | Geneva, Switzerland |

## Health, Research, and Consumer Institutions

| | |
|---|---|
| Action Policy Group | Duxbury, MA, USA |
| Battelle | Washington, DC, USA |
| Centre for Medicines Research | Carshalton, Surrey, England |
| Centre for Pharmaceutical Medicine | Woking, Surrey, England |
| Degge Group | Arlington, VA, USA |
| HealthEcon | Basle, Switzerland |
| Interdisciplinary Research Centre for Public Health | St. Gallen, Switzerland |
| International Life Sciences Institute | Washington, DC, USA |
| National Council on Patient Information and Education | Washington, DC, USA |
| Sonnenreich & Roccograndi P.C. | Washington, DC, USA |
| Swiss Re-Insurance | Zurich, Switzerland |
| The Patients' Association | London, England |

## Media and Public Relations

| | |
|---|---|
| Basler Zeitung | Basle, Switzerland |
| Die Zeit | Hamburg, FRG |
| Financial Times | London, England |
| Michael Foley Associates | Geneva, Switzerland |
| Nippon Broadcasting Corporation | Tokyo, Japan |
| Pharma-Kritik | St. Gallen, Switzerland |
| The Three Pigeons | Radnage, Bucks, England |

# Part I

# The Wolfsberg Dialogue

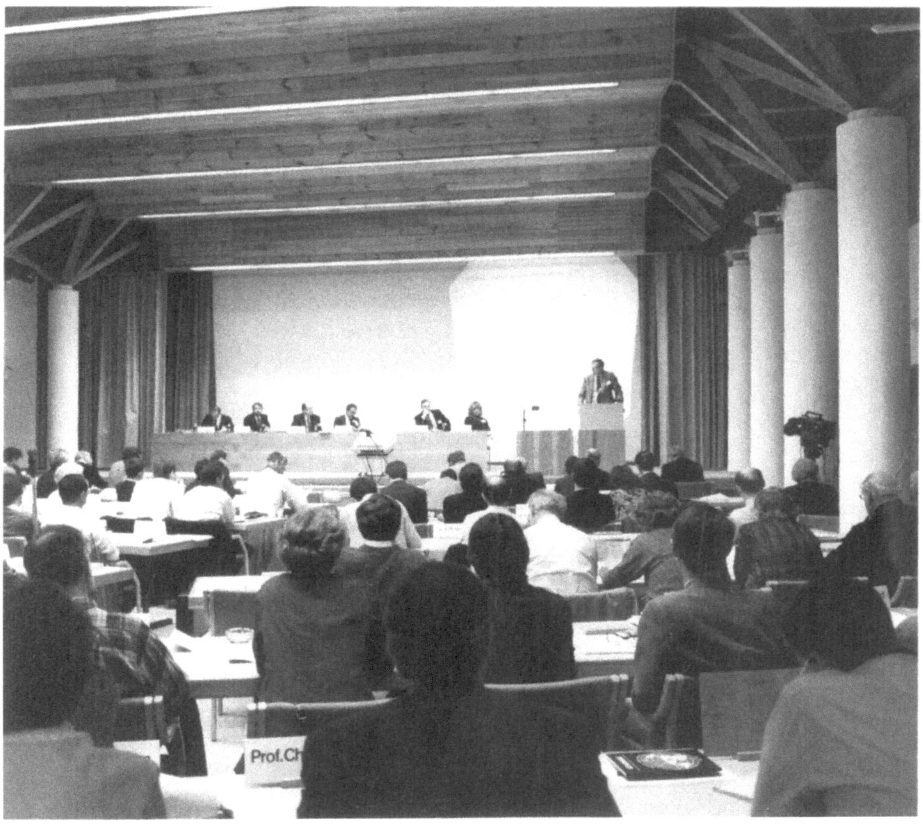

# 1. From Questions to Missions and Actions

The 1990 meeting in Wolfsberg, Switzerland, was neither the beginning nor the end of an international effort to understand the risks and benefits of pharmaceutical products. It was, rather, a further step in a process to improve drug safety and the health of people throughout the world.

For over a decade, Wolfsberg has served as a setting for international exchanges on health care issues. In 1979, the conference center hosted a meeting on cost sharing in health care. Among the topics covered were consumer participation in decision making, and how health standards and efficiency in health care spending could both be improved. The seminar attempted to evaluate the impact of cost-sharing policies on trends in health care services, and it also compared the expectations of individuals as consumers of, and as payers for, health care services.

In 1982, Wolfsberg was the site for a meeting on the economic and medical evaluation of health care technologies, including drugs. The World Health Organization provided assistance at this conference, both technical assistance and support in setting up the dialogue between the medical profession, economists, and the producers. Then, in 1987, the Wolfsberg conference theme was the "Socioeconomic Evaluation of Drug Therapy." At that time, the medical profession was still reluctant to adopt or even to accept socioeconomic evaluation techniques; the prevalent presumption in much of the world was that the medical profession had both the skills and the knowledge to decide what was best for the patients. The rationale of good medical practice seemed to be based on a set of expectations expressed by the public, elaborated by the media, and articulated by the medical opinion leaders. The 1987 conference participants, however, concluded that safety-related, efficiency-related, and cost/benefit-related information was an integral part of good medical practice and could improve doctors' decision making.

Responding to the changing orientation, the 1988 Wolfsberg meeting focused on "The Perception and Management of Drug Safety Risks." This shift in focus from cost/benefit to risk/benefit concerns was not surprising. The public had become increasingly active in its efforts, and demands, to have a say in drug safety issues. Leaders from the pharmaceutical industry, academia, medicine, and the media realized that progress was likely to occur only if a means were developed to bring the various opinion leaders together. These leaders needed an overview of the status quo, feedback from people with scientific and practical experience with drugs, and some insight into patient concern. They needed clear definitions of some very central issues in order to identify the problems and the public's perceptions about them. For these leaders, Wolfsberg provided one important mechanism, a forum for dialogue; it was clear that other initiatives would be needed.

From the 1988 conference the Wolfsberg Questions emerged, which focused on risk analysis, risk perception, risk communication, risk/benefit appraisal, and risk management. Through their formulation of these questions, participants educated themselves on concepts and concerns in each other's fields, shared some of their own knowledge, and began to pin down the important problems. They gave attention to the scientific side, especially pharmacology and epidemiology, as well as to the communication side, which emerged as more important than many had originally perceived.

Risk analysis concerns expressed during the 1988 conference centered on the consistency of methodologies used, including what could be done to improve the existing adverse drug reaction reporting systems. The problem of defining risk perception and assessing its effects also troubled the 1988 participants, as did the issues of informing physicians, patients, and the public about risk, and of communicating drug risk and benefit information to the media. Drug regulatory authorities, physicians, patients, and the public shared their different views of how to weigh drug risks against drug benefits. The topic of risk management was animatedly discussed, and the means by which manufacturers could improve the drug risk/benefit ratio was of great interest throughout the discussions.

These concerns were all covered in the Wolfsberg Questions. The questions were taken home, internationally, and had two years to be debated, refined, extended, and considered from all sides. The 1990 Wolfsberg conference picked up the momentum generated in 1988 and sought to build upon it. Experts from academia, government, media, industry, medicine and international health and consumer organizations met at Wolfsberg again. They now had a mission: to take the knowledge gained at and since the 1988 conference, to apply it to the drug safety problems within their means, and to share the responsibility for finding and implementing solutions.

The 1990 Wolfsberg conference participants were committed to an open dialogue about ethics and drug safety, about generating and communicating knowledge on drug risks and benefits, about the patient's rights and responsibilities, and what makes good drugs and good business. The issue was no longer how risks and benefits of drugs should be defined and discussed, but what can be done about them, what action is needed, and who is going to take the initiative.

The men and women who gathered at Wolfsberg in 1990 are aware that the public is unlikely to let them forget their mission. They also have enough knowledge and insight to know just how complex and difficult their task is. Sharing the responsibility to improve drug safety is critical if effective action is to be taken.

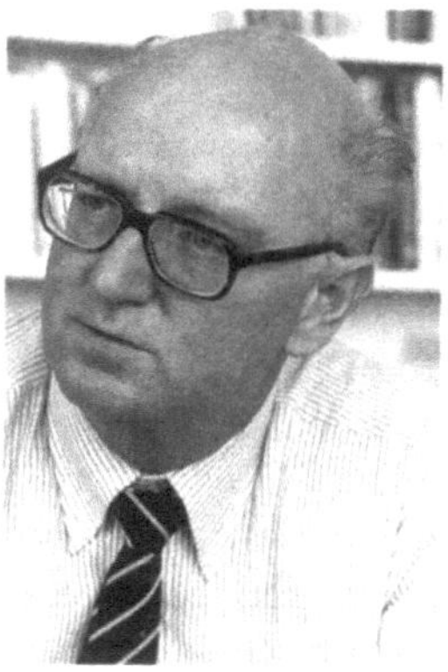

# 2. The RAD-AR Agenda

W. P. von Wartburg

Exactly 2 years before the 1990 conference and in the same setting, some 25 pharmaceutical manufacturers and a number of journalists assembled for a Wolfsberg conference which resulted in the formulation of an initiative. We believed that industry had a responsibility to improve drug safety for the benefit of the public. In 1990 the second Wolfsberg conference on drug safety welcomed not only members of the pharmaceutical industry but representatives from regulatory authorities, academia, the medical professions, the media, patients, and the public. These groups were represented here by delegates from all over the world. There were participants not only from the United States, Japan, and Europe, including one from the German Democratic Republic, but also from Australia and the People's Republic of China.

In the initial stages of trying to establish an agenda for this meeting, we were in favor of a consensus conference. However, it soon became clear that a consensus must be preceded by searching discussion. Accordingly, we shifted the focus and decided on a dialogue conference. Before the dialogue is presented in the following chapters, I would like to provide a little background on the RAD-AR initiative. RAD-AR stands for Risk/Benefit Assessment of Drugs, Analysis and Response. The objective of RAD-AR is to enhance drug safety through improved understanding and communication of the relationship between risks and benefits.

One of the factors which defined the need for such an initiative was society's growing concern about risks in general. Salmonella in eggs, hormones in poultry, listeria in cheese, and pesticides in drinking water are just some of the problems that people are confronted with in their daily lives. Often, however, the concern expressed is disproportionate to the actual risk involved. Nobody knows how to quantify the risk and decide whether it is acceptable or not.

Risk is, I believe, an aspect of a healthy society, but it is one that must be dealt with wisely. If we are inundated with risks, it is difficult to discriminate between those which are more or less severe. It is in this context that drug risks enter the scene. There is an increasing awareness in large segments of the population of the risks of pharmaceuticals. Although we are interested primarily in the benefits, we must also acknowledge that no effective drug comes without its attendant risks.

Traditionally, drugs are perceived as being largely risk-free. Those who are involved in producing, regulating, and prescribing drugs are aware of the existence of adverse drug reactions, but this awareness does not extend to the general public. These differing perceptions of drug safety determine, in turn, how drug risk is qualified and quantified. An acceptable level of risk is increasingly a question of politics, not just a question of how many mice have reacted in a particular way in a toxicological experiment. Growing risk awareness on the part of the authorities and the public begs a number of responses. It must be understood that there is no efficacy without the risk of side effects. However, those risks should be assessed in relation to the benefits they bring. It must further be understood that actual risk and the way the public perceive it are often at variance.

The evidence to support these statements must be found through action. This can take the form of comparative studies. The risks of drug therapy, for example, should be compared with the risks of nontreated disease or with the risks of medical intervention, such as surgery. Such studies have rarely been undertaken. Epidemiological studies are needed to improve assessment of risk in drug therapy on a worldwide scale. Risk perception studies such as these have already started but need to be implemented on a broader scale. In these ways, the RAD-AR multicompany program is a response by its various partners to the increasing awareness of risk.

We have always said that RAD-AR activities should be international in scope, and this stems from the fact that drug safety issues are increasingly international in their nature. Adverse drug reaction reports and epidemiological studies that are done on a national scale are recorded internationally almost immediately. Consumer organizations voice their concern through international networks; the media, likewise, operate in a global village, and regulatory authorities also act in consultation with other nations. This indicates a response to the internationalization of all the drugs that are marketed on a worldwide scale.

The basic purpose of RAD-AR, as defined in Wolfsberg in 1988, was to initiate an international exchange of experience concerning drug safety issues; to improve measures for the prevention and containment of drug safety problems; and to find unified approaches in furthering the discipline of pharmacoepidemiology. Progress has been made. The recent formation of the International Society for Pharmacoepidemiology came partly as a result of the RAD-AR initiative. We now have a stronger voice and more "critical mass" in communicating drug safety issues, and there is a network of parties concerned with drug safety in the making.

The RAD-AR agenda since 1988 has included a string of meetings in London, Washington, Tokyo, Basle, New York, Talloires, and Geneva. All of these were part of a step-by-step program that has involved many working parties in a growing number of countries. The momentum for these activities has been maintained by increasing concern about safety issues. I am convinced that, in a similar way to the cost containment issue that came to the fore 7 or 8 years ago and is now of worldwide importance, the risk management issue will increase, not decrease, in importance. In view of this, we would all be well advised to redouble our efforts in this area.

To put risk into a manageable context, it must be seen as an aspect of society's evolution. It is present in nature and likewise in the whole history of man. Risk and risk taking are also ingredients of innovation. Creativity entails risk. Research implies the risk of failure. In this way, risk is an essential part of human solidarity. Some take risks so that others may benefit. As I said before, society needs to consider risk management carefully, so that it can assure its future by concentrating on what is important and not worry fruitlessly. If we look at risk and therapeutic progress, we see the same pattern. Evolution in medicine, as in society, often implies risk. In this case, the risk is to patients, whether it is in placebo-controlled, double-blind clinical trials, innovative surgical techniques, or unexpected adverse drug reactions. This is a factor of the evolution of medicine, and we must simply learn to live with it and adapt to it as best we can.

Clearly, there are also ethical dimensions of risk in medicine. How much protection, for example, is enough? To what extent should society be protected from certain risks related to medicine? How can risks be distributed fairly? Should they be distributed so that one part of the population is subjected to them while another receives the benefits, or can the two be linked in certain populations? Do we live in a society which is paternalistically organized, where somebody tells us which risks we should or should not take? Or do we live in a society which is structured around freedom of choice, where people, on the basis of what they know or of their own free will take certain risks, even in therapeutics?

When talking about risk management, there are three crucial elements to be considered: analysis, assessment, and communication. Drug-related risks to the public health must first be analyzed. How is this done with reporting systems? Risks must then be assessed. What kind of value judgments are brought to bear on this process? Finally, the results must be communicated to the medical professions and the public in a way that can be clearly understood. Only if these three phases of analysis, assessment, and communication are followed through can one talk about proper risk management. The process of proper management requires the participation of the industry, medical professions, regulatory authorities, and the media, as well as that of patients and the general public.

When trying to identify risks during the analytical process, we can point to a great deal of premarketing testing. Animal testing can provide data on such factors such as toxicity, mutagenicity, and teratogenicity. Such data, however, can give no reliable evidence on the risk of adverse drug reactions which may show up later on. We have only limited information on the risk of unexpected side effects by the time a drug comes on the market and is being prescribed to patients. This indicates that we need ways of identifying drug risks after the approval process. Monitoring systems that are particularly intensive in their scope during the first few years go a long way towards fulfilling this need. A number of ways to quantify drug risks after regulatory approval do exist. There are systems for spontaneous reporting of adverse drug reactions. There are epidemiological data banks. Experimental or observation-based prospective studies can be carried out, as can case-controlled studies.

Having identified the risks, one must ask what are the benefits. One cannot talk about risk, and the acceptance of appropriate levels of risk, without balancing it against the benefits of medical intervention. These benefits may be of a social, medical, or even an economic nature. In addition to proving the medical benefits, there is also a growing need for the kind of clinical evidence based on quality-of-life studies, cost/benefit studies, and cost/effectiveness studies. These types of social and economic data have to be taken into consideration on the benefits side. This continuous process of evaluation should take place at the levels of the manufacturer, the physician, the regulatory authority, and the patient. It implies a weighing up process that culminates in an assessment of the risk/benefit relationship of a specific drug from the perspective of the decision maker involved.

Benefits and risks of alternative treatments should also be taken into consideration, as well as the degree of risk awareness or risk acceptance present in the people exposed to a drug. We all have different values and priorities, and if one goes beyond the medical boundaries and looks into the legal, social, and ethical dimensions, these differences become more marked.

If a judgment on the risks and benefits has been made and if the relationship between the two elements has been assessed, then the next priority is to communicate the results, not only to the medical profession but also to the other parties involved in the process. Communication of facts is the basis upon which informed choices can be made and erroneous perceptions changed. Effective communication is, I believe, the key to risk acceptance and management by patients and the general public. If we take a close look at the extent of communication that exists between the medical profession and patients, as well as between the industry and the medical professions or regulatory authorities, we will quickly see that the need to generate new data to assess the risk/benefit relationship is parallelled by the need to improve communication to all those groups concerned with drug safety.

Trends in medical communication are changing as a result of a changing health environment. They show a move from old publics, represented by the medical professions, the scientific communities, and regulatory authorities, to encompass new publics that include patients, society at large, politicians, the media, and consumer representatives. The second group will not replace the first, but it has staked its claim to better health-related information. This trend is also characterized by calls for more patient-oriented information phrased in simpler, more accessible language, in contrast to the expert, scientific language currently employed. Finally, there is a shift from old behavior which is reactive and selective, to new behavior which is pro-active, involving collective communication and dialogue, as opposed to monologue.

If we believe in these trends and support them, I am convinced we will achieve better understanding and management of the ever-present risk/benefit relationship of drugs. The medical professions will benefit from better routine and spontaneous reporting of adverse drug reactions. We will have greater quantities of data which will permit us to make rational choices and judgments.

Manufacturers will have to adopt a more open position regarding adverse drug reactions, and communicate their findings in a pro-active way, updating patient package information as necessary.

For the regulatory authorities, better management means establishing a mandatory reporting system and being more open about its results. They should also aspire to find the optimal level of acceptable drug risk, instead of leaving no risks in medical hands. For the media, it will mean aiming at more comprehensive factual reporting of relative risks and benefits, rather than concentrating on the risks and blowing them out of proportion. It will also mean avoiding overly sensational stories that might mislead patients into stopping a course of treatment or into taking drugs that are more dangerous for the individual. Finally, for patients it will mean the possibility of more informed choice, not just informed consent but access to information leading to choice. All of the above will optimize the rational use of drugs from which we benefit.

As I said at the beginning, I had hoped that the 1990 Wolfsberg meeting would be a consensus conference, but I was probably being too demanding in that respect. Instead, the conference participants entered into a dialogue with the hope that it would pave the way towards a consensus for action. Representatives of all the important parties in drug safety were assembled, including manufacturers, members of the media, academics, representatives from many branches of the medical profession and regulatory authorities, as well as consumer representatives. Together they worked to identify the various expectations and needs we have in this complex area of drug safety. They also worked toward formulating an agenda reflecting a continuing dialogue for understanding, mutual respect for differing aspirations, and agreement on important needs and recommendations for future action.

# *Part II*

# *Welcoming Addresses*

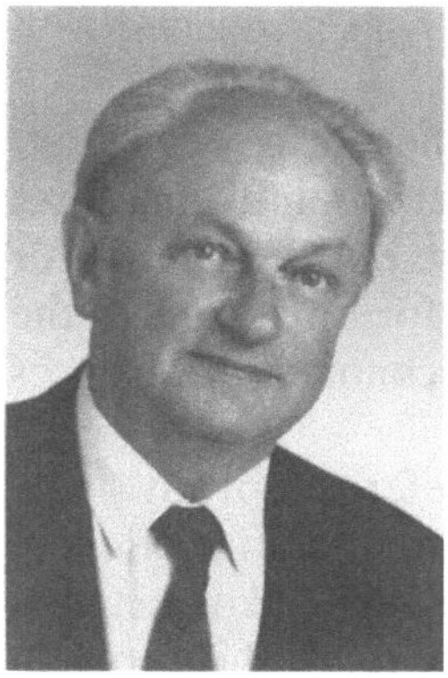

# 3. Council for International Organizations of Medical Sciences

Z. Bankowski

It is an honor and a great pleasure for me to welcome you, on behalf of the Council for International Organizations of Medical Sciences (CIOMS), to this international dialogue conference organized in the framework of the RAD-AR initiative. The main aim of the conference, as expressed in its title, is to improve drug safety through the joint efforts of all those who are partners in this very complicated but crucial task of ensuring progress in medicine. I am particularly pleased by the presence of all major constituencies responsible for drug safety, namely, representatives of the national drug regulatory authorities, drug manufacturers, and health professions, as well as scientists, journalists, and representatives of consumer organizations.

To the best of my knowledge, this is the first time that such a multidisciplinary and multisectoral conference will consider drug safety from ethical perspectives. The presence of outstanding ethicists is a guarantee that we shall be well guided in this fascinating but difficult approach.

Any consideration of the advances made in medicine during the last half-century shows how closely they have been linked to the development of new drugs. Consider the sulfonamides, vaccines, beta blockers, penicillin, and other antibiotics, and biogenetic drugs, only a few examples, and their remarkable impact on the therapy and prevention of diseases. Medicaments and vaccines will always be essential elements of medical progress. This is the main reason why the pharmaceutical industry, the developer and producer of drugs, is a natural partner of medicine; its contribution to the progress of medicine cannot be overestimated.

The use of every drug has both beneficial and harmful effects, however. Historically, societies have drawn up rules, codes, and legal measures for ensuring the rational and safe use of new knowledge and technological progress in the service of man. Traditionally, physicians have the main responsibility of safeguarding the ethical principle of beneficence to patients. Ethical codes and guidelines have been developed to help them fulfil this responsibility. In ensuring the safety of drugs, the health professions share responsibility for their beneficial use and the reduction of risk with pharmaceutical manufacturers, who produce and distribute drugs, and drug regulatory authorities, who have a mandate from their governments to protect society from risks associated with their use.

Some 10 years ago, CIOMS began to bring together drug regulatory authorities and drug manufacturers to discuss and to develop jointly measures that would assure more benefits and fewer risks in the use of drugs. Also, for more than 25 years now, CIOMS has provided a forum for discussion of the moral and ethical issues implicit in the application of new technological advances to the practice of medicine.

The ethical issues of drug safety go beyond the terms of reference of any single body or organization responsible for drug safety. A truly collaborative effort of all those involved and responsible is urgently needed. The RAD-AR objective is to improve drug safety in a collaborative effort and to approach this problem from an ethical point of view. Hence, CIOMS strongly supports the RAD-AR initiative, which aims to maximize benefits and minimize harm for all users of medicaments.

May I express, on behalf of CIOMS, best wishes for the success of this conference. May I also express our willingness to contribute our international experience to this collaborative initiative in drug safety.

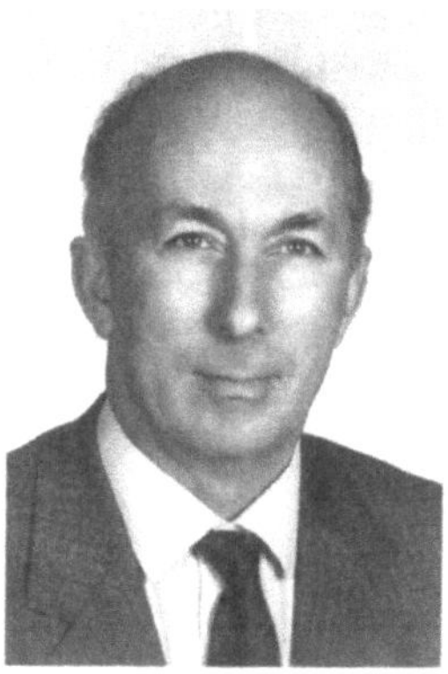

# 4. International Federation of Pharmaceutical Manufacturers Associations

R. B. Arnold

Those of us who were at the Wolfsberg meeting 2 years ago will recall that, apart from a strong showing of distinguished academics in the field of epidemiology, most of the participants were from companies in the pharmaceutical industry, together with a few of us representing international associations. Most of us were there to hear for the first time what the acronym RAD-AR represented. Both the list of participants and the agenda for the meeting starting today show just how much progress has been made since 1988. Few people in the major industrialised countries of the world who are professionally concerned with the issue of drug safety are now unaware of the RAD-AR initiative. Important meetings in Stratford, Washington, Tokyo and other places have contributed to that awareness.

The choice of those who have been asked to welcome you today is highly significant. Dr. Pfanner of the IKS in Switzerland represents the regulatory agencies. It is particularly encouraging that a number of important regulatory authorities have been willing to be actively involved in the RAD-AR debate. The presence of Dr. Bankowski, both to welcome you and to lead the first working session, not only underlines the recognition of the ethical dimension of the issue under discussion but also represents a link between WHO, the regulatory agencies, academia, and the pharmaceutical industry. The fact that I am here representing the International Federation of Pharmaceutical Manufacturers Associations (IFPMA), which also co-sponsored the October 1989 Tokyo meeting, indicates the wide degree of interest in the RAD-AR concept throughout the research-based industry and the very encouraging level of committed support from important companies.

Over the past 2 years, the RAD-AR initiative has passed through its early growth phase and become a vigorous adolescent. It is now crucial that the RAD-AR concept be further developed by a broad spectrum of the research-based pharmaceutical industry, by the regulatory authorities, and by the international agencies, especially CIOMS and WHO. Academia will provide the mortar which binds this aggregation together. Only by the acceptance and direct involvement of all the key players will RAD-AR succeed.

The major task now will be to work out a practical mechanism for the further development, operation, and supervision of RAD-AR by a consensus of the interested parties I have identified. I am confident that this Wolfsberg conference will be a decisive step to that end.

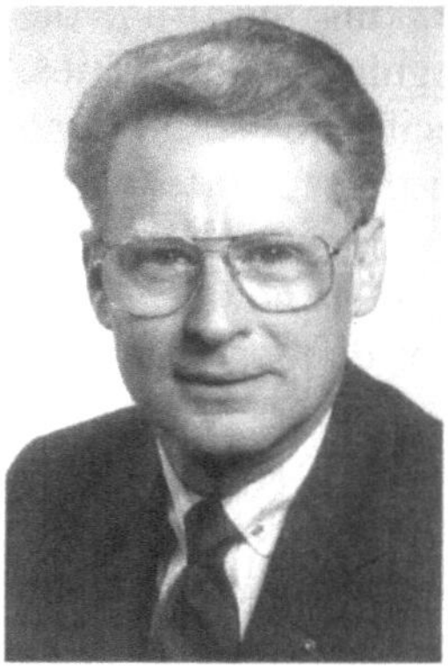

# 5. Intercantonal Office for the Control of Medicines

J. Pfanner

It is a great pleasure and a privilege to welcome you on behalf of the Swiss regulatory agency, the Interkantonale Kontrollstelle für Heilmittel (IKS). The focus of the RAD-AR initiative, namely, the risk/benefit assessment of drugs, has always been the most important and the most demanding task of drug regulatory agencies, not only in Switzerland but in all countries. I am pleased that during the last 2 years our office has undertaken several important steps to improve drug safety.

One of them was the establishment of a pharmacovigilance centre within IKS, which until then had not been directly involved in monitoring adverse drug reactions. Another Swiss centre of pharmacovigilance, called SANZ, has, however, existed, to which physicians and pharmacists could report cases of suspected adverse reactions. This centre is a foundation supported by the pharmaceutical industry, the Swiss Medical Association, and the Swiss Pharmaceutical Association. The new concept for monitoring and evaluating voluntary adverse drug reaction reports in our country proposed by the IKS envisages a closer collaboration between the regulatory agency, the present pharmacovigilance centre SANZ, and academia, represented by the divisions of clinical pharmacology at the university hospitals in Switzerland.

About 2 years ago, in most of these divisions of clinical pharmacology, a drug information service was established to supply interested physicians with expert information on pharmacotherapy. A substantial proportion of the inquiries concern adverse drug reactions. According to the new IKS pharmacovigilance concept, the divisions of clinical pharmacology will, in addition to SANZ, serve as peripheral or satellite centres that collect the information, perform the first evaluation, and pass the information further to the new drug monitoring centre in our office. In addition to improving the coordination of efforts and the communication between the industry, medical profession, and academia, the IKS pharmacovigilance centre will be responsible for international contacts with the adverse drug reaction centres in other countries.

In view of our interest and activity in the field of drug safety, I appreciate very much that efforts, such as the RAD-AR initiative, are also coming from the industry. The improvement of the risk/benefit ratio of drugs is in the interest of all parties involved: the consumer, that is, the patient taking the drug; the medical profession; the pharmaceutical industry; and the regulatory authorities. Until recently, each of these parties had followed its specific goals; although much has been achieved during the past two decades with respect to better use of drugs, the efforts were not always coordinated.

This dialogue conference represents an opportunity to seek new ways for better coordinating our efforts. This unique opportunity for dialogue between several groups with different interests will help to open doors for better communication between them. All parties involved should be able to profit from the expert knowledge, information, and the experience of their partners in the important field of drug safety. It is our joint responsibility to assure the safe and efficient use of drugs.

# 6. RAD-AR Consortium

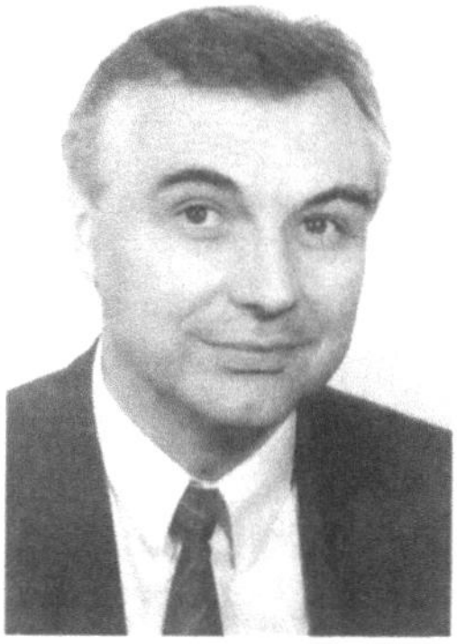

P. SIMON

It is a special privilege for me to address this eminent gathering of people who have at least one thing in common: the desire to foster health and when necessary restore it by the rational use of the most appropriate means. People representing various fields have come together here for a dialogue aimed at the improvement of drug safety. As a representative of the RAD-AR consortium, I have the great honour of welcoming you all to this decisive and promising conference and of exhorting you to assume joint responsibility with the pharmaceutical industry to achieve this objective.

Two years ago, a number of well-known research-based pharmaceutical companies gathered here at a similar conference to discuss this collaboration and lead the way with the new RAD-AR initiative. However, it is only today that a substantial number of representatives of the regulatory authorities, of the academic world, of the health professions, of patient and consumer associations, of the media, and of international organizations are joining in this dialogue. In short, representatives of practically all the professions and functions who share responsibility in this complex process of pharmacotherapy are here. In these next few days, there will not be many occasions when we will not hear a viewpoint or opinion being expressed, because all those sharing responsibility in risk/benefit assessment and management are present.

Let us, therefore, *listen* to each other and honestly strive to *understand* each other's position. These are the first two prerequisites for progress in this common field of ours, as they were defined by the rapporteurs of the 1988 Wolfsberg conference. The other two, *formulate a message* and then *communicate* it, can also be achieved in the next few days if all of us are prepared to be open and sincere.

In the report of the 1988 meeting [1], under the heading "Responding to the Issues", there is a long list of proposed activities, a mine of positive ideas that should occupy us all in the coming years. I suggest that this year's meeting take stock of which of these proposed activities have actually been realized in the last 2 years and which of them are still awaiting realization, establishing priorities as well. We are not starting from zero in these efforts, however. For example:

- The three Basle companies, Ciba-Geigy, Sandoz and Hoffmann-La Roche, together with the Swiss federal regulatory authority and in accordance with the intentions of patient and consumer organizations, took the initiative to introduce *patient package leaflets* in layman's language. This was at the beginning of the 1980s.
- Earlier, in 1976, the same three companies, together with the biggest Swiss consumers' association as co-editor and distributor, produced an explanatory leaflet for consumers on *"The Rational Use of Drugs"*, which over the years has been widely distributed throughout the world.

These are only two of many practical and successful initiatives which give me hope that we can conceive and implement further concerted action. I extend an invitation to my colleagues from the RAD-AR consortium companies to use this meeting as a starting point for further activities of this sort, with the support of all our partners present here, by identifying steps which can take us the furthest toward our common objective: *the optimization of pharmacotherapy as an improved service for the patient.*

The patient, our ultimate customer, is "out there". His or her health, or indeed fate, often depends on all of us, from industry and its regulators down the "responsibility road" to the prescribing, and, hopefully, counselling, physician and the dispensing pharmacist. More and more the patient is no longer quietly waiting there, waiting for our eventual consensus as to how we can benefit him or her best. Let us take the patient's more active involvement as a fact that merits our very serious consideration.

## References

1. Horisberger B, Dinkel R (eds) (1989) The perception and management of drug safety risks. Springer, Berlin Heidelberg New York Tokyo

# *Part III*

# *Ethical Perspectives*

# 7. The Discipline of Ethics

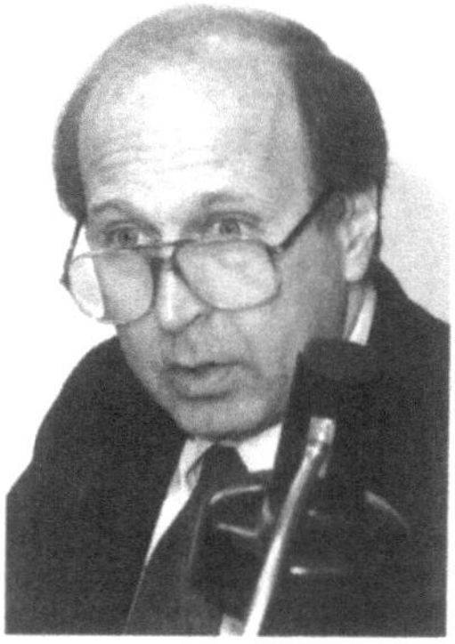

S. Gorovitz

There is much talk about ethics in public discussion and also in various professional circles, but there seems to be very little explicit discussion of what ethics is. It might be useful to start there. Ethics is about interpersonal relationships, about how people and the institutions they constitute ought to behave toward one another. Ethics is therefore rooted in concern with peoples' individual and collective needs, aspirations, and values, and it requires a sensitive understanding of what those are. What is often overlooked is that ethics is autonomous. Ethical questions cannot be resolved simply on the basis of an appeal to the facts of psychology, economics, law, sociology, or any other discipline. It is its own enterprise. Ethics is not a list of right actions and wrong actions, or a set of moral prescriptions and prohibitions. It is, instead, a discipline concerned with principles and with the quality of moral reasoning.

Ethics is notoriously hard, but not in the same way as quantum physics, which is hard for different reasons. Ethics is hard because people studying ethics are only interested in the hard issues. Easy questions do exist, however. There is nothing ethically challenging, for example, about the moral question of whether in developing a new drug one should impose it on an unconsenting population of experimental subjects. Since it is so easy to make that judgment, we spend little time thinking about it.

The discipline of ethics tends to focus instead on difficult ethical problems. The more difficult the problems are, the more they capture the interest of people who are concerned with ethics, so one can get the impression that ethics is interested only in cases that are so hard as to be almost impossible. But hard does not mean impossible. It is possible, often, to deal with a difficult ethical problem and reach a reasoned and defensible conclusion. Also, it is possible to learn something instructive from cases which are so easy as to seem to be uninteresting.

Although ethics is not a list of right and wrong actions, it is, nonetheless, about right and wrong and the difference between them. There are competing ethical theories; that is, there are theories of what makes the difference between what is right and what is wrong. Among the most familiar examples are consequential ethical theories that explain the difference between right and wrong in terms of the consequences of actions. The most prominent of these is utilitarianism as exemplified by John Stuart Mill, the theory that the right thing to do is that which produces the greatest good for the greatest number. Nonconsequential ethical theories are very different, such as that of Immanuel Kant, who held that the difference between right and wrong actions was not a function of their consequences, but of the actor's obligations and motivation.

There is not time even to provide an inventory, let alone an examination, of all competing ethical theories here. I emphasize, however, that ethical theories themselves come under scrutiny from the point of view of ethics. Anyone seriously pursuing the discipline of ethics must evaluate each competing ethical theory against certain basic criteria. It must be intelligible or it will fail to provide any ethical guidance. It must correspond to deeply held and widely shared moral judgments or it will lack credibility. And it must have universality, reflecting respect for all persons as morally equal.

That final criterion, the universality criterion, has real significance for how we make moral judgments and moral choices. One example in the context of pharmacology is simply this: if it is wrong to behave in a certain way toward experimental subjects in the United States, it is no better to behave in that way toward experimental subjects in the Third World. The fact that an administratively convenient research population may be available in a Third World country does not exempt those in charge of the test protocol from adhering to the same sort of ethical requirements and respect for persons that are essential in this country.

At the Wolfsberg conference in 1990 many different constituencies were present: members of the pharmaceutical industry, providers, regulators, and everyone of them at least potentially a patient. In the light of that diversity, I proposed the following brief exercise as a way of illustrating one mode of moral thinking: Consider a question having to do with the crucially important element of control. It has been emphasized that people attach importance to exercising jurisdiction over what becomes of them. We are all aware of the difference between voluntarily assumed risk and imposed risk. The imposed risk, though it may not be of greater magnitude, is of much greater moral severity than a voluntarily assumed risk. Experiments in cognitive psychology demonstrate that control is often taken to be more important even than outcome optimization. People will relinquish some percentage of likelihood of success in exchange for greater participation in determining the outcome, even knowing that is what they are doing.

Now take the question of how much information, of what sort, ought to be provided by whom to whom in regard to drugs that are complex in effect, substantial in potential benefits, and significant in risks. How might we think about that? Notice that the question had the word 'ought' in it. How do we think about questions about what 'ought' to be? That is at the heart of ethics.

I do not have time to review Plato, Aristotle, Aquinas, Kant, Mill, Hume, Moore, Ross, and all the rest as background, but let me refer to the work of one contemporary moral philosopher, John Rawls of Harvard University, who wrote a massive book (not quite like the PDR, but still massive) called "A

Theory of Justice." One idea from Rawls is especially useful as a heuristic device, and we can imagine its application in our context. Assume that we have a particular drug in mind. The questions arise: How shall we handle information about this drug? What should be told to the physicians? What should be told directly to the patients? What should be required of physicians that they tell patients? What should be released to the media? What should the regulators know, and what should the legislators know? As we debate these questions, there is a natural tendency for each of us to think about each question from the perspective that we bring to the debate. A stockholder in the company that manufactures the drug might have a somewhat different perspective from a vulnerable patient who both wants and fears it, or a physician who understands that the provision of information to patients itself has certain costs and risks. How you think about it tends to be a reflection of who you are and what particular values and perspectives you bring to bear.

Assume that an unexpected and indeed unprecedented storm strikes the Wolfsberg Conference Center, picks it up, and spins it around, with the remarkable effect that there is induced in each of us a kind of selective amnesia. When the storm abates and the building settles back down right onto its foundation, the conference participants are all a bit confused and befuddled. That is, each still knows whatever he or she knew about pharmacology. Each knows whatever he or she knew about principles of constitutional law, physics, history, and all the other disciplines. But there are things each of them has lost as a result of this strange event. First, there is something even worse than jet lag, a kind of severe disorientation. No one can see or hear very clearly, so when someone speaks, the others can tell well enough *what* that person is saying, but they cannot discern *who* it is. They cannot distinguish one person from another. Second, they have selective amnesia. They can remember nothing that distinguishes themselves from anyone else. So they know there are manufacturers, providers, media people, and regulators present, but, oddly, they cannot tell, beset by this veil of confusion, which they themselves are.

In "A Theory of Justice", Rawls puts forth the thesis that a just society is a society operated in accordance with those principles that would be adopted by a set of people negotiating, seeking to protect their own interests, to be sure, through what he calls such a "veil of ignorance." If you do not know whether you are a patient, manufacturer, health care provider, regulator, or legislator, then the decisions that you make about what ought to be done will necessarily be protected from the distorting parochialism of your own prior perspective. To say that is to say that the right decisions are those that you would be able to endorse no matter which role you fill. When your head cleared, when the buzzing stopped, when the veil of ignorance lifted, and you found that you were a patient or manufacturer or regulator, it would not make any difference, because the views that you advocated were supported by reasons that were wholly independent of the special considerations associated with those different perspectives and roles. That is a way of saying that the decisions were entirely fair. That is one way of reflecting this general criterion of universality that applies to all ethical principles. That is, it must be no respecter of special interests.

In the following discussions it would be useful to try to adopt that mindset, to consider each point of view with this question in mind: Would I be as enthusiastic about this if I were in some very different role than the role that actually brings me here?

The context of health care especially requires moral reflection. Each person's ability to function well and autonomously, to pursue a lifeplan, even to sustain life, is profoundly affected by his or her own circumstances of health. Given the intimacy of medical interventions and the fragility of health and even of life itself, the choices that are made in health care settings typically are laden with moral significance, often beyond the degree that is perceived by those immediately involved. Those decisions have an impact, often profound, on the values and interests of those they affect. It is especially important, therefore, for everyone in health-related professions to be ethically sensitive, well informed, and rigorous.

# 8. Ethics and Health

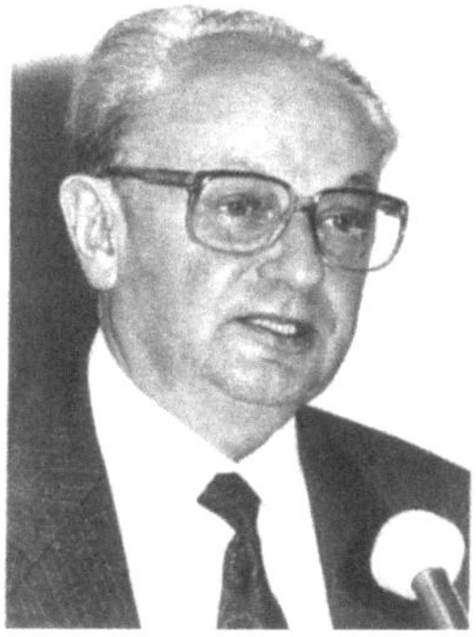

Z. BANKOWSKI

The extraordinary progress of biomedical sciences and medical technology during the last three decades and the application of the results in medical practice confront our societies with new ethical dilemmas. The number of books and articles in daily and professional journals bear witness to the importance of ethical questions and society's preoccupation with them. The terms "ethics", "health", "medical ethics", "bioethics", and "health policy ethics" appear more and more often, and usually in confusing texts. Therefore, for a better understanding, it is useful to provide a brief description of these terms.

*Ethics* is the branch of philosophy dealing with the distinction between right and wrong, with the moral consequences of our actions. Ethics provides principles of right conduct such as those governing the actions of an individual or of a professional group.

*Health*, according to the World Health Organization (WHO) definition, is a state of complete physical, mental, and social well-being and not merely the absence of disease or infirmity.

*Medical ethics* concerns the obligations of the physician toward the patient, and some obligations towards other physicians. Medical ethics provides the principles that govern professional conduct in medicine.

*Bioethics* is the term used to distinguish traditional medical ethics from ethical issues that arise from recent progress in biology and medicine.

*Health policy ethics* concerns ethical issues relevant to the organizing, financing, and delivering of health care services.

## Medical Ethics

The central role of ethics in the practice of medicine cannot be too highly rated. Medicine presupposes certain fundamental values such as the preservation of life and the relief of suffering. These values distinguish medicine from other sciences and imply some special responsibilities, particularly for the physician and other members of the health professions.

The most important obligations of the physician toward the patient are fidelity to the patient's interest, truth telling by the physician, and confidentiality of patient information. In a physician-patient relationship where there are emotional and physical intimacies, patients often entrust their bodies and sometimes even their lives to physicians, and therefore trust must exist. Medical ethics provides the basis for this trust. To assure patients that their interests are the most important, to promise to keep their confidences, and to deal honestly with them are fundamental values of medicine to which physicians must adhere.

Ethical problems arise when these values conflict with one another or with other interests. For example, there may be conflict between fidelity to the patient's best interest and the physician's financial interests, or conflict between the obligation to tell the truth and the obligation to protect the patient's well-being, e.g., in a case where the physician fears that an honest description of a hopeless prognosis would seriously upset the patient.

Because of the physicians' central role as decision makers about the health and welfare of their patients, the dilemmas they face are the primary concern of medical ethics. This role of decision maker has created a degree of paternalism, in that the physicians are qualified by their expertise and are obligated by this relationship to their patients to take the responsibility for decision making. The patient expects his physician to possess both technical knowledge and ethical wisdom.

## Bioethics

For more than 20 years now, CIOMS has provided a forum for the discussion of moral and ethical issues implicit in the application of new scientific knowledge and technological advances to the practice of medicine. Its programs in this area culminated in the establishment of International Guidelines for Biomedical Research Involving Human Subjects (1982), Principles of Medical Ethics Relevant to the Protection of Prisoners Against Torture (1983), and International Guiding Principles for Biomedical Research Involving Animals (1985). International Guidelines for Epidemiological Investigations are presently being prepared. Our approach in CIOMS is multidisciplinary and involves consultations with a broad range of biomedical specialists, as well as with legal experts, civic and religious leaders, and nongovernmental organizations concerned with human rights.

Recent progress in biomedical science, the resulting development of new medical technology, and the growing possibility of its applications provoke a certain anxiety. In order to explain society's concern, it may be useful to describe briefly the methods of biomedical experimental research and their application. Investigation begins with the construction of hypotheses which are tested in a laboratory and with experimental animals. For the findings to be clinically useful, experiments must be done on human subjects and, even when carefully designed, such research entails some risk to the subjects. This risk is justified not by any personal benefit to the researcher or the institution at which research is conducted, but by its benefit to the human subject involved, its potential contribution to human knowledge, to the relief of suffering, or to the prolongation of life. Long-term, the benefits are likely to be collective.

Society, together with the medical profession, is developing measures aimed at protecting against possible abuses. Thus, immediately following the Second World War, the judgments passed by the Nuremberg Tribunal on those who ran the Nazi concentration camps articulated the standard for carrying out human experimentation, emphasizing the subject's voluntary consent. Furthermore, represented by the World Medical Association, the medical profession took an important step further to reassure society: the Helsinki Declaration of 1964, elaborated and revised in 1975 and 1989, provides ethical principles for research involving human subjects. It adheres entirely to the concept of voluntary informed consent and imposes other protective measures such as a review of research protocols by independent ethical review committees.

These issues were further expanded by CIOMS, which has published international ethical guidelines for such research. Besides prior review of research protocols, the ethical review committee at the hospital, university, or other facility where the research is conducted may only approve research when the expected benefit/risk ratio is favorable to the subjects, and when the subjects' informed consent has been obtained.

Today's new technologies raise highly complex bioethical questions. One example comes from the resusciation of an individual whose cardio-respiratory system has failed. When the vital functions are artificially restored and maintained but the patient remains unconscious, is the body still a living person or merely a corpse that appears to have life? A similar quandary is posed when an infertile couple uses in vitro fertilization. Who are the parents of the child resulting from such fertilization of an ovum donated by Mrs. A, fertilized by Mr. B, implanted in the uterus of Mrs. C and handed over at birth to Mrs. D and Mr. E?

The sperm and the ovum, and the fertilized ovum resulting from their in vitro union, can be manipulated to a hitherto unknown extent. Artificial insemination by a donor other than the husband is an established procedure; a husband's sperm can be frozen and stored for future use, even after his death. Similarly, the fertilized ovum can be frozen and stored for later use, and women "lease" their wombs to carry other women's embryos. Genetic engineering is already capable of changing some inherited characteristics, and genetic selection is feasible, based on prenatal diagnosis.

Research at present under way on molecular genetics, and particularly on human genome mapping and sequencing, presages a new scientific era, perhaps a revolution, in the medicine of the 21st century. It opens up the possibility of changing the ways in which certain genes function in order to prevent or to treat many diseases and disorders. The particular dilemmas raised by genetic screening and counseling include the ownership of genetic information and the advantages and pitfalls associated with genetic counseling and engineering.

Who owns genetic information? The traditional moral viewpoint has been that professional secrecy is in both the patient's and the doctor's interests. But, today, ought we not to be concerned to make genetic information available to the relatives (or the potential spouse) of the patient? If the health and well-being of relatives or of future offspring are at issue, does the obligation to keep a secret then turn into an obligation to tell? It now seems that the totality of one's physical existence exceeds the limits of one's body, and consequently the traditional right to secrecy may turn into a duty to share information with the family or even with others in society.

There is also a right not to know. For one reason, false positive test results give inaccurate predictions. Secondly, some people are unable to cope with the burden of knowledge. Thirdly, information obtained from predictive testing can be misused. A fundamental principle of patient autonomy would seem to be that it is the basic right of the person to be tested or not to be tested, and to choose whether to be informed fully or only in part. Here is an area of interaction between the developments in biomedical science, ethics, and health policy making that cries out for further elaboration.

Predictive screening is warranted only if a free and informed decision is possible and if adequate facilities are available for long-term follow-up of those identified as disease-gene carriers at an early age. Another reason for concern is the risk of social discrimination by employers, insurance companies, and so on against someone known to have some genetic predisposition.

These and similar questions seem to go beyond the terms of reference of the medical profession alone. Can we consider that the neurologist or the cardiologist is the only person to decide who is alive and who is dead? Are the geneticists, obstetricians, and embryologists the only people to answer the questions about the moral status of human germinal material, eggs, sperm, and embryos, whether in the human body, in the laboratory test tube, or even frozen in laboratory containers? Society is largely unprepared for, and unconcerned about, such rapid scientific and technological developments. The ethical issues to which they give rise need to be examined thoroughly in the light of social norms, legal codes, and human values.

## Health Policy Ethics

In the face of the enormous power of medicine for both good and harm, each nation must develop health policies, i.e., strategies for the optimal use of its health care resources. Many, perhaps most, health policy decisions raise ethical questions. Policies having to do with who shall receive health services, how resources shall be allocated, what criteria should be used in setting priorities, what constitute acceptable forms of health care, when health care should be begun or ended, even the matter of who should be involved in making policy decisions, all have inherent ethical components. Different national, cultural, and religious traditions yield different ethical value systems, and their interactions with health policy making will therefore vary from country to country.

Many factors other than ethics influence policy decisions. Political, economic, cultural, religious, and organizational issues can obscure, distort, displace, or promote ethical considerations. Of considerable importance and interest is the dynamics of policy making, whereby ethical values are taken into account or lost from sight as policies are formulated.

The ways in which health policy, ethics, and human values interrelate are described by the American physician and philosopher, Edmund Pellegrino:

> "*The health policy* of a nation or a community is its strategy for controlling and optimizing the social uses of its medical knowledge and resources. *Human values* are the guides and justifications that people use for choosing the goals, priorities and means that make up that strategy. *Ethics* acts as the bridge between health policy and values. It examines the moral validity of the choices that must be made, and seeks to resolve conflicts between values which inevitably occur in making those choices. Ethics, therefore, orders human choices in accordance with normative principles" [1].

A health policy, therefore, ultimately reflects the values of a human community, the fundamental beliefs and commitments that a community or a nation attaches most closely to its identity and integrity. Through the expression of its values in the choices and priorities of its health policies, a community exerts its influence over the enormous momentum of technological advance.

Ethics is itself grounded in sociocultural, philosophical, or religious convictions. These convictions are a society's measuring rods for right and wrong, good and evil. They are often incommensurable and irreconcilable from one culture to another. To examine these convictions or to disagree with them is often perceived as a moral assault because they are so integral to a person's or a nation's self-image. It is this that makes transcultural ethical dialogue so difficult.

Health policies are rarely derived from explicit and systematic analysis of the moral values that shape them. Much of the art of national and international politics consists in structuring decision making in such a way that value issues are *not* confronted. The aim is to keep peace between, and within, divergent belief systems. However, once framed, a public policy unerringly reveals the values that drive a society. This is especially the case in health policies, which so often deal with those in the "shadows" of life, the very young, the poor, the sick, the aged, or individuals who are biologically or socially vulnerable or damaged. Different peoples value these groups differently. When resources are limited, tragic choices must be made that may be to the disadvantage of one group or another.

In every culture there is an unavoidable ethical problem inherent in the very conception of policy formulation. This is the inevitable tension that any policy generates between individual and social good. While most policy makers strive to serve both, there is always some point at which further improvements in a society's good intolerably undermine the worth of each individual's life within that society.

According to Pellegrino [1], three general considerations should motivate health policies and health policy makers:

1. To attempt to control the social and economic impact of the unrestrained use of advanced medical technology in treating individual patients. The results of health policies are now becoming apparent in many countries: prolongation

of the process of dying, increasing the numbers of patients surviving in persistent vegetative states or with lifelong disabilities and handicaps that require large expenditures of human and fiscal resources.

2. To achieve a more equitable distribution of the benefits of medical knowledge. What constitutes a just principle of distribution will vary from country to country, but each country must confront the issues involved in deciding on some principle of allocation of its resources among health goals, and between health and other social goals.
3. To use medical knowledge in an anticipatory way for the collective good of present and future generations. Some examples with very serious moral implications are policies that would make sterilization or limitation on procreation compulsory for carriers of defective genes; denying life-support measures to defective infants or older patients; and manipulating genetic material to control the future physical and behavioral characteristics of the human species along previously determined lines.

Each of the above three purposes arises out of the unprecedented possibilities of modern technology, and each presents some conflict between social and individual good, between traditional medical ethics and social ethics.

Health policy inevitably involves critical choices of ethical and other values, and these, in turn, are drawn from different national and cultural traditions influencing health policy decision makers. The influences on those responsible for health policy are diverse, ethical, cultural, political, economic, religious, tribal, bureaucratic, and personal. In any case, the policy maker will make a decision that represents his or her resolution of those diverse influences.

Value systems, the systems of principles or standards that determine what is valuable or important in life, play at least four different roles in health policy making [2]:

1. Value systems provide a framework for choosing among policy alternatives. It requires taking different feasible options and deciding which among them is the most valued pursuit, according to the ethical and other values of the group.
2. Value systems provide the framework for choosing who the policy makers will be. To choose the decision maker is to choose the value system according to which decisions will be made.
3. Value systems are critical even in providing the medical and other facts upon which health policy decisions must be based. The cultural system of beliefs and values is critical not only for choosing which policy alternative is the most valuable and choosing which persons should be vested with policy making authority, but also for deciding which facts will be taken into account and how they will be used for purposes of policy making.
4. Value systems are critical in determining what the possibilities are for intercultural cooperation in health policy. In something as fundamental as health care policy, there is tremendous opportunity for cooperation even among those whose basic cultural systems are radically different. There may well be intersections of these cultural traditions that facilitate, indeed require, collaboration across traditions.

To provide a forum for an international and transcultural discussion of these issues, CIOMS convened an international conference on "Health Policy, Ethics and Human Values, an International Dialogue." Participants included health policy makers, ethicists, and philosophers from different cultural and religious groups, including secularists. The concerns of the conference coincided with those of WHO, particularly as regards equity, social justice, community participation, and the dignity of individuals in sickness and health, as expressed in the goal of health for all. The conference helped to clarify the differences in attitude and to identify the common ethical approaches of different philosophies, cultures, traditions, and religious and nonreligious groups. It strongly recommended a continuing international, intercultural dialogue to improve understanding of the relationship between health policy making, ethics, and human values in different cultural settings.

To follow up the conference recommendations, in 1985 CIOMS undertook a program also entitled "Health Policy, Ethics and Human Values, an International Dialogue". Its objectives are:

1. To strengthen national capacities for addressing and making decisions about the ethical and human values issues involved in health policy.
2. To contribute to improved understanding of the concepts inherent in WHO's goal of health for all, particularly in terms of its values content.
3. To develop transcultural and transdisciplinary approaches and methods for working in this field.
4. To use improved understanding of the approaches of various societies to the ethical and human values aspects of health policy, as a way to promote deeper human understanding of human values across cultural and political lines.

### *The Health Professional's Role in Forming and Implementing Policy*

The formation and implementation of health policies require the closest technical and moral cooperation of health care professionals and policy makers. According to Pellegrino [1], the physician has at least five separate levels of moral responsibility to be exercised in the judgments and choices essential to policy formation and implementation: as an agent of his patient's good, as a technical expert, as a morally responsible citizen, as an agent in the implementation of policy, and as a morally accountable human being. At each level the physician interacts with policy makers, who themselves have the same range of moral obligations.

*The Physician as the Patient's Advocate.* The physician who offers to treat or help a person who is ill is bound in a special way to the patient. He invites the patient's trust that he will be competent and will place that competence at the patient's disposal. Except for the most extraordinary reasons, e.g., the risk of serious immediate harm to others, the physician has an inescapable primary obligation to work for the patient's good, and not in his own or others' interests.

*The Physician as Technical Expert.* When he is not locked into a trust relationship with a particular patient, the physician is obliged to participate in policy formulation because he has the technical knowledge which policy makers need to make rational choices among alternatives. This is an obligation he owes to society, since his knowledge is not proprietary. A clear separation must be drawn between the physician's role as an expert in medical science and his presumption of expertise in value decisions. In this respect he faces the same problem all experts face, how to separate what is known factually and objectively from what he would like to see enacted as policy.

*The Physician as Citizen.* The physician's duty to act as a technical witness in policy formation does not exempt him from his obligations as a citizen. Thus, he must favor policies that are morally sound, and oppose those that are immoral. As long as he does not take advantage of his position as a technical authority, he can and should take the measures open to all citizens in his society to work for those health policies that will benefit his patients or society at large. In this the physician has the same moral obligation as any other citizen and with no more or less authority.

*The Physician Implementing Health Policies.* Sooner or later, health policies must be implemented in the care of individual patients. Here the physician faces his most difficult moral conflicts and the most direct challenge to his traditional ethic of beneficence. Several positions have been taken with respect to this moral dilemma: the physician as primarily an agent of social or fiscal policy; the physician as arbiter of the application of health policies; the physician as protector of the patient's autonomy. Whichever position one chooses, the central moral issue remains: when there is conflict of moral values in implementing a health policy, whose good should come first, the patient's, the physician's or society's as expressed in a health policy?

*The Physician as Moral Agent.* The physician, like any other person, is morally accountable. Therefore, he cannot carry out a health policy, for example, mandatory sterilization of carriers of genetic disorders, or refusal of care because of the patient's inability to pay, that he considers fundamentally immoral. He has a moral responsibility that transcends his role as an agent of public policy.

These five levels of moral activity are intermingled in the most intricate relationships in actual health-related decisions. The complexity of these role relationships illustrates the urgent need for the careful reconstruction of professional ethics to address the new dilemmas and conflicts that medical technology and the implementation of health policies introduce into the physician's role.

Health policy makers have the same five moral roles in policy formation and implementation. They are the agents of individual and social good. They too are technical experts. They too are morally responsible citizens, agents of policy implementation, and morally accountable persons. Policy makers have not traditionally had professional codes to guide their ethical decisions. Perhaps the time has come for them, too, to recognize explicitly the obligations they owe their fellow humans for the moral quality of their actions and decisions.

Today, it is possible, and indeed necessary, to examine these questions not only as the ethics of care, but much more extensively as the ethics of health policy and biotechnology as a whole. The intention is not to undervalue moral and ethical aspects at the individual level, but rather to view them within a wider frame of reference.

## References

1. Pellegrino E (1985) Keynote address. Health policy, ethics and human values. In: Bankowski Z, Bryant JH (eds) Health policy, ethics and human values, an international dialogue. Council for International Organizations of Medical Sciences, Geneva
2. Veatch R (1985) Value systems: Their roles in shaping decisions. In: Bankowski Z, Bryant JH (eds) Health policy, ethics, and human values, an international dialogue. Council for International Organizations of Medical Sciences, Geneva

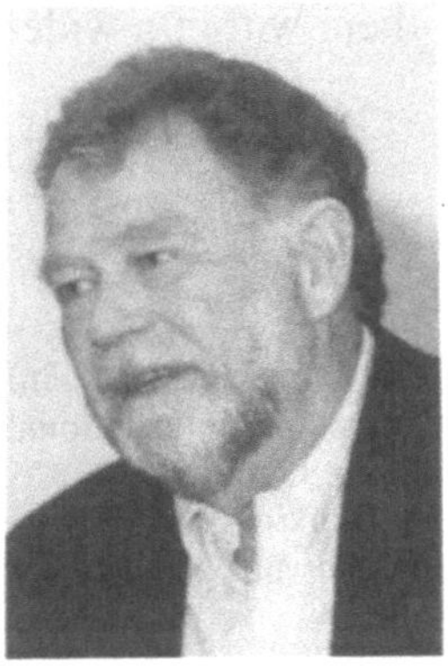

# 9. Biomedical Ethical Perspective

E.W. D. YOUNG

The idea which gave birth to this conference is brilliant in its simplicity. Drug safety can be improved. Or, to put it the other way round, the deleterious effects of prescription drug use can be minimized. If this is to happen, scientific data must be constantly generated about the risks and benefits associated with various pharmaceutical products. The knowledge thus acquired has to be evaluated, appraised, and assessed. It must then be communicated or disseminated. Finally, this knowledge has to be used as a basis for action, whether by the people who buy and consume these products or by those who formulate public policy. And improving drug safety is the joint responsibility of a wide variety of different people, all of whom are represented in this conference: drug manufacturers, researchers in the academic community, regulators, physicians, pharmacists, the media, patients or consumers, and their advocacy groups.

This may be a simple concept, but implementing it is fraught with complexity. The theme that brings us together in this conference soon will lead us into a moral maze, if not a moral minefield! My task is simply to offer a guiding biomedical ethical perspective on the theme: "Improving Drug Safety: A Joint Responsibility." I begin by discussing briefly some basic principles.

In the Hippocratic literature, the primary ethical principle guiding the practice of medicine was that of *nonmaleficence:* the duty not to harm the patient, or to alleviate the patient's suffering. It is summed up in the maxim *primum non nocere* or "first of all, do no harm." Those were the days when benefiting patients was rather a hit-and-miss affair. Hence the principle of *beneficence* (requiring the attempt to benefit the patient) was secondary to that of nonmaleficence until the dawning of scientific medicine in the late 19th and the early 20th century. Only when it became possible predictably to do some good did beneficence assume primacy.

Until the middle of the 20th century, medicine was guided by these two primary ethical principles: beneficence and nonmaleficence. Since all interventions are not only possibly beneficial, but also potentially harmful, assessing the ratio of risk or harm to benefit and deciding that the potential risks or harms of an intervention are *not disproportional* to the likely benefits is a necessary ongoing duty required by these two principles. The process of risk/benefit assessment begins with animal models but, as Bruce Ames et al. [1] point out, not only do different species of animals react differently to the same drug, for example, but "quantitative extrapolation from rodents to humans ... is guesswork that we have no way of validating." Only large epidemiological studies can give us accurate scientific data about the risks and benefits of pharmaceutical products.

After World War II and the revelations of the Nuremberg trials, leading to the promulgation of the Code of Nuremberg and then the Helsinki Declarations, *autonomy* became an equally important principle in the research setting. In the United States, it became as central as beneficence and nonmaleficence in the clinical setting after 1950, for various reasons [2]. Although the need for human research subjects to participate in experiments only with their voluntary and informed consent is now universally recognized, autonomy in the clinical setting is valued unevenly in different cultures. In the United States, it is valued extremely highly, largely because of the consumer movement extending its concerns to the provision of medical care. The relationship between physicians and patients in the United States is now more collaborative than paternalistic. In other societies, autonomy has a lower priority, and the relationship between providers and consumers tends to be more paternalistic, the traditional form of the physician-patient relationship.

Under conditions of scarcity, whether the scarcity is absolute or relative, actual or perceived, concerns about *distributive justice* inevitably emerge. As long as there is more than enough food to go around, it does not very much matter whether the person sitting next to me at lunch has a bigger helping on his plate than I have; during a famine, or on a lifeboat with limited supplies and no knowledge of how long it will be before rescuers arrive, it may matter very much indeed. When everybody cannot have all they want, how is what is available to be fairly distributed?

In the United States, this question has been asked seriously since the early 1980s, when the federal government attempted the first of several cost-containment measures with respect to medical care. Under the Diagnosis Related Group system of reimbursement introduced by the federal government in 1983, hospitals would no longer be reimbursed for the *actual* costs incurred in caring for patients, but only on the basis of *average* costs. If, after a hysterectomy, a patient required 9 days of hospital care, the institution would only be compensated for the average, for example, 5 days of care. Once they started losing money under this system of reimbursement, hospitals in the United States were no longer able to provide free hospital care to the uninsured or the uninsurable. There are now some 33 million people in the United States without the means to afford private health insurance, and ineligible for federal or state health care programs. This has led many in the United States to become increasingly concerned about justice.

The principle of justice, distributively understood, forces upon us questions about access to potentially beneficial products and about their cost. The phenomenon of AIDS patients in the United States being prevented from obtaining a drug like AZT because of excessive bureaucratic regulation and exorbitant cost became a hotly contested issue and indicates the importance distributive justice has assumed in contemporary ethical discussions.

As a principle, justice imposes the duty of calculating the cost/effectiveness of a drug or other intervention in exactly the same way that the two primary traditional medicomoral principles give rise to the duty of risk/benefit assessment. A drug may be effective and safe, but be too costly to produce or market because the demand for it will be too small. Is it fair that those who could benefit from such a drug be deprived of it because of an unfavorable cost/effectiveness assessment? As Professor Leisinger makes clear, this is a major ethical issue in the developing world [3].

Additionally, autonomy and justice are always potentially in conflict with one another as the rights of the individual are pitted against the common good. Again, different societies adopt varying solutions to the problem of individual versus collective goods. In the United States, we err perhaps on the side of giving too much weight to individual autonomy (as may be seen from our inability to enact effective legislation controlling handguns, which now cost us $ 16 billion annually in direct medical costs and in lost earnings). Equally, the countries of Eastern Europe clearly went too far in the direction of collective control; the freedom of the individual has asserted itself with astonishing rapidity in recent months and with still quite unpredictable results.

This has led me to postulate a fifth moral force, the notion of *community*, mediating between autonomy and justice (Fig. 1). Community inevitably constrains autonomy (I am not free to disregard traffic laws or not to pay taxes). Equally, community demands justice, for if we do not treat one another fairly, the fabric of our society, even of our civilization, is destroyed. The form concerns for the community take will differ from one country to another. In some, limitations on individual autonomy will be minimal and so will the requirements stemming from the principle of distributive justice. In others, there will be maximal limitations on individual freedoms and a maximal emphasis on the equitable distribution of scarce resources. In Switzerland, for example, it appears that the community exercises stronger constraints on individual freedoms than is the case in the United Kingdom. Conversely, as an example, the sense of community in Sweden results in a wider array of publicly funded services (such as free university education, efficient mass transportation systems, and the subsidization of the arts) than in the United States.

None of the first four principles is a moral absolute, always and universally taking precedence over the others. This means that it will be impossible to realize any of them perfectly. In my view, the fact that principles are realistically unattainable is not a sufficient reason for abandoning them. I regard these principles more as guiding lights or as lighthouses than as harbor lights. That is to say, they do not represent destination points so much as provide us with a direction to follow. This also means that these principles are in constant tension, and sometimes even in conflict with one another. The ranking of these principles in order of priority is an ongoing exercise in ethical judgment.

There are three important variables which will affect the value accorded and the weight given to each of these guiding biomedical ethical principles as we apply them to the issue of improving drug safety. The first is that at different

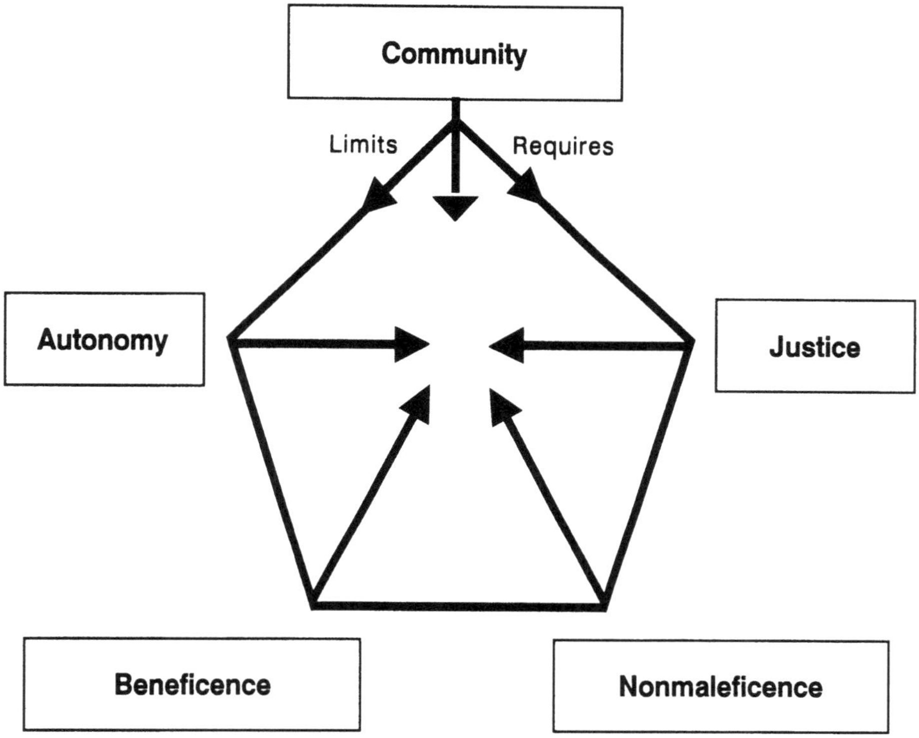


**Fig. 1.** Interacting biomedical ethical principles in the 1990s

stages in the process of moving from knowledge generation to knowledge utilization the balance between principles necessarily shifts. The second is that different principals (or players) will view and value these principles differently, and that even the same principals might view and value these principles differently at different times (when a disease is first diagnosed, for example, as compared with its terminal stage). And the third is that these principles will be viewed and valued differently in various political, cultural, and national contexts. Each of these variables requires further elucidation.

## The First Variable

*At different stages in the process of moving from knowledge generation to knowledge utilization, the foundational biomedical ethical principles will be viewed and valued differently.*

Let us make the assumption underlying the structure of this conference that there are four stages necessary to the process of improving drug safety: the *generation* of reliable scientific data about the risks and benefits of pharmaceutical products; the *evaluation* of these data and the assessment of the ratio of risks to benefits; the *communication* or dissemination of this information; and, fourth, the *utilization* of this knowledge, either by consumers or by those responsible for the formulation of public policy.

It is fairly obvious that at each of these four stages, the foundational principles will be assigned different priorities. It might be argued that in the early stages of this process, drug efficacy matters more than drug safety. Later, the reverse might be true: even more important than that a drug works is that it should be safe. I have asked conference participants to join me in the first of three experiments in descriptive ethics. I instructed them to use their own judgment to rank the principles of beneficence, nonmaleficence, autonomy, and justice from 1 to 4, at each of the four stages from knowledge generation to knowledge utilization (see Fig. 2). In this ranking 1 represents the principle considered to be *most* important; 4 represents the principle regarded as the *least* important. The results of all three experiments are presented in a later chapter (see "Guiding Principles"). Obviously, this was not a scientifically valid experiment. For it to have empirical significance we would, among other things, have had to make available to all participants in their preferred language (Japanese, Chinese, Greek, French, German, Italian, English, Polish, etc.) copies of this form and definitions of the terms used. Nevertheless, the results are of interest, if only because they illustrate the points I make in this chapter.

| | Knowledge Generation | Knowledge Assessment | Knowledge Communication | Knowledge Utilization |
|---|---|---|---|---|
| Beneficence | | | | |
| Nonmaleficence | | | | |
| Autonomy | | | | |
| Justice | | | | |

**Fig. 2.** Experiment 1. Rank the importance of the biomedical ethical principles at different stages from the generation to the utilization of knowledge

## The Second Variable

*The various principals (or players) will view and value these foundational biomedical ethical principles differently, and patients might value them differently at various stages in the disease process.*

The ranking of the foundational biomedical principles not only will vary at different stages in the process of moving from knowledge generation to knowledge utilization, but also will depend upon which principals (or players) are determining the priorities. Obviously, academic researchers, manufacturers, regulators, physicians, pharmacists, members of the media, patients or consumers of pharmaceutical products, and consumer advocates all have different values or biases. Seldom are these made explicit. Usually they are implicit, and therefore hidden, as much from the principals themselves as from other interested parties.

A good example of how the various principals will value our guiding ethical principles differently was provided in a recent United States newspaper article [4]. The headline read "Scorned Thalidomide Researched Anew." The article pointed out that "researchers have discovered that [thalidomide] is a spectacularly effective agent for combating rejection of foreign tissue and for alleviating the symptoms of several diseases in which the immune system turns against the body." It went on to state that "despite thalidomide's promise as an agent for suppressing the immune system, scientists involved in the research say that it has been extremely difficult to persuade drug companies, physicians, and government agencies to cooperate in the experiments." However highly scientists may have come to value thalidomide's efficacy, this is likely to be outweighed by the biases of others based on concerns about its safety.

According to which of the many principals involved is at the center of the pentagon (Fig. 1), the ranking of the guiding principles will differ. To illustrate this point, I asked the conference participants to take part in a second exercise in descriptive (or analytical) ethics. Each participant was given a copy of the form shown in Fig. 3 and was asked to circle the group he or she represented, whether manufacturer, researcher, regulator, physician, pharmacist, representative of the media, patient (or consumer), or consumer advocate. Researchers were invited to add, if either was appropriate, the word "chemist" or the word "epidemiologist". Participants were allowed to circle more than one group if they wished, since they could be both a patient and a member of one of the other groups. Those who identified themselfves as patients were asked to characterize the problem for which they required prescription drugs as either mild, moderate, or major. Then, from the perspective or perspectives they had indicated, they were to rank the same four biomedical ethical principles in importance from 1 to 4, where 1 represented the principle believed to be *most* important and 4 that of *least* importance.

As Shulman [5] points out, in the United States "the courts have relieved pharmaceutical manufacturers of the obligation imposed on manufacturers in general to communicate directly with patients about the risks inherent in their products. At common law, the manufacturer's duty to warn is owed instead to

| | Drug Manufacturers | Academic Researchers | Regulators | Physicians | Pharmacists | Media Representatives | Patient (Mild Problem) | Patient (Moderate Problem) | Patient (Major Problem) | Advocacy Groups |
|---|---|---|---|---|---|---|---|---|---|---|
| Beneficence | | | | | | | | | | |
| Nonmaleficence | | | | | | | | | | |
| Autonomy | | | | | | | | | | |
| Justice | | | | | | | | | | |

**Fig. 3.** Experiment 2. Rank the importance of the guiding biomedical ethical principles from perspective of category in which you fit

the physician." He continues: "Two exceptions to the learned intermediary rule have emerged. ... The first involves mass immunization programs. ... Second, in MacDonald v. Ortho Pharmaceutical Corp., the Supreme Judicial Court of Massachusetts imposed a common law duty on manufacturers of oral contraceptives to communicate risk information directly to the user." What this suggests is that pharmaceutical manufacturers in the United States are likely to be more interested in the principles of beneficence and nonmaleficence than in respecting and upholding the patient's autonomy or assuring equality of access.

Academic researchers are anything but a homogeneous group. They range from chemists and pharmacologists, on the one hand, who are likely to be interested primarily in the potential benefits of a new drug, to epidemiologists, on the other, who are more concerned about accumulating data on possible side effects, risks, and harm. It is, however, likely that neither group of scientists will be predominantly interested in respecting the autonomy of the consumer or in making it possible for all who need a new drug to receive it. I predict that the primary focus of regulators will be on the risks or harm associated with new products; the benefits stemming from them will be of secondary interest. Regulators are likely to be interested more in (paternalistically) protecting consumers than in enhancing their autonomy, although in the United States they are beginning to be responsive to concerns about access.

Physicians might be expected to be the patient's primary advocate, and, therefore, to be interested more than any other party in enhancing patient autonomy. In fact, it appears that around the world the predominant form of the physician-patient relationship is paternalistic rather than collaborative. This is changing rapidly in the United States, where increasingly physicians view their patients as partners in a joint quest for wellness. Overall, however, one would have to rate beneficence and nonmaleficence above autonomy on physicians' evaluation of these principles. Alarmed at escalating medical care costs, many physicians are now expressing concerns about justice and equality of access to expensive drugs.

Historically, pharmacists have been more knowledgeable about drugs and drug interactions than physicians, and have been more concerned about educating consumers with a view to enhancing autonomy. Pharmacists are likely to be concerned primarily about the risks and secondarily about the benefits of drugs.

The media, interested almost by definition in the extraordinary rather than the ordinary, the unusual rather than the usual, are prone to exaggerate both the benefits and the risks of new pharmaceutical products. Either form of exaggeration can be "the kiss of death" to a new product. The overstatement of benefits gives rise to adjectives like "miracle", "magic", and "wonder" as applied to drugs. It is evident in a recent headline in *The New York Times,* which read: "New Antidepressant is Acclaimed but not Perfect" [6]. The strong implication is that there are perfect drugs, a notion as fallacious and as dangerous as the suggestion that any medical intervention is risk-free. Equally, information about risks is often enlarged upon in the media. Sensationalism sells newspapers or brings people back to the television set. These concerns supersede any interest in patient autonomy. With some few exceptions, the media do not use their vast power to educate consumers so as to enable them to make better choices. Certainly this is the case in the United States. So autonomy is probably valued third by the media, with concerns about equality of access fourth.

Strange as it may seem, I suggest that patients value autonomy and justice less highly in their decision to use drugs than what they know about benefits and risks. Also, benefits and risks are likely to be valued differently by different patients. Someone with acne probably will be unwilling to assume a large risk for the sake of a promised benefit. However, the AIDS patient might be willing to assume massive risks for the sake of even marginal benefits. At different stages in an illness, even the same patient might rank benefits and risks differently. At the time of diagnosis, a patient with a potentially fatal cancer might be willing to assume serious risks for the sake of promised benefits; in the terminal phase of the illness, however, when the quality of the time remaining is of paramount importance, there may be less willingness to experience devastating side effects for the sake of marginal benefits.

Where the patients are children, it is astonishing how even well-educated parents will be cavalier about the risks to which they expose their offspring. As Jane E. Brody [7] puts it:

> A study of 500 mothers by Dr. Marshall H. Becker and colleagues at the University of Michigan School of Public Health revealed that half kept seven or more types of drugs on hand for their children, often more than one drug in each category. Four out of five of those interviewed said they would medicate their children for fever without consulting a physician.
>
> A panel of six pediatricians who reviewed the drug choices concluded that the mothers had a lot to learn about the effectiveness, the desirability, and possible hazards of the medications they gave their children.

Advocacy groups are likely to be concerned, above all else, with enhancing patient autonomy and, next, with improving access to costly or scarce pharmaceutical products. Only then are concerns about risks and benefits, respectively, likely to emerge.

## The Third Variable

*These foundational biomedical ethical principles will be variously viewed and valued in different political, cultural, and national contexts.*

The principles earlier described are context-invariant. The principals, also identified earlier, upon whom these principles impinge, are relatively constant. However, they will accord these principles differing weights (or values) according to where they are, whether in Italy or the United States, Belgium, Biafra, Brazil, Uganda, or the USSR. Are we talking about a Marxist or a capitalist country? A Roman Catholic or a Protestant community? A developed, developing, or under-developed nation?

H. Tristram Engelhardt, for example, has some interesting observations on bioethics in the People's Republic of China [8]. He writes, with respect to consent:

> As far as we could determine, consent to medical and experimental procedures involves a full presentation of the likely risks and benefits of the procedures to be used. ... When consent is obtained in difficult cases *the family becomes the focus*. In a commune hospital we were told that the physician often went to the family and that everyone then spoke with the patient about the virtues of the treatment of choice. This approach reflects two aspects of the Chinese resolution of disputes. First, community social pressure is the first and usually very effective mode of obtaining agreement. Second, the family plays an important role in securing patient consent, even with adult patients.

Clearly, this is quite contrary to the American way of doing things! In the United States, on the basis of the principle of respect for autonomy, it is the patient rather than the family who, together with the treating physician (and often more than the treating physician!), is the primary decision maker.

So, in addition to the variables of where one is in the process of moving from knowledge generation to knowledge utilization, and of who is ranking the various biomedical ethical principles, there is a third force influencing how these principles will be viewed and valued: that of the geographical context within which the evaluation takes place. In countries where life expectancy is relatively short, those with immediate needs will be unimpressed by warnings of harm that becomes apparent only with the onset of aging and will grasp instead at the promised present benefits. In countries where individuals are expected to live longer, long-term risks are less likely to be ignored for the sake of immediate gains. In one culture, truthfulness in the encounter between physician and patient will be of paramount importance; in another, a concern to respect the person who is ill will loom larger, especially if he or she is an elder or a leader (like Japan's Emperor Hirohito) and out of respect, the true diagnosis and prognosis may be withheld. In the political context of the AIDS crisis in the United States, gaining immediate access to new drugs has come to be seen as more important than slowly and patiently generating information about risks and benefits.

Not only are different countries likely to come to different conclusions about the ranking of the basic biomedical ethical principles, but even within the same country the emphasis will vary according to the prevailing cultural and political context.

As a final experiment, I asked conference participants to take a blank piece of paper and, first, to indicate whom they thought ought to be at the center of the pentagon of principles (Fig. 1): the manufacturer, the physician, the patient, the physician and the patient, etc. Second, they were asked to state the country they represented and were reminded that it was important in the working groups for them to take into account the national, cultural, and political context in which ethics was being applied.

I expected and predicted that most participants would respond that the patient ought to be at the center of our concern. This would have important implications for policy decisions, whether within the pharmaceutical industry or by regulators, as much as it has for the physician-patient relationship.

## Conclusion

I have proposed a framework of guiding biomedical ethical principles for the theme of this conference, "Improving Drug Safety: A Joint Responsibility." I have also suggested that the principles of beneficence, nonmaleficence, autonomy, and justice will be variously viewed and valued: first, according to where one is in the process of moving from knowledge generation to knowledge utilization; second, according to who is doing the ranking; and, third, according to where one is in terms of the national, cultural, and political context. I have also proposed that in different countries concerns for the community will limit autonomy and require justice more or less severely.

In my view, these three variables make it impossible to offer a standardized biomedical ethical prescription for assuring drug safety. One generalization, however, may be in order. Respect for the autonomy of the patients who ultimately must choose whether or not to use a given pharmaceutical product is assuming more and more force as a guiding ethical principle, not only in the United States where this has been true since the end of World War II, but in other developed countries as well.

It remains to be seen whether or not the trend towards expanding the range of choices available to the consumer or the patient will in and of itself improve drug safety. In the meantime, applied ethics has to take account of the realities of the context in which moral problems emerge, as well as the differing perspectives and values of the various principals, on the one hand, as much as the relatively context-invariant ethical principles, on the other, in the attempt to formulate policy. While not necessarily providing us with absolutely right or wrong answers, this approach will, at the very least, point us in the direction of responsible and honest responses to the challenge to improve drug safety. That may be as much as we can reasonably hope for, and more than we expect.

## References

1. Ames BN, Magaw R, Gold LS (1987) Ranking possible carcinogenic hazards. Science 235 Apr 17: 271–280
2. Young EWD (1989) Alpha and omega: ethics at the frontiers of life and death. Addison-Wesley, Reading, Mass
3. Leisinger KM (1989) Poverty, sickness, and medicines. An unholy alliance? IFPMA, Geneva
4. Blakeslee S (1990) The New York Times. Apr 10
5. Shulman SR (1989) Public health and the law: the broader message of accutane. Am J Public Health 79 (11): 1566
6. Angier N (1990) The New York Times. Mar 29
7. Brody JE (1990) The New York Times. Apr 12
8. Engelhardt HT (1989) Bioethics in the People's Republic of China. In: Veatch RM (ed) Cross cultural perspectives in medical ethics: readings. Jones and Bartlett, Boston

# 10. Corporate Ethics

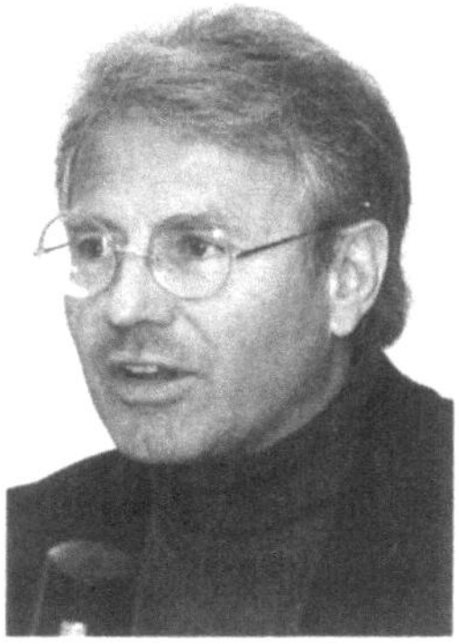

K. M. Leisinger

*"Would you tell me, please,*
*which way I ought to go from here?" said Alice.*
*"That depends a good deal*
*on where you want to go," said the Cheshire Cat.*

Lewis Carroll
Alice in Wonderland

## Introduction

Businesses are rarely indicted for corporate manslaughter, as occurred after the 1987 accident of the ferry "Herald of Free Enterprise," in which nearly 200 passengers died. It is also unusual for a business to evaluate the use of a product safety feature merely by comparing its costs with the economic costs of injuries and deaths that would otherwise result. And yet this has also been done. One automobile company, calculating that a particular safety improvement would cost $ 11 per vehicle on each of its more than 12 million cars and trucks on the road (in 1977), and that these costs far outweighed the economic costs of the otherwise predicted 180 burn deaths, 180 serious burn injuries, and 2100 burned vehicles, finally decided against the additional safety investment, in obvious disregard of the serious consequences [4].

A recent publication on the pharmaceutical industry paints a similarly dark picture. A specific pharmaceutical company which "knowingly and willfully put corporate greed before human welfare, suppressed scientific studies that would ascertain safety and effectiveness, concealed hazards from consumers, the medical profession, and government, and assigned a lower value to foreign lives than to American lives" blamed almost every other major drug company for having done one or more of these things, some of them even repeatedly or routinely [19].

Despite the fact that these examples are, as far as I know, exceptions to the rule, they illustrate why the phrase "business ethics" is increasingly thought a contradiction in terms.

## The Concept of Corporate Ethics

Questions about the ethics of business, its decisions for right or wrong, have been asked for many years. They are heightened whenever a blatant example of irresponsible behavior of "big business" hits the news. Over the last 10 years, in dozens of conferences, seminars, and meetings, people from the business world and from academia have come together to discuss the intellectually appealing subject of corporate ethics. Literature on the subject is growing rapidly, as are courses at universities [1, 5, 6]. Despite all this explication, however, corporate ethics continues to be a source of confusion and sometimes cynical humor among academicians and practitioners alike. The task of defining and implementing "business ethics" has been likened to nailing jello to a wall [16].

In general, ethical questions ask, "What, in a given situation, constitutes morally good and just behavior? What is right and wrong?" These questions burden us all with the responsibility of understanding moral principles and of developing, evaluating, and applying criteria for our behavior. Corporate ethics, by extension, is the effort to answer these questions for one's business relationships both inside and outside the firm.

A distinction must be made between the institutional dimension of corporate ethics, which is demonstrated by the corporation as a whole, and the personal dimension, which is demonstrated by the executives. On the one hand, corporate decision making depends widely on a company's institutional constraints, or on its conventions and the competitive forces it faces. On the other hand, not anonymous giants but people make decisions.

Business ethics is applied ethics. And this is exactly the problem: it is intellectually fun and edifying in the abstract to read books about ethics and give lectures on the subject, but the devil is in the nuts and bolts of moral reasoning in daily practice, especially under serious constraints of money and time.

Whenever it is asked whether a corporation can have a conscience or whether it can be expected to behave "ethically", the answer is usually affirmative. Today's conviction is that society has the right to expect ethical behavior from business [23]. But the underlying question remains: What, under specific circumstances, is "right conduct" or "ethical behavior" for a business corporation? What exactly is the "basic human good" to which individuals and corporations are supposed to contribute, and at what price or other social cost? Answers to these questions are often not only inherently complex, but also depend on complex cultural and personal values. Ethical judgments are easy to arrive at in extreme cases of misconduct, difficult to make more generally.

Although there is no need for a special pharmaceutical ethics, there are some important structural differences between the pharmaceutical industry and other firms. The resulting ethical challenge for the pharmaceutical industry is pronounced: drugs are not commodities in the sense of other consumer or investment goods. They are used because people are sick or in pain, or because they have physical or mental disorders, or because they are dying. Consumer sovereignty, the freedom to choose or refuse a product, is limited in this industry's market.

Similarly, drug safety and risk/benefit assessments that the pharmaceutical industry makes have particularly fateful properties: if their specialists or managers err, they err not just for themselves and their company; they err for the sick people, who are at their mercy. Even when the pharmaceutical industry is governed by comprehensive laws, it must be conscious of the special position it holds arising from its involvement in public health.

## The Perception of Corporate Ethics

In the past 10, 15 years, society's image of private industry, and particularly of large companies, has become shaped by skeptical unease. Many believe that a company cannot simultaneously have high principles and high profits. In fact, the view is increasingly common that many companies are ethically irresponsible, pursuing their profits unscrupulously at the cost of the environment and the safety and health of consumers [3]. This view has also had repercussions for the public's image of executives. In a Gallup poll on the ethical standards and honesty of various professions in the United States, corporate management ranked very low, behind clergymen, pharmacists/chemists, doctors, dentists, college teachers, engineers, policemen, bank clerks, TV reporters, journalists, newspaper reporters, and lawyers [12].

But also within management circles there is widespread doubt if not discontent: in 1977, a study published in the Harvard Business Review reported that 43 % of the executives interviewed felt compelled to resort to practices they considered shady but apparently found necessary for their companies' survival and hence their own careers [2]. Also, more recent studies confirm that executives, predominantly in marketing, experience conflicts between their own ethical beliefs and their perceived obligations to their organizations [24]. European surveys confirm the international scope of the issue [18]. This sad state of schizophrenia has been traced back to the fact that executives are appraised almost exclusively according to their financial short-term results, being rewarded for increases in sales, profit improvements, and cost reductions, and without thought of long-term social consequences.

## A Pragmatic Approach to Corporate Ethics

Although many assume otherwise, there is not an either/or relationship between ethical corporate conduct and profit. The pure pursuit of ethical objectives runs a high risk of ending in practical catastrophes in the business environment. And, vice versa, the pure pursuit of profit can end in ethical disaster. However, neither of the two extremes is at issue in most everyday business.

How can a business enterprise respond to the challenge of corporate ethics? Corporate policies, ethical codes of conduct, and more comprehensive personnel and management development policies are some pragmatic approaches to this end. But what is needed in the first place is a fair amount of common sense.

## Moral Common Sense

Some might argue that common sense is innate, even though it seems that we are often too preoccupied to consider it. Yet, particularly in the world of business, good common sense is invaluable in tackling complex problems. The following rules of thumb, which Goodpaster [10] referred to as "moral common sense,"

may appear rather unsophisticated, but they reflect sound and prudent basic principles of the class of good people to which we hopefully belong:
- Avoid harming others
- Respect the rights of others
- Do not lie or cheat
- Keep promises and contracts
- Obey the law
- Prevent harm to others
- Help those in need
- Be fair
- Reinforce these imperatives in others

Yet, however fair these precepts are, life is not so simple to address, of course; these basic rules do not provide full moral guidelines for every case. The rule "obey the law", for example, might not suffice to prevent harm. Many Third World countries do not have state-of-the-art legislation in product safety or environmental protection; or they are, as Gunnar Myrdal [20] called them, "soft states," where existing laws are not enforced. These and other circumstances require that we take a deeper look at our moral obligations.

Even when the quality of law and its enforcement is high, there is room for ethical reflection. At their best, civil and criminal law reflect the greatest common denominator of acceptable behavior. And because law does not encompass all moral judgments (in fact, for that matter, can sometimes be wrong), ethical behavior goes beyond law. Technological innovations in particular often run far ahead of legislative procedures. Thus, acting legally is at best the ethical minimum and should not be taken as acting morally.

Transnational corporations may face still more complexities. Anthropologists and experts in jurisprudence have shown that moral and legal codes may vary from country to country and from culture to culture. Practices legally and morally frowned on in one place may comply with the law or even be seen as virtues elsewhere. Nevertheless, issues that concern the basic well-being of people and the environment cannot be dismissed by invoking ethical relativism; in some cases there are preferable values that can and should be determined and applied. Responsibility that is perceived as a result of better information or greater insight must lead to corresponding action, even if local law does not compel it. Particularly in areas like product, industrial, and environmental safety, standards that embody state-of-the-art knowledge and the highest morality must be brought to bear consistently, wherever in the world they apply and regardless of whether they are required otherwise.

Widespread poverty, illiteracy, and the resulting poor health conditions in many parts of the Third World are an additional ethical challenge to private enterprises. Those living in poverty do not have sufficient purchasing power to create an attractive market, and their inability to read and write limits their access to adequate information. Pharmaceutical corporations that have built up their knowledge in research and development over the years could make a major contribution to solve health problems in developing countries. Instead, many succumb to the temptation to concentrate scarce and expensive research, marketing, and information resources on markets that produce higher returns [15].

The obvious necessity to follow the rule "help those in need" has no appeal for those taking the bottom line as the guiding beacon. Masters in business administration could offer arguments based on the school of thought associated with Peter Drucker [7] and Milton Friedman [8]. According to this philosophy, the true and only social responsibility of business is to use its resources and engage in activities to increase profit, as long as one stays within the rules of the game, to wit, engaging in free and open competition without deception or fraud. These thinkers maintain that the principles of the free and competitive marketplace automatically moralize corporate behavior, quite independently of any explicit action. Morality, responsibility, and conscience reside, according to this school of thought, in the invisible hands of the free market system, not in the hands of particular organizations, and even less in the hands of their managers. Drucker's and Friedman's thinking is based on that of Adam Smith, and deserves serious consideration. But it should be kept in mind that Adam Smith was a moral philosopher in the first instance and an economist second, a background that hardly applies to the average executive. More importantly, we should remember that our economies do not demonstrate the perfect market conditions, the complete transparency, and the rational consumption patterns that economic models may assume.

The invisible hands of the system, in my conviction, need support by explicitly considered moral common sense rules. Ethical reasoning is even more important if one considers the extent and irreversibility of the potentially harmful effects of modern technologies, for example, of nuclear power plants or genetic engineering, and the cumulative character of their impacts [11]. The hard truth remains "that corporate misconduct, like the lowly cockroach, is a plague that we can suppress but never exterminate" [9].

## Corporate Policies and Codes of Conduct for Sensitive Matters

Not everything legal is legitimate, and better knowledge and deeper insight should lead to appropriate measures regardless of existing regulations. A multinational corporation, which has to function in different legal and social frameworks and which strives for uniform ethical standards, is well advised to develop corporate policies for its sensitive activities, marketing, environmental protection, activities in the Third World, animal rights, research policy, and so on. These policies must find their practical expression in corresponding internal codes of conduct. Both policies and codes of conduct must embody complete and specific state-of-the-art knowledge and be realistic with regard to implementation. Not only should they reflect the philosophy of corporate management but should, prior to their adoption, be seriously challenged by external, independent review. Corporate policies and codes of the kind to which I am referring should be the result of discussions among the best expert minds and brains both within and outside the corporation, even if the relationship between the two has been adversarial in the past. Policy formulated along ideological or fundamentalist lines does not improve the quality of solutions.

Industry dialogues with medical and social scientists, government, medical practitioners, the media, and health, consumer, and public interest groups can help to seek shared understanding. The process of wrestling with problems that have no simple solutions and the willingness to be challenged by people who have different experiences and who base their ethical judgments on different values increases the quality of all kinds of results, not just corporate policies. Such dialogues, if they are to be meaningful, must be enlarged beyond the narrow range of self-interest. While such dialogues will, of course, not automatically lead to comprehensive agreement on ethical matters, they broaden understanding and the available information. All those involved should be able to dispense with claims to superiority, to reconsider their own positions, and, if necessary, to accede. Dialogues illustrate the continuing value of the old Socratic distinction between "certainty," a subjective conviction that is no longer subject to doubt, and "truth," which is objectively identical with the real facts. None of us possesses the definite and complete truth, however certain we may be. All of us are, at best, on the way to a greater truth. It may be painful to admit this, but it is important to continue to search for new and more appropriate solutions, even when we are convinced that we have all the answers. Individual or collective assumptions and perceptions often act as fences that keep some things inside and other things outside our awareness. Openness and pluralism are required, though not arbitrariness or cheap tolerance to avoid arguments. True dialogue, in this case, differs from manipulative persuasion and modern advertising by dealing critically both with the necessity of acting in an economically reasonable manner and with wider public interests.

Only recently has the awareness of ecological problems found expression in the concrete protective measures that specialists and so-called green groups pled for long ago. In the meantime, many years characterized by ecological indifference have passed. This social learning period could have been shortened to the benefit of everyone through proper dialogue. This truth applies to many other sensitive matters, including questions about the safety of pharmaceutical products.

Company guidelines on sensitive matters are obviously not standardized instructions on ethical dealing that can always clearly determine what is ethically acceptable. No code of conduct can possibly cover every single ethical dilemma encountered in daily business practice. Rich [21], in particular, pointed out that an ethical question is one to which there is no clear, soothing, and harmonious answer, no answer that will leave a clear conscience. There are diverse and sometimes conflicting determinants for ethical decisions, stemming from individual, social, professional, and organizational norms. However, reasonable guidelines give the employees of a company a clear basis for setting some priorities and, when necessary, for weighing commercial interests against moral concerns, especially for decisions that must be made under time and financial constraints. The guidelines must contain meaningful and clearly stated provisions, and sanctions must be enforced for noncompliance. It must become clear within the organization that a person can be demoted or discharged for violating codes of conduct, even if the result of the person's misconduct was beneficial in economic terms, and, vice versa, that the intrinsic value of ethical behavior may lead to promotion even if its short-term economic effect was negative. Codes are more useful if they are complemented by complaint review procedures, ombudsman services, and education and certification programs [17].

Corporate policies and guidelines are indispensable for a successful and pragmatic approach to business ethics, but they are not sufficient. As Johann Heinrich Pestalozzi said 200 years ago, no type of government is any good if the people are a real bad lot. Likewise, one could say that the best policies and codes of conduct are only as good as the executives who implement them and that the decisive element is the human element.

## Personnel Policy

Max Weber, the eminent German sociologist, once observed that people who must decide on matters that affect many people's lives will, unless they have lost all reason, find themselves forced to evaluate their ethical motivations and the likely consequences of their decisions based on their knowledge and conscience. Moral rules for business people, again, are not significantly different from those for others, but responsibilities certainly increase with increasing knowledge, abilities, and complexity of technology. We need executives who are fully aware that they are accountable for the consequences of their actions (or omissions), people who try to live in keeping with fundamental ethical ideas.

Personnel policy must therefore aim at recruiting people who are more than expert in special topics. Expertise in conventional business disciplines such as marketing, economics, or general management in no way guarantees proficiency with moral issues. Yet being responsive to the values, convictions, and needs of others is the foundation for sustained business, and should in some way be considered in hiring personnel.

Another aspect of sound personnel policy has to do with leadership and human relations within the company. Here, as elsewhere, the application of the Golden Rule is appropriate: Act in the way you hope others will act toward you. If we stretch this Golden Rule beyond direct personal relations to include information gathering and processing, involvement in decision making, considering conflicting points of view to build consensus, and other forms of earnest company internal dialogue, we will have to arrive at participative forms of management rather than elitist authoritarian decisions.

## Management Development

All major corporations have highly sophisticated management development programs to continually upgrade their executives' skills. And yet, only a few programs cover ethics, and those that do are then directed to top management, not to middle and lower management where (perceived or real) pressures are higher [14]. Admittedly, the subject of ethical reasoning is difficult; virtues like modesty, sensitivity, social responsibility, and the ability to take a larger view of life are not as easily taught as marketing or finance. But, moral philosophy, social psychology, and other resources can help us determine a reasonable approach. Because such disciplines do not supply mechanical solutions or definitive procedures for decision making, practical wisdom and sound, experienced (and ethically sensitive) judgment continue to be indispensable.

On the issue of moral reasoning, it might be thought appropriate to bring in religious points of reference, but there is no need to subject company ethics to ecclesiasticism and every reason to be sensitive to the wide range of employees' religious beliefs. Moreover, in view of the erosion of traditional religious direction found, for example, among management executives in German industry [13], too much emphasis on religious points of reference could be regarded as a Sunday sermon and jeopardize the whole matter.

I am not so naive as to assume that we common folks are able to live up to the ethical ideal of the Sermon on the Mount. If we were, cheating, oppression, exploitation, and other contemptible behavior would have vanished from the earth. Yet, if we are convinced that profit is not the only end, that we also have fundamental responsibilities to society, then we must add to the content of conventional management development. Holistic training within the framework of management development must be sustained, a "quick bleach job" in the subject of ethics will not do justice to its complexity, nor will it result in a change of attitude. Yet sustained endeavors are worth the effort, since they increase the value of decision making and facilitate group efforts, and thus improve the effectiveness of the company.

Such an investment in people can improve the ethical quality of a firm. A corporate environment that supports higher ethical standards in individual decisions is likely to make them contagious. Every manager can encourage ethical behavior in his or her sphere of activity, first of all by setting a good example.

## Broader Measurement and Reward Systems

If we are going to be serious about business ethics, we must not only select executives accordingly and add to management development, but also reconsider performance appraisals. Empirical data show that executives faced with ethical dilemmas tend to opt for the profitable course of action rather than the ethical one, where these are not the same [24]. This has partly to do with the prevailing incentive and appraisal system. As long as we measure employees by short-term financial results only, we risk forcing them to choose between their self-esteem and clear consciences on the one hand and their careers and financial benefits on the other. Performance appraisal criteria must increasingly cover social, ecological, and other ethical objectives in addition to economic and technical ones, regardless of how hard they are to quantify. Accomplishments in product safety, environmental protection, ensuring truth and accuracy in information, and fairness in hiring, firing, and promotion, to name a few areas that are not immediately related to economic efficiency, must be visibly rewarded.

For ethical accountability, we need measurement and record keeping. The measurement of ethical performance could, of course, be elevated to the philosophical heights of the Kantian categorical imperative: did we act in such a way that the action could be taken as a universal law or rule of right behavior? In most instances, however, a much simpler test will suffice: would we feel comfortable explaining to a national television audience why we made this decision?

An important virtue to be considered in appraisal and reward systems is the courage to stand up for one's beliefs. The analysis of several great disasters of recent years shows that long before the Challenger tragedy, the Chernobyl disaster, and the Exxon-Valdez accident, critical voices had been raised about the problems later so terribly revealed. But these warnings were ignored or swept aside. We need to keep in mind the ultimate truth of President Andrew Jackson's dictum: "One man with courage makes a majority."

The law has signaled what is expected of corporate decision makers. In the 1970 court proceedings against a company involved in the Contergan case, the state court of Aachen (West Germany) made the responsible employees liable for their lack of courage. It was the opinion of the court that "In view of the severely harmful implications ... you could have been expected to accept possible personal difficulties. This is not an excessive demand. The health of many people was put at stake" [22].

The selective employment of people who are aware of their responsibilities and sensitive in their judgment, and training and performance appraisals that encompass ethical as well technical content can help ensure that managers are developed people rather than performing robots who do not care what happens to the rest of the world as long as they know how to feather their own and their companies' nests.

## Good Ethics Are Good Business

Why should a company consider ethics in directing its behavior, on top of law, self-interest, and convention? For increasing numbers of people the answer is obvious: more aware of the problems of industrial development, they believe greater corporate responsibility is necessary to save present and future generations from avoidable harm. Simply doing business productively and efficiently no longer suffices today to convince broad segments of society of the legitimacy and value of private corporate dealings. A growing part of our society wants to know not only *how much* a corporation earns, but also *how* these earnings are achieved. The moral quality of corporate activities has gained importance.

Commercial success is thus no longer simply determined by annual profits. There are stronger customer requirements: to be socially responsible, to use energy and other resources wisely, and to protect the environment. Profits to the companies are like food to people: an absolute necessity, without which they die. But only a few, sick people would consider eating the central or only purpose of life. The reputation of a company is one of its most valuable assets, even if it does not appear directly in the balance sheet. The verdict of the public depends significantly on the company's perceived contribution to socially valued ends.

Though to some degree such perceptions are a question of public relations, image campaigns and advertisements cannot manufacture or maintain a reputation if, in practice, the company trades unethically. A company acquires or gambles away its reputation by the way it trades, by the direct contact (through people, products, and services) it has with the public (customers, employees, shareholders, neighbors, and others). Communication programs can only have a strengthening or explanatory effect; they cannot provide the basis for successful commercial trading. Corporate ethics programs are something quite different from image campaigns. A corporation's image can be seriously damaged if the public perceives its ethics programs as merely a cover for reprehensible actions or as aggrandizement of actions that are clearly ethically required.

Applied business ethics will become a greater and greater component of corporate identity. Employees who regard themselves as one with their company in spirit, outlook, and principles have greater motivation to work. The number of consumers who are well informed about what goes on behind the scenes is increasing, and they will make their choices accordingly, as will serious investors, who will not want to be shareholders in a suspect company. Sooner or later it must be recognized that applied business ethics is a matter of enlightened self-interest: frictions within a company can be avoided or diminished, cooperation encouraged, and the corporate image improved.

Ethical conduct in business is additionally important in protecting entrepreneurial freedom: as long as business ethics are low or perceived to be, politicians and government agencies will have to respond. Disclosures of unethical behavior, or carelessness or of gross negligence through investigative reporting and accidents will inevitably lead to more and more stringent legislation. Corporate leadership must take the initiative to achieve certain ethical standards, or its later choices may be severely curtailed.

Business ethics are likely to provide a solid new basis of competition beyond the standard forces of classical markets. For many reasons including a more affluent and informed society, the opportunities and problems of technology use, and others, company ethics may become, and in many instances already are today, decisive in consumer choice. These considerations are seen in young people's choices of their employers. Swiss polls suggest that the perceived ethics of a corporation plays a more important role than salary alone when choosing a job. Trends like this may, admittedly, change drastically, particularly if a recession should occur. But despite this possibility, for an increasing number of people, as both employees and consumers, ethics do matter. This trend will become a business problem for those who ignore it. It will be a business opportunity for corporations who take ethics seriously.

The concern with business ethics is not a passing craze that will simply disappear. It is much more enduring, and increasingly an issue in maturing industrial societies. It is likely to become as integral to corporate decision making as financial and legal matters are today. And, it must be said, beyond the potential high corporate gains of such an approach, to achieve sustainable and enjoyable development for ourselves and our children we have no other choice.

## References


1. Beauchamp TL, Bowie NE (eds) (1988) Ethical theory and business. Prentice Hall, Englewood Cliffs
2. Brenner SN, Molander EA (1977) Is the ethics of business changing? Harv Bus Rev Jan/Feb: 57–71
3. Business Week (1989) 29 (May 29)
4. Davidson DL, Goodpaster KE (1984) Managing product safety: the Ford Pinto. In: Goodpaster KE (ed) Ethics in management. Harv Bus School Publishing Division, Boston, Mass, pp. 111-119
5. De George RT, Pichler J (eds) (1987) Ethics, free enterprise and public policy. Prentice Hall, Englewood Cliffs
6. Donaldson T, Werhane P (eds) (1982) Ethical issues in business. Prentice Hall, Englewood Cliffs
7. Drucker P (1981) What is "business ethics"? The Public Interest 63: 18–36
8. Friedman M (1970) The social responsibility of business is to increase its profits. The New York Times Magazine 13.9.1970: 32 ff
9. Gellerman SW (1986) Why "good" managers make bad ethical choices. Harv Bus Rev Jul/Aug: 85–90
10. Goodpaster KE (ed) (1984) Ethics in management. Harv Bus School Publishing Division, Boston, Mass
11. Jonas H (1984) Das Prinzip Verantwortung. Versuch einer Ethik für die technologische Zivilisation. Suhrkamp, Frankfurt
12. Jones TM, Gautschi FH (1988) Will the ethics of business change? A survey of future executives. J Bus Ethics 7: 231
13. Kaufmann FX, Kerber W, Zulehner PM (1986) Ethos und Religion bei Führungskräften. Kindt, München
14. Laczniak G (1983) Business ethics: a manager's primer. Business Atlanta 33: 23–29
15. Leisinger KM (1989) Poverty, sickness, and medicines. An unholy alliance? IFPMA, Geneva
16. Lewis PV (1985) Defining "business ethics": like nailing jello to a wall. J Bus Ethics 4: 377–383
17. Lowrance WW (1985) Modern science and human values. Oxford University Press, New York, Oxford
18. Management Wissen (1988) 12: 52–65
19. Mintz M (1985) At any cost. Corporate greed, women, and the dalkon shield. Pantheon, New York
20. Myrdal G (1968) Asian drama. An inquiry into the poverty of nations. Penguin, Harmondsworth
21. Rich A (1985) Wirtschaftsethik. Mohn, Gütersloh, FRG
22. Schmidt-Salzer J (1982) Entscheidungssammlung Produkthaftung, vol. IV. Schweitzer, Berlin
23. Sherwin DS (1983) The ethical roots of the business system. Harv Bus Rev Nov/Dec: 183–192
24. Vitell SJ, Festervand TA (1987) Business ethics: conflicts, practices and beliefs of industrial executives. J Bus Ethics 6: 111–122

# 11. Discussion

A member of the audience began the discussion by posing an ethical dilemma with regard to the universality of ethics. The example involved the speaker's supervision of an Indian researcher who wanted to conduct a randomized trial in a developing country with a drug produced by a major international company and marketed heavily and solely in developing countries on the somewhat questionable grounds that it improved psychomotor development in low birth weight children. The trial was to meet rigorous scientific and ethical standards, and the control group would not be placed at a medical disadvantage. The dilemma arose with respect to the issue of informed consent. Were the trial to be conducted in the United States or Australia, for example, participation would

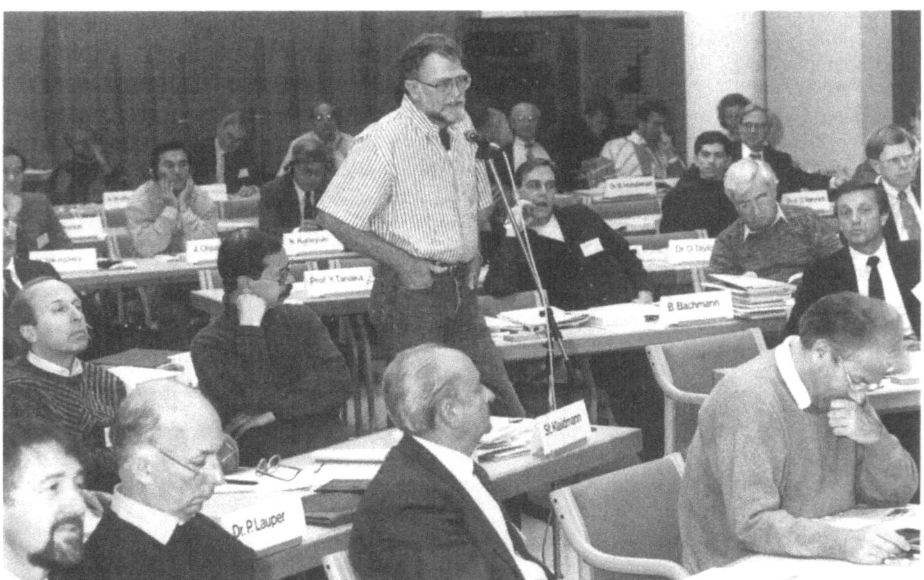

have required informed consent. The researcher maintained, however, that it was ethical for him to proceed without the participants' informed consent, because otherwise he could not conduct the trial and because, on balance, more good than harm would result from the trial. Although the trial subsequently was conducted with his approval, the speaker expressed concern over the ethical dilemma he had faced and invited the comments of the panelists.

In the view of Professor Gorovitz, the argument that more good than harm will result from an action was a very weak justification. Although it is useful to have such information, if indeed it is true, in general it does not constitute a sufficient reason for taking an action. In the case of the dilemma posed, however, Professor Gorovitz emphasized that this does not necessarily mean the trial should not have been conducted. The important point about the universality of ethics, he continued, is that no one has interests that are morally discounted. The fact that a particular population may not have the cognitive or psychological resources to participate in the institution of informed consent does not make its interests less important. It may only mean that we must identify different means to protect those interests. The ideal of informed consent simply does not apply in many situations, including those involving emergency medicine and diminished mental capacity. But that does not mean that informed consent should be circumvented for reasons of convenience. Researchers who introduce the notion of presumed or retrospective consent in their protocols when informed consent is difficult or impossible have a responsibility to protect in other ways the interests of the research participants.

Professor Young, addressing the same issues, expressed his concern about moral imperialism. People in developed countries should not assume that their values and institutions are always to be preferred over those found in other countries. Professor Leisinger wondered why the drug in this example was not being marketed in industrial countries, but only in those countries in which informed consent was viewed as inappropriate. He emphasized that special care was required in conducting medical trials under circumstances of extreme poverty in which a small fraction of the society determines what is good for the rest of the people. Dr. Bankowski added that CIOMS has developed guidelines for the conduct of research involving human subjects, particularly in the context of developing countries, to identify practical alternatives to informed consent. These guidelines recommend that a proposal for such research be closely scrutinized both by an ethical review committee in the country in which the study originates (usually in North America, Western Europe, or Japan) and by a similar committee, even if it has to be created, in the developing country.

A member of the audience asked the panelists if they could suggest any short-term incentives to increase the attention to corporate ethics in the pharmaceutical industry, even if such ethical attention is externally driven by a regulatory agency. He expressed concern that in recent years the marketing practices of the pharmaceutical companies in the United States have become increasingly aggressive and wondered whether competition and market conditions were breaking down corporate ethics.

Professor Leisinger emphasized that the marketing challenge is a difficult one. Multinational companies must balance the need to be locally successful with the need to be internationally acceptable. Yet the research, development, and experience advantages of such firms should make it unnecessary for them to resort to questionable marketing practices in local settings. He also noted that, although good ethics is good business in the long run, it also is true that unethical corporate behavior often leads to boycotts and other responses by consumers in the short run. To enhance the attention given to corporate ethics by pharmaceutical company employees, these companies should actively and visibly promote and otherwise reward employees whose daily codes of conduct reinforce corporate ethical standards.

A member of the audience observed that most people in positions of corporate responsibility want to view themselves as ethical and to do what is right, and that companies can indeed encourage such behavior through internal incentives. At the same time, however, no approach to ethics in business or in any other segment of society will work with a population that is fundamentally uninterested in behaving rightly. Another speaker added that the more ethics is made a legitimate and respected topic of reflection and discourse, the greater the likelihood people will act morally because it is the right thing to do. It was suggested that media could play a role in encouraging such behavior.

Virtue ethics was introduced as a potentially useful alternative approach to encourage greater attention to corporate ethics by business people. In this approach, concepts like integrity, candor, and faithfulness to one's words and ideals are important; the right kind of person to be is given greater consideration than the right way to act. It was observed that business people more readily give attention to ethical issues when they are asked to reflect on what types of individuals they most admire, what kinds of people they would like to be perceived as being, and what choices they would make over time in order to be able to look back on their lives with pride and satisfaction. The applicability of virtue ethics to other professional fields, including government and medicine, was also noted.

A questioner from the audience asked what measures pharmaceutical companies are taking to change the practice of often conducting trials in Third World countries on products unimportant for these countries, while failing to conduct serious research on the unique pharmaceutical needs of people in these different cultures. Professor Leisinger agreed that inadequate Third World pharmaceutical research is being conducted. He stressed that the drug companies are seeking both to expand their research capacities in Third World countries and to give greater consideration to these kinds of international issues in corporate decision making, but that such corporate changes occur slowly.

The panel was asked to comment on how and why the ethics of the right-to-life movement in the United States and corporate ethics in the Federal Republic of Germany could prevent the marketing of the French abortion pill RU 486 in these two countries. Professor Leisinger responded by observing that many drugs are unavailable in the United States, with the right-to-life movement only one of several politically powerful groups able to influence the medical and pharmaceutical actions taken by the United States government. In Germany, the decision not to bring RU 486 into the market was reached only after extended discussions of ethical considerations among numerous corporate officials and reflected the company's best judgment at that time. Others in the audience also spoke on this topic, emphasizing the ethical dilemma involved in making corporate and national decisions about pharmaceutical products as well as recognizing an individual's right to choose whether or not to use drugs such as RU 486. Final comments addressed the ethical dimensions and implications of consciously using less than adequate standards for both medical/clinical trials and patient-directed drug leaflets.

# *Part IV*

# *Generating Knowledge About Drug Risks*

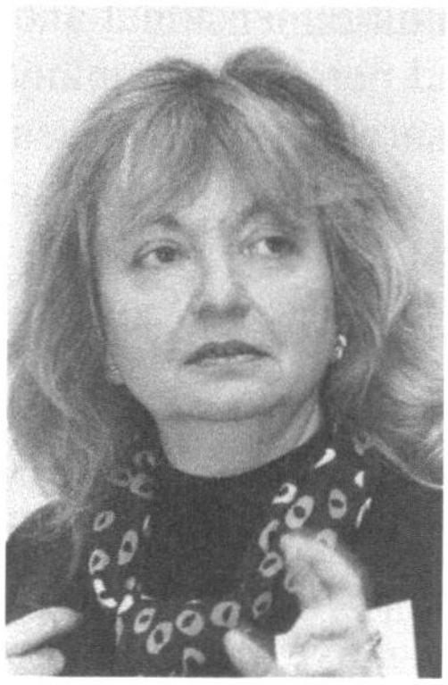

# 12. Categories of Risk and Worldwide Resources

J. K. JONES

## Introduction

The overall goal for understanding drug risk is to characterize and quantitate the risks of pharmaceuticals, and to use this information to manage drugs and to assure their optimal, safe use in populations. Management of the risks of pharmaceuticals is complex, and although the term "drug risk" is used very generally both the meaning of the term and the actual management of the risks are different for the manufacturer, the regulator, the physician and, ultimately, the patient.

The use of any single pharmaceutical product with established benefit will typically have an associated array of adverse effects. It would not be unusual for a drug to have five to ten known serious adverse effects and a number of other less clinically significant side effects. In the majority of developed countries, there are roughly 2000 different generic pharmaceutical entities on the market. Thus, the universe of important information about the risks of drugs could extend from the patient who is taking 1–5 different drugs (10–50 possible significant effects), to the physician with an average armamentarium of 25–50 agents (250–500 effects), to the much larger universes of the multiproduct manufacturer and national regulator.

At the present time, our understanding of the known risks of drugs and their management is rapidly evolving with the increasing interest and study of the area. This paper will outline some characteristics of drug risk in order to chart the directions of our pursuit and identify some of the pitfalls in the development of our understanding.

It will first provide some definitions and the context for this discussion. Then, some commonly used categories of risk will be considered, followed by a brief consideration of well-known factors which modify risk. Next, a multidimensional concept of risk will be illustrated to demonstrate one version of a "map" of overall risk. Finally, the current and future state of our worldwide resources will be described as they might be used to continue this overall process of understanding and charting the terrain of pharmaceutical risk.

The overall message is this: The study of drug risk is multidimensional and complex. It is affected by many factors, and described and perceived in many ways, but these factors are identifiable and potentially measurable (or have even been measured). So, our job in the last decade of this century and looking forward is to describe the scope of this task, get the tools, and proceed.

## The Definitions of Risk and Safety

The terms "risk" and "safety" have attained wider use in recent years, but have sometimes been used interchangeably. Clearly they are perceived to have different connotations, with "risk" sometimes indicating negative attributes, to be subtracted from "benefit", for example, and "safety" connoting a more positive characteristic. However, as noted by both Lowrance [1] and Urquhart [2], "risk" is a quantitative term which refers to a measurement. This measurement is done either experimentally, as an $LD_{50}$ in animal experiments, for example, or alternatively, from either a retrospective or prospective observation of clinical or epidemiological data. These data are then used for a prediction or estimate of likely risk. Urquhart has differentiated two definitions based on different needs. The "what if?" or "talking" definition describes risk as the combined probability and severity of an adverse happening, while a "pricing" (for insurance purposes) definition defines risk simply as the probability of an adverse happening [2].

The determination of "safety" does not involve a measurement, but a judgment based on the acceptability of risk, usually taking into consideration not only the measured risk, or risks, but also the benefits and alternative risks at the very least [1].

In the case of pharmaceuticals, both the measurements of risk and the judgments about safety are very complex and, at the present, plagued with considerable uncertainty; however, much progress has been made in the past decade, and the prospect for future significant progress is considerable. It is useful to outline some of the categories of risk as well as resources for their characterization as one approach to begin to minimize that uncertainty.

## Categories of Risk

The general description of drug risk has been notoriously difficult because it has many dimensions. In general, the range of possible adverse effects to drugs closely mirrors the spectrum of human symptoms and disease, with a few exceptions, and adds a few unique specific drug-caused entities, such as overdose, drug-crystal kidney stones or other drug deposits in tissue, and unique syndromes (e.g., the practolol syndrome). Further, except where the event is unique to a drug, it is often quite difficult to establish a causal association; this is almost always true for individual cases and not infrequently in large populations. In an effort to organize this diverse information for purposes of regulation and public health, various characteristics of these clinical events have been identified as organizing principles for decision making and policy purposes. As will be illustrated with some examples, each of these characteristics varies with one or more of the variables described above; furthermore, as a drug remains on the market, these factors also change over time.

*Pathological Type of Event.* Despite the fact that potential drug effects are myriad, certain discrete pathological categories of adverse drug effects are seen with a number of drugs and a body of information is continuing to accumulate [3–5]. Clearly prominent among these are liver dysfunction, birth defects, hematological abnormalities (e.g., neutropenia, aplastic anemia), serious skin disorders (e.g., Stevens-Johnson syndrome), neurological disorders (e.g., Guillain-Barré syndrome), and various cancers. Although some appear to resemble completely the related disorder, some are unique to the drug etiology, as appears to be the case for some types of drug-associated lupus erythematosus [6]. Although these disorders are often categorized according to body system, a classification partly attributable to the groupings used for computer coding of reactions, a number of events may be multisystem and/or the same drug will produce different manifestations in different patients, as is the case for some anticonvulsant-associated adverse effects in patients genetically at risk (S. Speilberg, personal communication). Both these factors complicate the generalization and description of drug risk to populations.

*Presumed Mechanism of the Event: Type A Versus Type B.* The categorization of drugs according to the presumed mechanism of the event is relatively widely used to denote dose-related (A) reactions versus so-called idiosyncratic, or non-dose-related (B) reactions [3]. It has frequently been noted that although type A reactions are the more common, type B reactions receive the most regulatory attention because of their often unexpected and dramatic nature. Also implied within this categorization is the fact that type A reactions can be predicted and prevented, while type B reactions cannot. However, although the two types are usually qualitatively different, type B reactions are typically those about which little is known. With extension of our understanding of the genetic differences in handling drugs, however, it is likely that a proportion of the type B reactions will, in essence, be dose-related reactions in genetically susceptible persons, as in the lupus syndrome associated with hydralazine and peripheral neuropathy in patients with a particular acetylating enzyme profile, e.g., slow acetylators [6].

*Latency of the Event: Acute Versus Delayed.* In addition to the diversity of their pathology, there is considerable variation in the timing of the manifestation of these events in relation to initiation of drug therapy. This is illustrated in Fig. 1, which shows a hypothetical frequency distribution of the time of occurrence of three types of events seen with a number of drugs after variable lengths of exposure. In some cases, effects which were latent may become manifest after drug discontinuation (e.g., vaginal carcinoma associated with diethylstilbestrol, DES); in others, the appearance of a later effect is based on continued exposure. Both of these factors may have an important impact on the quantitation of risk both in clinical trials and in later studies. For example, some common significant drug effects such as neutropenia and hepatic dysfunction may only occur after 6–12 weeks exposure to a drug. If the time window for a study does not include a

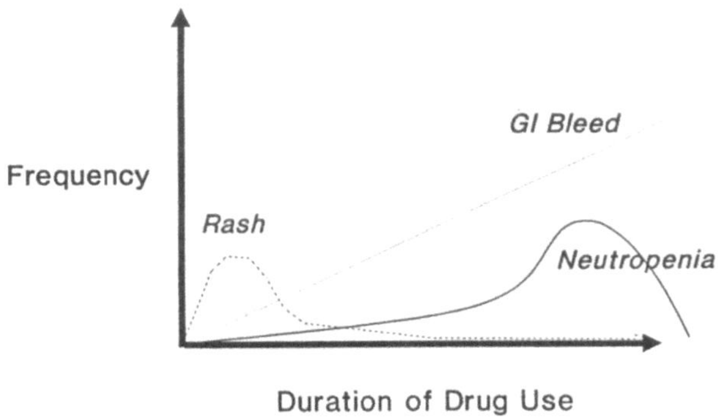


**Fig. 1.** The varying latency of drug-induced effects. Curves indicate a frequency distribution within the population experiencing the effect relative to length of exposure to the drug. *GI,* Gastrointestinal

sufficient number of patients exposed for an adequate time, no effects may be found. Accordingly, the typical latency of an event must be taken into account in a study, when possible. In many cases, these data are not well described except in sporadic reports; this underlines the need for careful description of the range of drug-induced diseases.

*Frequency of the Event: Common Versus Rare.* Knowledge of the frequency of a drug-induced event is a major tool for developing a judgement about the safety of a drug. Unfortunately, quantitative data on the vast majority of adverse effects of drugs are not available owing to the considerable difficulty in quantitating all but the most common effects determined in clinical trials, which are typically those occurring at a rate greater that 0.5%–1%. The majority of effects, particularly the severe, relatively rare effects, are seldom, if ever, detected at this time, so any quantitation in larger populations must be done using epidemiologic methods, usually after marketing. The large number of study patients needed to develop useful quantitative estimates of rate for many significant adverse effects of interest (e.g., anaphylaxis, aplastic anemia) [7] has precluded quantitation in most cases, although the current rapid increase in pharmacoepidemiology studies suggests this will improve in the coming decade.

The value of knowledge of the incidence of a particular event may sometimes be limited to the extent to which the event considers a number of factors which can markedly alter its actual frequency and/or its measurement in a population (e.g., as noted above, the duration of observation and the definition of the event in any study could exclude actual cases). Thus, although a particular event may occur in 1% of a population overall, its frequency may range from 0% in those who take a drug for a few days to more than 30% in those who take a drug for a longer period of time or who are in a special category of risk. This is certainly the case, for example, for oral prednisone, which has minimal risk if taken short-term in high concentrations, but a very high rate of gastrointestinal bleeding after long-term use and/or in the presence of nonsteroidal anti-inflammatory drugs, which can also cause this effect. For the individual patient, the frequency with which adverse effects occur can only be used as a rough probability estimate. Nonetheless, for all attempting to manage drug risk, some notion of rareness continues to be useful and has now been incorporated into the drug label for many United States products.

*Seriousness of the Event: Event Type Versus Outcome.* In recent years, the event type versus the outcome has been widely used in evaluating drug risk as a basis for action and urgency. However, even this characteristic has ambiguity. For example, the majority of described events, such as diarrhea, anemia, edema, and even arrhythmia, may actually range from trivial (in duration, distress, or outcome) to life-threatening. Accordingly, after initial attempts by working groups at the World Health Organization Collaborative Monitoring Center, the United States Food and Drug Administration (FDA), and other institutions to categorize events by seriousness, it was recognized that the outcome of a particular event was more helpful in defining a measure of seriousness[1]. Even here, the consideration of whether criteria of seriousness include use of a prescription drug to treat an event became somewhat controversial, and this criterion was recently dropped by the United States FDA.

With respect to understanding the risk of a drug in a population, the seriousness characteristic has some limitations. In general, the seriousness of an event is often event-specific, and if monitored for, recognized, and treated early is often less serious. Thus, the longer a drug is available and its spectrum of risks understood and characterized, the lower its risk may become.

One interesting example is the risk of pseudomembranous colitis associated with a variety of antibiotics. Prior to the understanding of its etiology and pathophysiology, it was viewed as an extremely serious condition. Today, it is a relatively common, treatable condition which, while serious and often resulting in prolongation of hospitalization, is manageable.

*Detectability.* The estimation of the magnitude of risk may also be affected by detectability. The likelihood of detecting a drug-induced event varies with the clinical setting, the type of event, and the patient, as summarized in Table 1. Each of these factors may vary widely, although they are potentially predictable for any given event. For example, clinical jaundice occurring shortly after starting a drug is very likely to be detected quickly; conversely, a stoic patient with multiple disorders who manifests only mild jaundice and elevated enzymes may not necessarily be detected for some time, unless followed by an observant clinician who either routinely monitors liver function tests and/or does this as part of therapy monitoring. Although such manifestations may be part of the spectrum of a single category of drug-induced event, it is evident that many factors could affect its detection, even in structured monitoring settings.

*Reversibility.* The extent to which an undesired drug effect is reversible if detected, the drug stopped, and the effect treated is potentially important in determining the safety of a drug. Thus, those drugs with even very serious effects which are promptly reversible with specific antidotes (e.g., narcotic antagonists) can probably be considered safer than those with clinically significant, irreversible effects (e.g., tardive dyskinesia, aplastic anemia). However, as with the

---

[1] The United States FDA's current definition of a "serious" adverse event is that the outcome is either death, hospitalization, and/or prolonged disability. Cancer, birth defects, and overdoses are also included.

**Table 1.** Detectability of a drug: factors affecting detection

| | |
|---|---|
| **Event characteristic** | |
| | Manifestation (unique, dramatic versus common sign or symptom) |
| | Affect on function (painful, debility versus asymptomatic) |
| | Timing (latency after exposure to drug) |
| | Time course (rapid versus gradual) |
| **Clinical Setting Factors** | |
| | Complexity of clinical setting |
| | Time physician has for patient |
| | Physician specialty and likelihood of noting event |
| | Likelihood event is routinely monitored (e.g., blood pressure, voice, T-cell count). |
| **Patient factors** | |
| | Number of existing disorders |
| | Threshold for discomfort/complaint |

other categories, this characteristic also varies. For example, some effects are reversible only if caught in time (e.g., acetaminophen hepatotoxicity), and, obviously, if an antidote is unavailable in a particular setting, reversibility is likewise purely academic.

*Preventability*. The likelihood of preventing a particular effect, at least in its most serious form, is a characteristic of drug risk more commonly seen in the legal arena. Consideration of this factor implies use of a drug under optimal conditions (e.g., the correct dose, the right time) in a patient with no identifiable risk factors for known toxicity, information which is typically contained within continuously updated product labels, or data sheets. A considerable proportion of the adverse events that occur are in part due to prescriber failure to exclude populations at known risk or to initiate and monitor drug therapy as recommended, as evidenced in a compendium summarizing drug litigation in the United States [8].

## Factors Which Modify the Risk of Pharmaceuticals in Man

As noted by Palminteri [9], general information about the benefits and risks of drugs cannot be mechanically extrapolated to a benefit/risk ratio in the individual patient. Thus, taken as a whole, each person exposed to a drug over time brings a unique set of characteristics which will determine the actual risk of any drug taken. These characteristics (which become variables in a population study) include most prominently:

- The indication for use of the drug
- Sex
- Other genetic characteristics
- Age
- Other diseases
- Other drugs
- Compliance or drug-taking behavior

The last three factors vary considerably over time in any given individual, which further affects this risk, as is carefully described by Fries et al. in their ARAMIS project [10].

## Estimating Overall Risk

When the risk of a drug is viewed over a population, which is the general view needed for understanding risk by regulators, manufacturers, and public health authorities, the relative impact of the different variables on the probability of risk becomes quite important. For example, it is now recognized that because the elderly have diminishing renal function, the risk of drugs excreted via the kidneys may be significantly increased in this population. For certain nephrotoxic drugs, risk is also increased with duration of exposure so that an overall map of nephrotoxicity associated with a drug in a whole population might be developed, as shown in Fig. 2.

As more structured information on drug risks in populations is gathered, it will allow progressively more refined definitions of true at risk groups of patients. This is already the case for some teratogens which otherwise have acceptable safety (e.g., isotretinoin, tetracycline) and for some drugs administered to the elderly (e.g., aminoglycosides and flurazepam) and to those with known allergies.

Proceeding further, there is the need to have an understanding of the overall drug risk calculated from all of the adverse effects in a population to weigh against the benefits. Figure 3 illustrates three (of many) dimensions which would describe overall drug risk. This task is very difficult, owing to the very factors pointed out in the introduction. Nonetheless, for some drugs, such as the widely studied oral contraceptives, we may be able to begin to approach such a task [11].

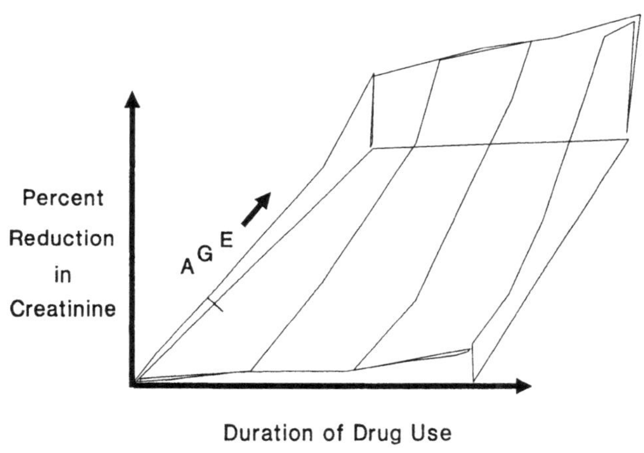


**Fig. 2.** A three-dimensional map of hypothetical risk associated with a nephrotoxic drug, such as aminoglycosides in a population where risk increases with duration of exposure as well as with age

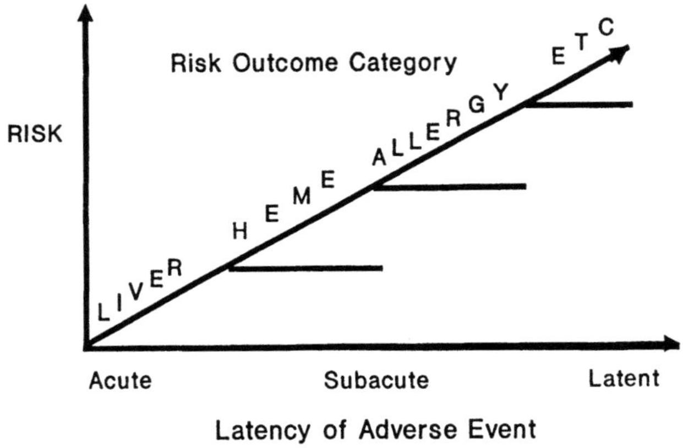


**Fig. 3.** A framework for consideration of overall risk associated with a pharmaceutical. Major categories of risk are considered by pathological category or body system and the risk over duration of exposure. Additional dimensions such as age (see Fig. 2) would comprise a further dimension of information

## The Prospects for Estimating Comprehensive Drug Risk

Although the task of truly understanding the overall risk of even a single drug is daunting, and even more so for the thousands of generic entities on the world market, the prospect for significant progress is good, for several reasons:

1. The marked interest in postmarketing surveillance which began in the late 1970s and has increased to the present, stimulated in part by the epidemic of drug withdrawals in the United States and elsewhere (see Fig. 4, which shows the timeline for the United States). This has resulted in a large amount of active research, which has increased the capacity for greater understanding, as well as knowledge of what is actually happening. For example, the concern over Bendectin or Debendox has resulted in a large body of epidemiologic data on birth defects in general.
2. The concomitant increased awareness of and development of data resources for the study of drug risk over the same time period has seen a rapidly growing effort in all types of data collection, notably the adoption of existing insurance systems for drug surveillance in the United States, the development of several types of systems in the United Kingdom, and great interest in

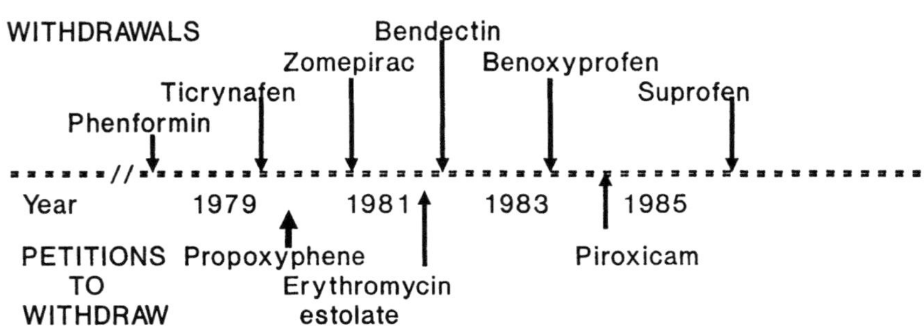


**Fig. 4.** The epidemic of actual and proposed drug withdrawals in the United States

**Table 2.** A summary of resources available for the study of drug risk worldwide by data type. Details of these data sources are described in the RAD-AR Data Resource Handbook [12]

| Type of data | Country | | | | | | | |
|---|---|---|---|---|---|---|---|---|
| | US | Canada | UK | FRG | Nether-lands | Switzer-land | Japan | Scandi-navia |
| Access to linked data on drugs/DX | √ | √ | √ | – | – | – | √ | – |
| ADR data and registries | √ | √ | √ | √ | √ | √ | √ | √ |
| Accessible data on drug use | √ | √ | √ | √ | √ | √ | √ | √ |

*DX*, Diagnosis

developments in several European countries and Japan, as summarized in Table 2. The RAD-AR series of Benefit Risk Data Handbooks, describing in detail all available data sources in the United States Canada, the United Kingdom, Europe, and Japan illustrate the current resources available [12]. In many cases, the use of these resources is just beginning and the prospects for generating a large amount of useful data are excellent. It is also likely, given the growing concern about health care costs and the need for documentation of benefits, that the data on outcomes generated from this sector will also enhance understanding of drug-related outcomes.

3. The increased interest and focus on characterization, both in epidemiological studies and in studies of mechanism, suggest the development of a body of knowledge about drug-induced disease which will help enhance future

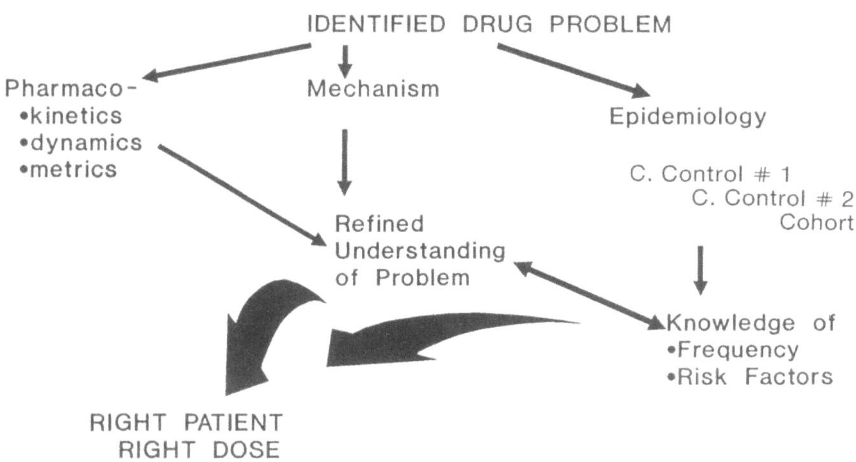


**Fig. 5.** A conceptual view of the integration of diverse information for understanding and managing drug risk. *C. Control,* Cohort Control

studies with more defined case definitions. It will also provide information about both the disorders and the populations in which they occur. These latter data will hopefully identify populations at risk and assist in preventing some adverse effects.

This paper has described some of the factors which must be considered for estimating drug risk and has outlined some limitations to this type of endeavor. A larger framework for considering the overall risk for a particular drug in a population is presented as a model for the future organization of information. Given the growth of data on larger populations and the prospects for automation of much clinical data collection, combined with the widening interest in the area, the likelihood of improved information on drug risk is great. This, combined with consideration of the biological and pharmacokinetic and pharmacodynamic attributes of drug products, as illustrated in Fig. 5, should help ultimately in increasing the likelihood that a drug will be given at the right time to the right patient at the right dose.

## References


1. Lowrance WW (1976) Of acceptable risk. Kaufman, Los Altos, CA, p. 8
2. Urquhart J (1988) Risk perception and management. In: Burley D, Inman WHW (eds) Therapeutic risk: perception, measurement, management. Wiley, Chichester, pp. 13–26
3. Davies DM (1977) Textbook of adverse reactions. Oxford University Press, Oxford U.K.: p 10
4. D'Arcy PF, Griffin J (1986) Iatrogenic diseases. 3rd edn Oxford University Press, Oxford
5. Naranjo C, Jones JK (1990) Drug induced disease: a symposium. Elsevier, Amsterdam
6. Relling MV (1989) Polymorphic drug metabolism. Clin Pharm 8:852–863
7. Strom BL (1989) Pharmacoepidemiology. Churchill Livingstone, New York
8. Patterson RM (1989) Drugs in litigation. The Mitchie Co., Charlottesville, VA
9. Palminteri R (1988) Benefit/risk ratio of new drugs: for whom? J R Soc Med 81:155–157
10. Fries J (1985) The ARAMIS (American Rheumatism Association Medical Information System) post-marketing surveillance program. Drug Inf J 19:257–262
11. Jones JK, Kennedy D, Piper J, Rosa F (1984) Judging risks versus benefits of oral contraceptives. Clin Pharm 3:521–522
12. Jones JK (ed) (1989/1990) The RAD-AR international drug benefit/risk assessment data resource handbook, Vols I (U. S., Canada), II (U. K.), III (Europe), and IV (Japan). Ciba-Geigy International Pharma and The Degge Group, Washington DC

# 13. International Risk Assessment

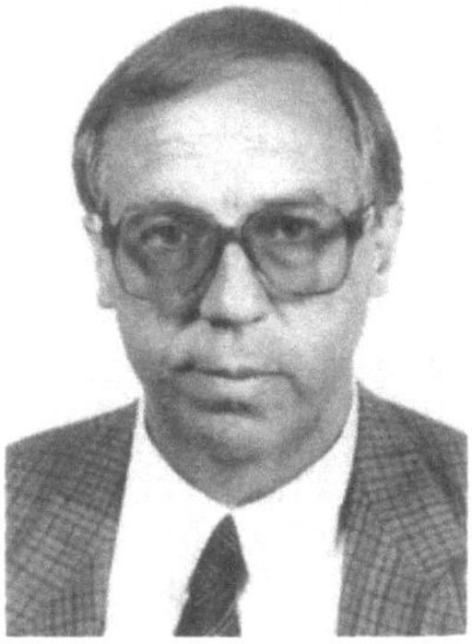

K. STRANDBERG

The internationalization of drug development and marketing as well as the rapid expansion of international cooperation between drug regulatory authorities, including moves towards supranational decision making, i.e., the European Economic Community (EEC), provide a scenario for the 1990s characterized by many more simultaneous introductions of new major drugs on the world market. This will result in massive exposure of patients of different ethnic origins, age, disease patterns, concomitant therapy, etc., to the new drugs without prior postmarketing surveillance (PMS) in other countries. By and large this evolution is a rational one with regard to development costs, need for rapid access to new medicines, and drug regulatory rigor. At the same time, however, it presents the question of how these drugs with a considerable scope of potential problems should be most effectively followed up in order to minimize health hazards. The responsibility for designing, executing, and monitoring necessary surveillance procedures must be shared by the pharmaceutical industry, the drug regulatory agencies, and the medical community.

Fortunately, there have been improvements in clinical trial design, methodology, and monitoring as well as more precise regulatory requirements for data base size and contents. These improvements have moved the process of drug development to a point where frequent short and mild-term adverse drug reactions to a new chemical entity (NCE) can be well characterized in populations prior to general marketing authorization. Generally, much greater care is taken today than 5–10 years ago in trying to maximize relevant data collection in clinical trials. This includes the introduction of, for example, population kinetics data, event monitoring, and patient subgroup analyses. Potential risk factors are, therefore, being screened better, allowing for more targeted studies when needed. In addition, the number of patients included in the clinical trial programs has increased over the years.

Premarketing studies indeed are capable of identifying frequent short-term adverse drug reactions (ADRs), in particular, and also frequent mid-term reactions. This has been repeatedly corroborated by PMS cohort studies and also by Inman's prescription event monitoring (PEM) studies. Our common problem, thus, relates more to the early identification of rare idiosyncratic

ADRs, long-term treatment-induced reactions, and problems emerging as a result of new patient groups being treated, e.g., increased susceptibility and new interactions.

Experience shows that many of the problems associated with the first category surface many years after the introduction of the drugs. In a recent survey [1] it was shown that the median market-life for NCEs withdrawn from the European market during the period 1982–86 was 9 years (Table 1). Only 15 % of these products were on the market for 2 years or less. Clearly, some of the problems for which the products were eventually withdrawn were known long before final action. Also, some of the withdrawals were questionable, but that is not the point. The point is that still new problems are identified for more common drugs long after their introduction. How can we deal with this situation more efficiently, considering that in the near future the gateways of drug introduction are going to be opened wide after marketing authorization has been granted on a worldwide scale? Indeed, this is the theme for this entire meeting, i.e., the collective move towards improved problem identification, analysis, decision making, and information.

Turning to the methodological issues, it appears quite clear that for the rare idiosyncratic reactions we will continue to rely on clinical observations by physicians motivated to pass on their information in the format of spontaneous ADR reports. Spontaneous reporting systems are also capable of detecting new possible interactions, whereas they are less suitable for identifying a higher degree of susceptibility in certain patient groups or changes in frequency rates of certain ADRs. Here, PEM studies might be helpful.

**Table 1.** Market life of products withdrawn between January 1983 and February 1987 in France, FRG, and the UK (from [1])

| Market Life (<2 years) | | Market Life (2–9 years) | | Market Life (>9 years) | |
|---|---|---|---|---|---|
| Product | Years | Product | Years | Product | Years |
| Indalpine | 2 | Antrafenine | 7 | Acetylsalicylic acid | 85 |
| Indomethacin-(Osmosin form.) | 1 | Cianidanol | 9 | Althesin | 12 |
| Isoxicam | 2 | Domperidone | 3 | Aminopyrine | 75 |
| Nitrefazole | 2 | Fenclofenac | 6 | Bendectin | 27 |
| Zimeldine | 1 | Feprazone | 8 | Clioquinol | 50 |
| | | Guanethidine (eye drops) | 9 | Clometacine | 10 |
| | | Indoprofen | 7 | Danthron | 25 |
| | | Isaxonine | 3 | Factor VIII | 14 |
| | | Nomifensine | 9 | Natural growth hormone | 25 |
| | | Suloctidil | 5 | Mercury amide chloride | 30 |
| | | Zomepirac | 3 | Oxyphenbutazone | 25 |
| | | | | Phenacetin | 80 |
| | | | | Phenylbutazone | 30 |
| | | | | Urethane | 50 |

In order to improve the spontaneous ADR reporting instrument overall, the following reporting elements must be analyzed separately: content, rate, delay, and analysis. I submit that with regard to the reporting physician there will be no major breakthrough for the first three elements, as long as it is not imprinted in medical schools or by leading authorities that the duty of every practising physician is to immediately report suspected ADRs according to current instructions. Certainly, feedback information is a key element in keeping it going, but my bias is that physicians' behavior in clinical practice is very much related to what impressed them during training. Thus, for the future it seems mandatory to align much more with academia. In this context it was very encouraging to learn that the Committee on Safety of Medicines (CSM) recently distributed a videotape outlining its activities to be shown to medical students during their term in internal medicine. I think this is a highly recommendable approach.

That motivation is the key element for a successful spontaneous reporting system has repeatedly been borne out by the fact that introduction of mandatory reporting has had no effect on reporting rates where it has been tried. Sweden is just one example which proves this. In other words, you cannot introduce motivation by legislation! Improved motivation will yield better reports, more reports, and more prompt reports. More countries should take up the French, Spanish, and British initiatives where regional clinical pharmacology centers are utilized to stimulate reporting by advising on ADR problems. Surely, this approach introduces the reporting system in a very practical sense to prescribing physicians.

We need more reports but, above all, reports of higher quality. At the same time it must not be forgotten that the alertness must be sustained beyond the early years of introduction of new medicines. Again, this calls for an understanding of the system and sustained motivation.

The next critical step is to handle the reports efficiently in order to identify possible signals as quickly as possible. This is of both national and international interest; my comments are here limited to the international situation. The most recent EEC Commission draft proposal on the "future system for the movement of medicinal products within the European Community" is here the most appropriate starting point for discussion. It correctly makes the point that the prime function of the system is to identify a potential health hazard as quickly as possible. Hence, the job cannot be left to understaffed regulatory agencies alone. This is how I interpret the proposal that copies of all serious ADRs reported to a Member State by health care professionals should be promptly sent not only to the central Medicines Evaluation Agency, but also to the manufacturer of the product(s) involved. This can, of course, be taken further, making access to material possible also for other interested parties, e.g., university researchers.

As a matter of fact, the EEC proposal is right on target compared with the seemingly endless debate on possible wider access of data in the WHO ADR data base, a major part of which consists of EEC Member States' reports. In this context, fortunately, a pilot project dealing with external requests for information from the WHO data base by a systematized country-by-country response was initiated last November. It will be interesting to find out what interest there is in accessing the data base outside the participating National Centers.

It remains to be seen how the EEC Member States will organize and operate their data base. From a technical standpoint, the WHO data base in Uppsala, today comprising more than 800000 reports, would have no problems in handling larger numbers of reports, format changes, selective retrievals, etc. There is now 12 years of experience in handling a large data base and clearly no need for duplication of efforts and costs. If the EEC proposal is successfully implemented, certainly data entry delays will be minimized and signal generation and analysis will be widened. In this respect, it is significant that the EFTA countries have expressed an interest in a common European surveillance system.

I will close with a few remarks on probably the toughest technical problem of all, namely, signal generation and analysis. It goes without saying that signal generation carries the moral obligation to initiate signal analysis. What constitutes a signal is largely still nebulous and in all likelihood an individual matter despite attempts to standardize by causality assessments, algorithms, index cases, etc. My view is that refinement of the methodology in this regard is of virtually no interest compared with the paramount need to quickly and reliably perform signal testing once a signal of a potentially significant health hazard has been identified, regardless of the criteria being used.

In this context, record linkage systems seem to offer at least cost-effective screening potential. On must be fully aware of the need at this point in time for speed. A major advantage of record linkage systems is just that. The problem is that such analyses may not be enough for validation or refusal of a signal. Case-control studies or cohort studies may be called for. However, and most importantly in the context we are discussing, record linkage studies are frequently likely to give a stronger indication than a signal alone. For regulatory bodies and pharmaceutical industry alike, this is important with regard to both problem solving as such and possible aroused public concern.

A more alarming problem, however, is the fact that there do not seem to exist enough data bases for the anticipated need. The problem is increased if new drugs are to be monitored continuously by record linkage studies in order to identify long-term treatment health hazards less arbitrarily and, hence, at an earlier stage.

The objectives for the use of medical data bases in an international perspective need to be defined. The potentials and limitations of the systems need to be clearly described, as do the safeguards required to guarantee that patient confidentiality and, hence, integrity will not be jeopardized. The fact that public concern about potential abuse of medical data bases in some countries still may not be overcome by these measures calls for an international consensus. This conference may be an excellent venue for discussing this option. If found appropriate, the forthcoming WHO meeting intended to shape the WHO International Drug Monitoring Programme for the future could be the ideal forum for a consensus statement. Hopefully, this would be accepted as a nonbiased declaration of what techniques are needed for improved international drug surveillance. Such a WHO statement would provide an extremely valuable platform for national explorations on how to participate at the global level. Here, it would be very appropriate to bring into focus all the current problems that can be studied only by an epidemiological approach. Again, it will be evident that most of these problems would take very long and be very costly to study using alternative methods – if indeed possible at all.

## References

1. Scrip Bookshop Report (1988) Drug withdrawal from sale: an analysis of the phenomenon and its implications. PJB Publications, Richmond, UK

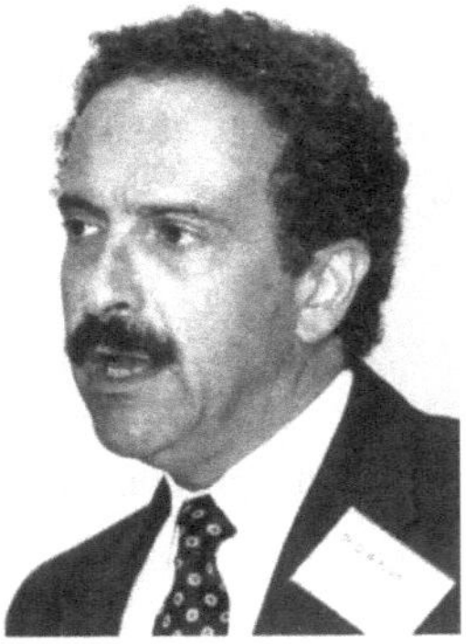

# 14. Resources Needed for Risk Assessment

G. A. FAICH

## Introduction

This paper addresses resource needs for assessing the risk of pharmaceutical products. My remarks are largely confined to the postapproval aspects of risk assessment and are based on lessons learned during the 6 years I have been charged with postmarketing safety monitoring at the Food and Drug Administration (FDA). There are three ingredients essential for providing resources for risk assessment:
a) data resources,
b) people, and
c) money.

Several beliefs underlie this entire presentation. First, for pharmaceuticals, I believe that assessment must precede communication; this seems obvious. Secondly, animal and mathematical models will not generally work in assessing pharmaceutical risk. This is because pharmaceuticals are generally used in the face of disease and are beneficial; most models, however, do not allow for the background of disease risk and the integration of these benefits. Also, since we have direct human experience with drugs, there is every reason to use epidemiologic techniques instead of speculative extrapolations from animals. Thirdly, for risk assessment to be meaningful, I strongly believe that it must be based on comparisons between drugs with similar indications and not attempt irrelevant comparisons with accidents of nature and other life risks.

## Resource Needs

Why have resources for risk assessment been delayed in coming? Probably the overall main reason is that there has been a lack of demand for risk assessments. Drug approval is primarily based on clinical trials, which have become the religion of drug development and approval [1]. A sad consequence of this is that nonexperimental observational data are often thought to be excessively complicated, confounded, uncontrolled, and heretical. Consequently, regulatory authorities and pharmaceutical manufacturers have not adequately contributed to developing risk assessment resources.

Postmarketing risk assessment is not a major regulatory focus except when a crisis arises; that is, routine comparative risk assessment is not a programmatic priority for regulatory agencies. Nonetheless, this area is bound to be increasingly important to physicians and third-party payers. Competitive consequences of comparative risk analyses will have a major influence on the need for risk data. For this reason, we must improve our methods and include anticipatory postmarketing studies as part of drug development [1].

## Data Sources

### *Adverse Drug Reactions*

Systems to collect and analyze spontaneously reported adverse drug reactions (ADRs) are the cornerstone of postmarketing surveillance [2]. It is well established that the collection of reports by manufacturers and regulators is crucial to the early detection of important new safety information about marketed products. Based on United States and World Health Organization data, it is also clear that ADR reporting is increasing in volume.

In order for ADR reporting systems to function effectively, regulators must develop clear guidelines for manufacturers about reporting requirements and methods [3]. It is also imperative that practitioners be stimulated to report ADRs. From the experience gained in pilot studies conducted in the United States, it is clear that such promotion must be done by simple means and focus on reporting serious reactions to newly approved new chemical entities [4, 5]. The rapid processing of reports using triaging and screening methodologies is the key to their use. In the United States, well over 60000 reports a year are received, and this volume is managed using a computer-assisted process and a sorting system to identify new and serious reactions.

ADR reporting systems should be viewed primarily as a method for developing signals of the possible association between a drug and a reaction. However, they must not be the last word in determining risk. Risk is the probability of harm, and its quantitation depends upon measuring the actual rate of occurrence of adverse events following an exposure. Because of underreporting and other limitations of all ADR reporting systems, the signals generated from these systems require additional independent studies to quantitate rates of occurrence. In recognition of these limitations in ADR reporting systems, the FDA routinely warns users to exercise caution in their interpretations of ADR reports (Table 1).

A major problem we all face is that information from ADR reporting systems will be used as indirect measures of risk if other data cannot be rapidly generated. To put it bluntly, poor data will be used if good data are not available. This is one of the central reasons that manufacturers and regulators should support approaches that go beyond ADR collection to assess risk.

**Table 1**

| Caveats for the use and interpretation of ADR reports |
|---|
| 1. There is usually no certainty that the drug caused the reaction<br>Suspicions, not absolute conclusions<br>The event may be related to the indication, not the drug |
| 2. Accumulated case reports are not reflective of incidences or estimates of drug risk |
| 3. Rates based on these are measures of reporting intensity, not actual occurrence rates |
| 4. Reporting is affected by numerous factors which limit the ability to make valid comparisons between drugs and statements about a single drug such as:<br>Length of time drug marketed<br>Size and training of manufacturer's sales force<br>Manufacturer reporting practices<br>Market share of the drug<br>Articles in the medical literature and lay press<br>Special promotions and advertising<br>Special studies or marketing studies<br>Regulatory action |

### *Linked Data Bases*

After signals appear from ADR reporting systems or other means, there is an urgent need to rapidly determine wheter they are likely to represent major risks. This determination can be made using linked data bases which have the potential to provide rapid, valid, defensible, cost-effective data [6, 7]. These data bases typically derive from patient management and claims files and have on many occasions proved to be extremely useful. In recognition of this, the FDA has been supporting a number of these through grants and contracts [8]. Ideally, these data bases would be used by experienced investigators and would combine information on a large number of exposures with longitudinal patient information. They would be easily accessible and linkable across separate data sets and would provide at the very least a second-level screening of preliminary signals.

It should be emphasized that there are major limitations to these data bases. These include their limited size, inadequate linkage, and the lack of experienced investigators. These data bases will *not* solve all risk assessment problems, but should be viewed as a preliminary means to conduct epidemiologic studies. Often, if not always, original patient charts will be required to validate information stored in the automated systems.

### *Drug Usage*

Drug usage information can be derived from linked data bases, commercial marketing sources such as Intercontinental Medical Statistics (IMS), and the manufacturer's estimate of usage. Drug usage information is important for assessing spontaneous ADR reports as denominator information. It also allows for studies of descriptive patterns of usage. Such patterns may signal risk concerns such as those found in the United States in the overuse of Accutane by women in child-bearing years. Surprisingly, many companies have a considerable amount of use information based on marketing surveys which may not be used by people in the same company who are charged with assessing postmarketing risk.

### *Ad Hoc Studies*

It is evident that, when important risks are suspected, structured epidemiologic studies may need to be conducted. Perhaps the most underdeveloped area in risk assessment is the appropriate use of anticipatory postmarketing observational studies. Such studies might allow for facilitated approval and, if properly targeted, will generate the data needed to answer risk questions which will arise after marketing.

For example, this type of study is now being conducted on topical minoxidil, a drug used to treat baldness. While the drug is not absorbed much under normal conditions, it is vasoactive when given orally. The FDA was concerned that case reports of myocardial infarction temporarily associated with drug exposure would be received and we would be unable to determine if the rate of these infarctions was increased by minoxidil exposure. Put another way, without a study it would be impossible to say if infarctions were coincidentally associated with exposure or not. For this reason the study was conducted. Preliminary analyses of the 10 000-patient postmarketing study appear to show no increase above the expected rate in cardiac events in users of minoxidil.

## Personnel

Data bases will be of little value without skilled professionals. I believe the key expertise needed for risk assessment is knowledge of epidemiology. Pharmacoepidemiologic training has only recently been supported by academia, industry, and government. In the past few years, there has been a much needed expansion in educational opportunities in this field. In the Western hemisphere, single course programs are now available at a number of universities, including Columbia, Harvard, Boston, McGill, and the University of North Carolina, to name a few. McGill has gone even further and developed master's and doctoral programs. Industry has provided some funding for these programs (e.g., Burroughs-Wellcome, Ciba-Geigy, Merck).

Within the United States government, most of the available training is "on the job". Some training support is available at the National Institutes of Health (NIH) and the FDA. In recent years the FDA has had at least nine trainees in pharmacoepidemiology and has been involved in conducting courses at universities and at FDA's own Staff College. Even with all this new effort to train pharmacoepidemiologists, there still remains a great shortage. This will only lessen when more funding for academic programs and project work is made available.

## Funding

Training of personnel, their gainful exploymeat, and development of data bases are dependent upon funding. Funding will only flow when the demand for risk assessments increases. This necessary demand is only now beginning to appear. The FDA has been the only core support source for pharmacoepidemiology in the United States. Funds have been greatly limited ($ 1.5–2 million per year) and have been used strictly for existing functioning data bases and not for data base or personnel development [8]. NIH and National Research Council funding almost everywhere is primarily geared toward specific questions often related to prevention and long-term mortality and morbidity (e.g., oral contraceptives, vaccines, AIDS, cancer therapies, hypertension, cholesterol lowering). These are certainly important efforts, but are not geared toward quantitating risk from most everyday therapeutics. Industry funding has been delayed in coming, but is now beginning to flow and will become imperative in the future. I feel industry will and must be the most important source of funding in the future.

## Barriers to Epidemiologic Approaches to Risk Assessment

I have identified our needs as data, people, and money. What are the barriers to providing for these needs (Table 2)? The greatest barrier is inertia – "we never did it this way before;" "it's not required" to get on the market; and the methods are "new, strange, and different from the clinical trial approach." I believe we need to be innovative and creative in our approach to safety, risk, and approvals. Clearly, familiarity can only come with use of epidemiologic techniques. Many epidemiologic studies may produce equivocal results and be slow to provide answers. Yet, growing sophistication in methods, newer data bases, and more targeted research should lessen these frustrations.

**Table 2**

| Barriers to epidemiologic approaches (regulators and industry) |
|---|
| 1. Perceived lack of rigor and validity |
| "Soft" data |
| Compared with trials (experiments, randomization, etc.) |
| 2. History of confusing results |
| Reserpine and breast cancer |
| Agranulocytosis |
| 3. Delay, cost |
| 4. Not driven by regulations – not required |
| 5. Data bases and epidemiologists not available |
| 6. Unfamiliarity with methods |

## Conclusions

Risk assessment, from my viewpoint, is dependent upon providing for data base development and use and training in pharmacoepidemiology and funding. We seem to have begun to move in this area, but much more needs to be done. Risk assessment will become increasingly important for approval, cost effectiveness, and competitive reasons.

## References

1. Faich GA, Lawson DH, Tilson HH, Walker A (1987) Clinical trials are not enough: drug development and pharmacoepidemiology. J Clin Res Drug Dev 1 (1):75–78
2. Faich GA (1986) Adverse drug reaction monitoring. N Engl J Med 314 (24):1589–1592
3. Sills JM, Faich GA, Milstien JB, Turner WM (1986) Postmarketing reporting of ADR's to FDA: an overview of the 1985 FDA guideline. Drug Inf J 20 (2):150–156
4. Scott HD, Thacher-Renshaw A, Rosenbaum SE, Waters WJ, Green M, Andrews LG, Faich GA (1990) Physician reporting of ADR's – Rhode Island. JAMA 263:1785–1788
5. Rogers AS, Israel E, Smith C, Levine D, McBean AM, Walente C, Faich GA (1988) Physician knowledge, attitudes and behavior related to reporting adverse drug events. Arch Intern Med 148:1596–1600
6. Faich GA, Stadel BV (1989) The future of automated record linkage for postmarketing surveillance: a response to Shapiro. Clin Pharmacol Ther 314:387–389
7. Ray WA, Griffin MR (1989) The use of medicaid data for pharmacoepidemiology. Am J Epidemiol 129:837–849
8. Food and Drug Administration (1987) Studies of reported adverse effects of marketed drugs; availability of grant; request for applications. Federal Register 52 July 10:26086–26088

# *Part V*

# *Generating Knowledge About Drug Benefits*

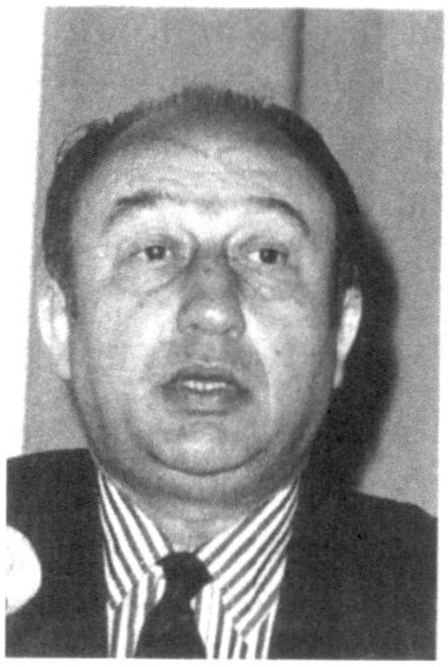

# 15. Quality of Life and Health Status: Innovative Outcome Variables for Research in Population Health

W. O. Spitzer

Quality of life and health status have acquired increasing importance as outcome variables in research, public health, and practice, where the ultimate latent objectives are to improve the lot of the sick and to protect the good fortune of those who are well. How well we do in those parallel objectives can no longer be assessed merely by measuring length of survival in patients or mortality rates in populations. This is not a new idea, since we have been aware of such imperatives for at least 15 years. During this time, clinical investigators, epidemiologists, social scientists, and statisticians have been developing measures of the attributes we term quality of life or quality of survival among patients. We have also invested much intellectual effort in quantifying the somewhat different concept of health status in population.

## Historical Foreword

One should not forget that long before quality of life measurement was in vogue, a handful of pioneers had introduced the revolutionary notion of function as an outcome variable of importance to the clinician and the social scientist. I shall mention only two of those giants: Karnofsky, who developed a measure of "performance status" [1, 2], and Sidney Katz, who produced an "Index of Independence in Activities of Daily Living" [3, 4].

When did the phrase quality of life, referring to human health and welfare, come into use? How is it linked to the concept of health status? The process of measuring health status is closely related to the assessment of health-related quality of life. When did measuring health move from the realm of philosophical speculation to the domain of attainable, relevant, and scientifically meritorious endeavor?

I must start with the World Health Organization (WHO) definition. In 1947, the WHO incorporated a definition of health in its constitution affirming that "health is not only the absence of infirmity and disease but also a state of physical, mental and social well-being" [5].

There is much disagreement about the usefulness of such a definition as a guide to research or to public health practice. There is also disagreement among thoughtful writers whether the WHO definition best describes health or rather perfect happiness. Lest we regard happiness as a trivial matter, one should not forget that Thomas Jefferson, when drafting the United States Constitution, included the pursuit of happiness as one of mankind's inalienable endowed rights. Moreover, it appears that the majority of methodologists in the health sciences and in the social sciences have adopted a policy of incorporating at least three dimensions in any scale of index purporting to measure health or quality of life: namely, physical function, mental status and ability to engage in normative social interactions. A good example is the McMaster Health Index [6].

When we search the medical literature using computer-assisted search facilities, we find that the relevant key word, quality of life, was not used before 1975. However, there were certain landmark papers before then.

First, a national survey done in the United States in 1957 was conducted by the Institute of Social Science under the auspices of the Joint Commission on Mental Illness and Health and reported by Gurin and associates [7]. The survey assessed clinical symptoms, emotional disturbances, and the type and nature of professional advice sought by respondents. It delved into determinants of happiness, reasons for worries, and outlook for the future of people in the samples surveyed.

Early acknowledgment of the importance of measuring quality of life is found in the 1960 Report of President Eisenhower's Commission on National Goals [8].

Referring to other early landmarks in the medical field, we have reached the 40th anniversary of Karnofsky's first publication. He introduced a scale which gained wide acceptance despite the shortcomings of the scale, which emphasizes physical functioning heavily [1, 2]. Although validation was cursory for several decades, Karnofsky's scale of performance status works well. It is used readily by clinicians, and it has been shown to have surprisingly good correlation with other indices designed to measure emotional well-being and social and physical function. Karnofsky's ideas and efforts may seem pedestrian and unimaginative today, but in 1948 his work was a radical departure from conventional approaches to assess the prognosis and progress of very sick cancer patients.

Somewhat later, in 1963, Katz gave us the Activities of Daily Living Scale [3]. A simple questionnaire, it seems, but it has face validity of compelling strength, and it is acceptable to investigators in a wide range of disciplines. It is understood well by clinicians and patients alike. Katz not only facilitated the operationalization, or the measurement of function, but channelled our minds to the importance of outcomes such as physical function in the context of daily life as part of the overall clinical evaluation of patients. I was one of those convinced early in my career by Katz's writing that levels of function should be measured and, more importantly, that they can be measured.

Some of the earliest papers to be found in the medical literature which deal with quality of life are editorials. In such an opinion paper Elkinton writes to the *Annals of Internal Medicine* in 1966:

"... what every physician wants for everyone of his patients old or young-is not just the absence of death but life with a vibrant quality that we associate with a vigorous youth. This is nothing less than a humanistic biology that is concerned, not with material mechanisms alone, but with the wholeness of human life, with the spiritual quality of life that is unique to man. Just what constitutes this quality of life for a particular patient and the therapeutic pathway to it often is extremely difficult to judge and must lie with the consciousness of the physician" [9].

Elkinton questioned the goal of curing disease such as that set up by the Johnson presidential commissions, which recommended 25 national centers to treat heart disease, cancer, and stroke and to find better treatment for those specific diseases. Instead he endorsed the goal of ancient Greek medicine, to help your patients to "die young – as late as possible" [10].

In another editorial, this one written in 1973 in the *New England Journal of Medicine,* Bunker and Wennberg [11] turned our attention to quality of life in relation to discretionary or elective surgery. They deplore the excessive use of mortality statistics to assess the appropriateness, accomplishments, and relevant merits of surgery, most particularly elective interventions. They discuss data, suggesting that lower rates of discretionary surgery may be associated with lower rates of disease-specific mortality. But they go on to say that "even if the hypothesis is found to be correct, it does not necessarily mean that fewer operations (than performed in Canada and the United States) are better. Death is, after all, only one index of the public health – or lack of it. It is to the improvement in the quality of life – to the relief of disability, discomfort and disfigurement – that elective surgery is primarily directed."

The increasing frequency of occurrence of the phrase quality of life in the medical literature attests to the growing interest in the subject by physicians and surgeons. Only four papers had quality of life in their titles between 1966 and 1970; there were 33 papers in the next 5 years (1970–1974). The specific subject areas included the contribution of the physician to the quality of life of people, quality of life of hospital patients (mainly in nursing journals), quality of life in schools and universities, quality of life in old age, and quality of life in poverty. In more recent years, one notes a trend to evoke quality of life as a target outcome for treatment in specific diseases, particularly the cancers, end-stage renal disease, hypertension, coronary artery bypass surgery, arthritis, hearing impairment, and specific mental illness. Quality of life is a target also in relation to nutritional requirements for people in developing countries. We see that whatever the phrase quality of life means to different writers, investigators, and lay people, it designates a prominent goal for health care in a very wide range of endeavors of patient care, health care systems, and social programs.

One might call the last 15 years the "modern era" in the field of health status measurement. We were ushered into this period by the work of several social scientists. They published in the health literature, facilitating access to the methodology for clinical investigators and epidemiologists. Papers began to appear in the early 1970s. The first wave authors included Bush and Chen [12]. In 1975, Marilyn Bergner and her colleagues first published reports about the Sickness Impact Profile (SIP) [13]. Further accounts of validation of the SIP were published the following year [14], and the Center for Health Services

Research at the University of Washington reported on final development and testing of the SIP in 1981 [15]. Kaplan, Bush, and Berry developed and published the Index of Well-Being in 1976 [16]. Ware, Brook, Davis, Stewart, and others developed and published the Rand General Health Perceptions Scale in 1979 [17].

My colleagues and I developed one of the few generic scales ever planned from the outset to be a quality of life measure. Reports of the calibration of research and validation appeared in 1981 [18]. Since then, we have witnessed an epidemic of scales and indices conceived to measure quality of life.

## Defining the Concept

There is considerable confusion in the health literature and in the literature of the social sciences about the attributes we are measuring as outcomes. The terms health status, quality of life, and functional status are used interchangeably. Investigators who 15 years ago started talking about their measurement instruments as health status measures now write about measuring quality of life. Similarly, the relative few who started out with the intent to measure quality of life sometimes drift into a stance of measuring health. What is said, what is written, and what is done seems to be determined at times by the theme of the conference one attends or the title of the book to which one contributes a chapter.

My view is that measurement of *health status* should be primarily for assessment of ostensibly healthy people, usually in the context of aggregates of unselected geographically defined populations or catchment area delineated clinics of a service program. It seems almost inevitable to me that the process of measuring health status will be primarily a research activity, since discrimination along the range from "perfect health", if that exists, to "probably compromised health" requires lengthy and elaborate measuring techniques unlikely to be administered reliably by clinicians in the course of patient care.

In my view, in contrast, the measurement of *quality of life* should be restricted to the assessment of a series of attributes among those definitely sick. The person classified by health-related or health-sensitive quality of life measuring instruments should have clear-cut manifestations of disease according to established explicit or at least implicit criteria of one or more diagnoses. Such scales can be modified in a minor way to increase discrimination at the end of the morbidity spectrum where people are very sick and in fact are terminally ill.

Figure 1 depicts the spectrum in which people can be found from state of near death and terminal illness to "perfectly" healthy. Measures of health status as we have known them and as they continue to be developed seem apposite on the right side of the bar shown in the figure, and health-related measures of quality of life are best applied on the left side.

There is a third group of outcome measures relevant to our discussion which can be referred to as hypothesis-determined functional measures. One now finds these tenuously lumped with either quality of life measures or health status measures. But these are measures of function generally designed for clinical

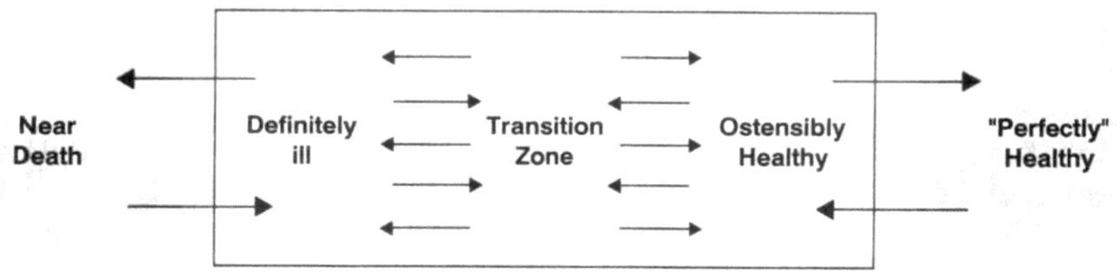


**Fig. 1.** Spectrum of health status states

investigation which evaluate the extent to which patients exposed to therapeutic, rehabilitative, or even preventive intervention can function in a restricted dimension demarcated by anatomical, physiological, or system targets. The demarcation is imposed by the intervention concerned. One wishes to know, for instance, what is the sexual function of those operated upon for breast cancer or prostatic diseases and for patients left with abdominal colostomies? How are selected activities of daily living changed following specific interventions of occupational therapy for amputees? How far can patients with chronic obstructive pulmonary disease walk after receiving intermittent assisted nocturnal breathing?

It is encouraging that investigators now recognize that functional outcomes must be included in trial assessing interventions that can affect function. What is regrettable is that many investigators assume that completely different generic or global scales of quality of life need to be designed de novo each time a new hypothesis is tested.

I hope that in the next few years investigators concerned with specific hypotheses about function will take one of a small number of available, validated, quality of life measures and append selected questions oriented to the hypotheses rather than reinventing the wheel for the generic index with each study. Conversely, methodologists concentrating on the development and calibration of global or generic measures of quality of life should construct them so that supplementary questions are easily appendable. Thus, results can be published simultaneously for general global function, with measures known by researchers and clinicians. Beyond that, for specific functions one can use measures relevant to the particular patients under study.

I will now point to common features of all the types of generic data gathering instruments I have discussed. In my view, we are not in the domain of either quality of life measurement or health status measurement unless we include physical function, social function, emotional or mental state, burden of symptoms, and perception or sense of well-being. These five groups of attributes seem to be found in most accepted and validated instruments. I would challenge those proposing a scale or index with less than those dimensions about the content validity of their measure.

Lastly, in examining what the attributes of quality of life and health status are all about, I am concerned with the frequently expressed assumption that their ascertainment depends entirely on reports by respondents of subjective perception. Indices can be designed so that clinicians can score the patient's quality of life or health status after observing or examining a patient even without eliciting information from the patient about how he or she feels at a given point in time. I have evidence from my work that this can be done so that scores taken from the objective assessment of the clinician and the report of the patient's subjective findings agree very well. Future work must permit both types of assessment if we are to advance the needs of ongoing patient care and health surveillance in populations. Otherwise, the logistics alone will be the barriers to implementation of quality of life indicators in clinical management based on sound clinical research.

## Number of Instruments

There are too many instruments purporting to measure health status and quality of life. As mentioned in the preceding section of this paper, I do not deny the need for appendices to generic scales which focus on outcomes determined by the hypothesis of a research question or by a particular clinical manoeuver. We are now hopefully at the peak of the epidemic of quality of life measuring schemes. This embarrassment of riches bewilders clinicians and even investigators. It does not favor in-depth work dedicated to validation, and it militates against understanding and acceptance of these types of measures for clinical research and clinical practice. The profuseness of the measurement instruments reported in the literature seriously inhibits comparison of the results and ascertainment of significance of the results across different studies assessing similar problems.

I believe that most of what needs to be done in health services research that requires measurement of health status can be accomplished with three, or at most four or five, thoughtfully developed and carefully validated measures of health status which are "on the shelf" now. I would be happy if, for the next decade or so, we narrowed our armamentarium to three finely-tuned good measures now in existence: the SIP [13–15], the Index of Well-Being [16], and the Rand General Health Perceptions Scale [17]. When it comes to quality of life, I am less objective about the subject and I will not presume to suggest which three or four scales should be candidates; but we only need three or four. At least one of these should incorporate utility function techniques for measuring quality of life. All approaches to quality of life measurement should bear in mind the need for applications that permit measurement of harm and benefit in large unselected populations. A crucially important application is in the field of postmarketing management of drugs in society. The lack of measurement of benefit to balance surveillance of harm has left an entire area of socially relevant endeavor at the mercy of sensationalists in the press or subordinate to the needs of bureaucratic self-protection.

## Validating the Instruments

Most measuring instruments designed or adapted to measure quality of life recorded in the literature are not validated in a satisfactory manner or are not validated at all. When I became intensely interested in this field 12 years ago, that was my greatest disappointment. The importance of validation is taken much more seriously by our colleagues in the social sciences. That is reflected by the prominence of calibrational work accompanying the introduction of measures of health status as was the case with the three important examples listed earlier [13–17].

In contrast, the scales and indices developed to use among sick patients to assess quality of life or quality of survival are generally submitted only to cursory attempts of calibration. Very frequently all that is attempted is face validity or content validity. Even those techniques are shoddily executed. Many clinical investigators have not taken the trouble to learn from several decades of conceptual and methodological developments of the social scientist in instrument development. They engage in unconventional and even bizarre correlations, which they call "validation," and then go on to declare their scale valid. We do not have a common or generally accepted consensus of what are scientifically admissible criteria of validity for new indices required in clinimetrics, health services research, or health economics research, although constructive proposals have been made [19].

When it comes to doing validity studies and declaring a verdict that a particular scale or index is valid, never have I seen more blatant examples of *post hoc, ergo propter hoc* reasoning. It is hard to find a report or hear an oral presentation in which an investigator presents his calibrational activities to validate a new measure and writes that the criteria he set forth in advance were not met and that therefore the index is not valid?

This is my view on what minimum criteria for validity should include:

1. The performance characteristics for content validity, criterion validity (if feasible), or construct validity should be declared in advance in a publicly archived protocol or in the indexed literature.
2. Content validity should be enhanced at the development stage by invoking the views of representative panels of patients, providers, and ordinary citizens.
3. Reliability should be verified at the hands of those for whom use of the instruments is intended.
4. When a gold standard exists, criterion validity should be performed with the types of respondents or patients among whom the scale or measure will eventually be used and under similar circumstances.
5. When a gold standard does not exist, construct validation should include at least one approach of discriminant validity and one of convergent validity. How much discrimination is to be attained and how much convergence is to be demonstrated should be declared in advance.

This list does not represent a complete or ideal set of tactics for acceptable validation. I put them forward as a minimum.

## Developing Gold Standards

We do not have a gold standard. Depending where you place the inception time, we have traveled for 15–40 years to develop the kinds of measures in which we are interested. When it comes to health applications, Karnofsky got us on the road in 1948. Earnest efforts invoking the best methods have been available for only about 15 years in the health field. Still everyone says or writes that we do not have a gold standard. It is almost amusing to note the plaintive bleat with which authors bemoan the lack of the gold standard. They then go on smugly to do sloppy calibrational work which tends to perpetuate the state of affairs.

I am convinced that we fail to have a gold standard, or that at least we do not have one that everyone accepts, because no one has made it his or her primary objective to develop one either for measures of health status or for measures of quality of life. Investigators have tried, for understandable reasons, to create scales and instruments that are accepted by respondents, patients, and clinicians. That means they must be relatively short and they must be usable in ways that do not require enormous research budgets for each application. Investigators who can and will direct their energies and skill to calibrational work leading to the creation of a generally accepted gold standard should be strongly supported. Investigators should be encouraged, if interested, to do the same in the realm of quality of life measures and in a battery of functional status measures potentially useful for common interventions for common ailments. I introduce the notion that what we really need is a reference library or a bureau of standards for quality of life and health status, which would serve us all. We would then end up with a situation where some scientists could advance calibration and others application in a complementary and synergistic manner.

## Conclusion

Our intended primary beneficiaries are the patient and the clinician. Without minimizing the importance of practitioners and scientists in the allied field of methodological development, our concern is that we find a way to translate what we have learned in the last 15 years and what we hope we will learn in the next 15 years to a parsimonious array of measurement techniques that can be used in clinical research and patient care. Directly or indirectly, since we have chosen to work in an applied field, the ultimate objective of measuring health status and quality of life is improved ways of caring for the sick and improved ways for protecting the health of those who are well.

"The office of medicine" wrote Francis Bacon in his *Advancement of Learning* "is but to tune this curious harp of man's body and reduce it to harmony" [20]. Although in the years since 1669 medicine has been getting better and better at the tuning, it still has some distance to go in getting to the harmony. Surely a better understanding of quality of life, with valid and practical techniques to measure it and clinically sensible methods of incorporating the measures into our therapeutic strategies, will get us closer to the harmony of which Francis Bacon wrote.

*Acknowledgement.* Adapted from a paper originally published in *Journal of Chronic Diseases* (1987) 40:465–471, used with permission of Pergamon Press.

## References

1. Karnofsky DA, Abelmann WH, Craver LF, Burchenal JH (1948) The use of nitrogen mustards in the palliative treatment of carcinoma. Cancer 1:634–656
2. Karnofsky DA, Burchenal JH (1949) The clinical evaluation of chemotherapeutic agents in cancer. In: MacLeod CM (ed) Evaluation of chemotherapeutic agents. Columbia University Press, New York, pp. 191–205
3. Katz S, Ford AB, Moskowitz RW et al. (1963) Studies of illness in the aged. JAMA 185:914–919
4. Katz S, Downs TD, Cash HR, Grotz RC (1970) Progress in development of the index of ADL. Gerontologist 10:20–30
5. World Health Organization (1947) The constitution of the World Health Organization. WHO Chron 1:29
6. Chambers LW, Macdonald LA, Tugwell P et al. (1982) The McMaster Health Index Questionnaire as a measure of quality of life for patients with rheumatoid disease. J Rheumatol 9:780–784
7. Gurin G, Verhoff J, Feld S (1960) Americans view their mental health. Basic Books, New York
8. President's Commission on National Goals (1960) Goals for Americans. The American Assembly, Columbia University Press, New York
9. Elkinton JR (1966) Medicine and the quality of life (editorial). Ann Intern Med 64:711–714
10. Anonymous (1968) In: Strauss MB (ed) Familiar medical quotations. Little Brown, Boston, p. 271b
11. Bunker JP, Wennberg JE (1973) Operation rates, mortality statistics and the quality of life. N Engl J Med 289:1249–1251
12. Patrick DL, Bush JW, Chen MM (1973) Toward an operational definition of health. J Health Soc Behav 14:6–23
13. Gibson BS, Gibson JS, Bergner M et al. (1975) The sickness impact profile: development of an outcome measure of health care. Am J Public Health 65:1304
14. Bergner M, Bobbit RA, Pollard WE et al. (1976) The sickness impact profile: validation of a health status measure. Med Care 14:57–67
15. Bergner M, Bobbitt RA, Carter WB, Gibson BS (1981) The sickness impact profile: development and final revision of a health status measure. Med Care 19:787–804
16. Kaplan RM, Bush JW, Berry CC (1976) Health status: types of validity and the index of well-being. Health Services Res 11:478–507
17. Brook RH, Ware JE, Davies-Avery A et al. (1979) Overview of adult health status measure fielded in Rand's health insurance study. Med Care 17 [suppl]:1–131
18. Spitzer WO, Dobson AJ, Hall J et al. (1981) Measuring the quality of life of cancer patients. A concise QL-Index for use by physicians. J Chronic Dis 34:585–597
19. Hutchinson TA, Boyd NF, Feinstein AR et al. (1979) Scientific problems in clinical scales, as demonstrated in the Karnofsky Index of Performance Status. J Chronic Dis 32:661–666
20. Bacon F (1640) The advancement of learning, book II. Lichfield for Young and Forrest

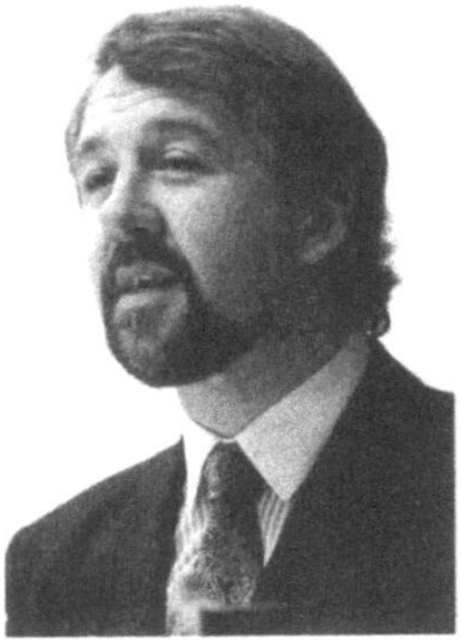

# 16. The Socioeconomic Evaluation of Medicines: A New Dimension

S. R. Walker

In moving from traditional endpoints to innovative outcomes in determining the benefits of medicines, five aspects should be considered, namely, the key issues to be addressed, the need for such a change direction, the benefits of the socioeconomic approach, the opportunities available in estimating benefits, and the principles to be considered and implemented.

## The Issues

This symposium raises a number of key questions:
- What is quality of life and how is it relevant to drug safety?
- How can quality of life be measured in large populations exposed to marketed drugs?
- How can benefits be quantified with reference to harm so that nonexpert policy makers can understand the resulting ratios?
- Are socioeconomic benefits essential determinants in drug development?
- Will psychosocial benefits become a factor in the drug approval process?
- How do we go from concept to measurement in quality of life?
- Can socioeconomic benefits be combined with clinical benefits?
- Are quality of life measurements of value when combining benefits with risks in assessing outcome?

Since the 1950s the double-blind controlled clinical trial has become the standard by which the efficacy of a new medicine is determined. However, while traditional endpoints are still crucial in measuring the benefits of new and existing therapy, the question is now whether we need innovative outcomes to more fully appreciate the benefits of medicines from the standpoint of the patient, the physician, and the pharmaceutical company.

Details of the historical background to the development of socioeconomic measurements of health outcome and the effectiveness of drug therapy (Fig. 1) indicates that, since the 1950s, the controlled clinical trial has answered the question, "does the treatment work?." The introduction of cost/benefit analyses

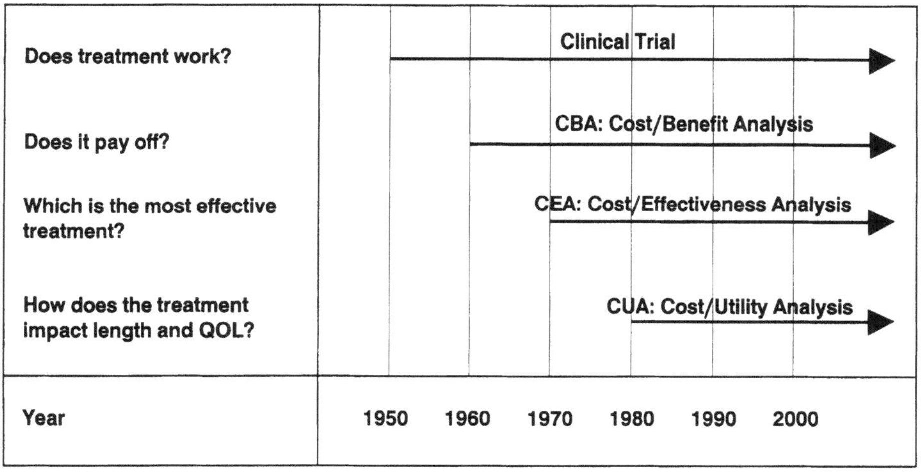


**Fig. 1.** Measuring health benefits. *QOL*, quality of life

in the 1950s and 1960s provided the framework for measuring the overall economic benefits of medical care and setting them against the corresponding costs by answering the question of whether the treatment pays off. During the 1960s and 1970s, the economic emphasis swung away from cost/benefit analysis to the concept of cost/effectiveness analysis which questioned which the most effective treatment is using given resources. However, since 1980s, the principle of cost/utility analysis has introduced the concept of utility as a measurement of value to complement the financial aspects and answer the question of how the treatment impacts on the length and quality of life.

It is useful in any discussion of quality of life to define what we mean by certain terms, for to be involved in valid quality of life studies requires a clear definition of the terminology which is broadly accepted and understood by those involved in this research. *Health status* is a measure of an individual's function in terms of physical, social, and mental well-being, while *quality of life* is more related to how a person feels and functions in his or her everyday life. *Quality of life* has been defined as a concept encompassing a broad range of physical and psychological characteristics and limitations which describe an individual's ability to function and derive satisfaction from so doing. However, with regard to measuring the benefits of medicines *health-related quality of life* is probably the key term, and this is defined as the level of well-being and satisfaction associated with an individual's life and how this is affected by disease, accidents, and treatment.

## The Need

It was Ware et al. [1] in 1981 who indicated there were a number of reasons for studying health status which could well apply to quality of life, namely, measuring the effectiveness of medical intervention, improving clinical decisions, assessing the quality of care, estimating the needs of the population, and understanding the causes and consequences in differences in health. The need to move from solely traditional endpoints to innovative outcomes is underlined by the fact that today's goal is perhaps not so much seeking the cure for a disease, but rather an improvement in function, the resolution of symptoms, and the opportunity to limit the progression of the disease and to improve a patient's quality of life.

In a recent article, Buxton and Drummond [2] identified three main reasons why quality of life data are so important in assessing the impact of medical intervention. They stated, first, that while it is still possible to identify new interventions that extend life such as medicines for AIDS most modern drugs are concerned with improving the quality, not quantity, of life. Therefore, measures are required to assess the impact of intervention for chronic conditions such as rheumatoid arthritis and cardiovascular disease. Second, most medical interventions are not entirely beneficial. They have associated risks of adverse effects which need to be considered alongside their therapeutic characteristics. Third, some interventions have serious associated risks that could reduce life expectancy, but offer, in return, improvements in the quality of life, e.g., open heart surgery. Alternatively, some interventions may extend life yet have serious unpleasant adverse effects, e.g., cancer chemotherapy. In such situations one wants not only to measure quality of life but also to assess how individuals trade off length of life for improvements in quality. The measurements of utilities – the relative evaluation of alternative outcomes – permits this assessment, and the quality-adjusted life year (QALY) is now the most familiar of such measures.

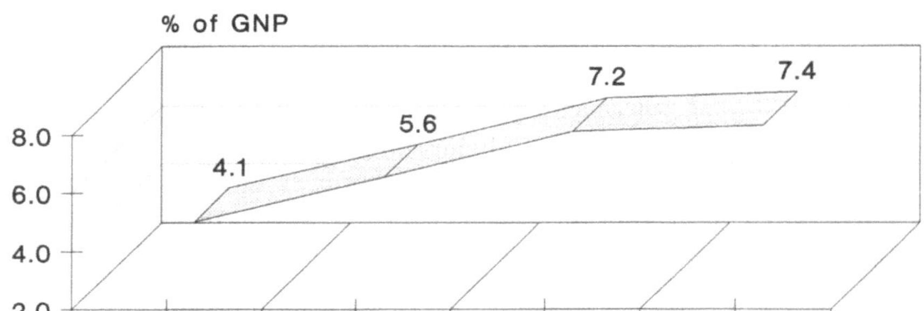


| | 1960 | 1970 | 1980 | 1985 |
|---|---|---|---|---|
| Germany | 4.7 | 5.5 | 7.9 | 8.1 |
| Japan | 3.0 | 4.6 | 6.6 | 6.6 |
| Sweden | 4.7 | 7.2 | 9.5 | 9.3 |
| UK | 3.9 | 4.5 | 5.7 | 5.7 |
| USA | 5.2 | 7.4 | 9.2 | 10.8 |

OECD Mean

**Fig. 2.** Trends in health care expenditure

Currently the trends in health care expenditure in major countries such as the United States, the United Kingdom, Sweden, Japan, and Germany underline the increasing importance, as well as the increased cost, of meeting the health care needs of patients in these countries (Fig. 2). In addition, a number of current government initiatives have provided a further stimulus to those involved in the evaluation of new medicines to make sure that we have the most appropriate means of determining their benefits. Some of these initiatives include global budgets for hospitals, cash limits on health authorities, clinical budgeting experiments, positive and negative lists of medicines, monitoring of physicians prescribing costs, and the limiting of reimbursement for medicines.

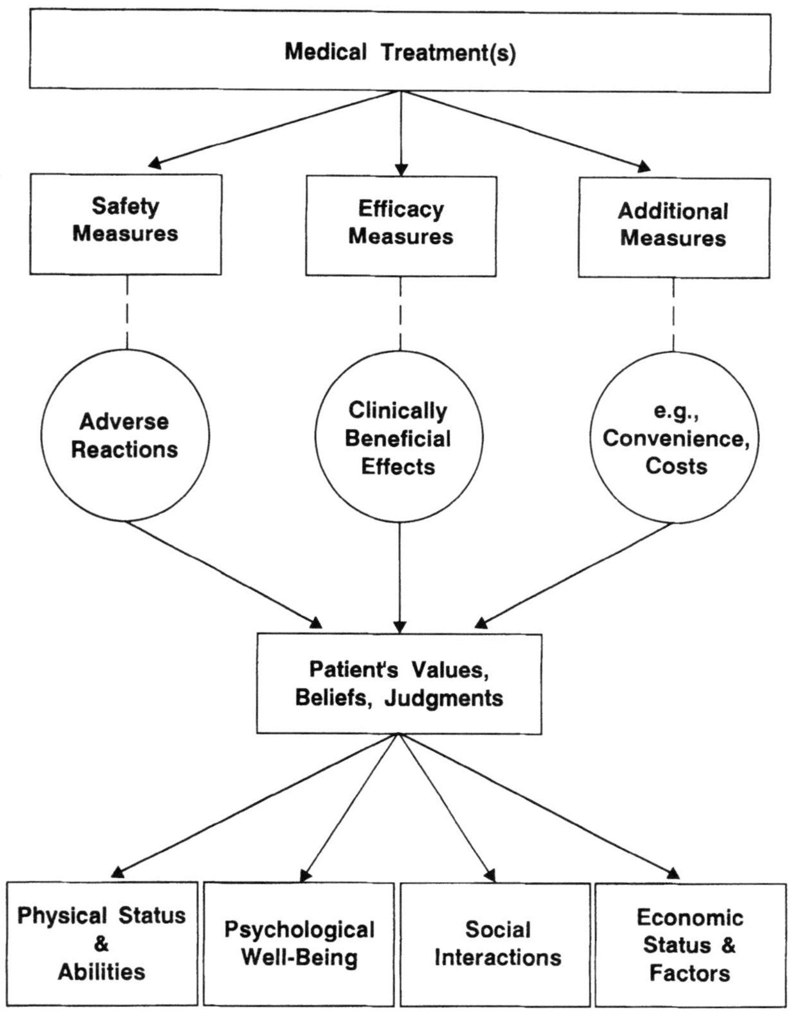


**Fig. 3.** Evaluation criteria of medical treatment(s). (From [4])

Quality of life measurements, therefore, offer the direct assessment of those features of medical interventions which are typically measured indirectly and give the overall impact on the patient of a combination of effects which could be both adverse and beneficial. This latter point is illustrated in Fig. 3.

Currently there is a need for further studies on:

1. The role of quality of life assessment incorporated within medical practice, as this ultimately can affect both perception and actual measures of therapeutic efficacy
2. The importance and nature by which the type of disease in certain cultural settings affects assessment of quality of life using standard instruments
3. How the measurement of quality of life can be practicably translated into information which can be broadly and consistently useful for understanding the benefits of pharmaceuticals

## The Benefits

The potential benefits of measuring health-related quality of life should concern a number of groups, namely, patients, physicians, pharmaceutical companies, regulatory authorities, and health authorities. For the patients, the opportunity for them to express and assess the impact of their disease and subsequent treatment on life style is often of more importance to them than the impact of treatment on clinical parameters. The immediate benefits on their quality of life, again, is often of more interest than the long-term gain, which may include extension of life. For physicians, the ability to have alternative methods of measuring outcome may, subsequently, influence their prescribing patterns. For pharmaceutical companies these innovative measures are of value in the comparison of different therapies, the assessment of the outcome of treatment, and the drug development process, as well as in providing data which may allow the repositioning of medicines and a reassessment of the balance between benefits and risks. The regulatory authorities are becoming increasingly interested in health-related quality of life measures. Buxton and Drummond [2] stated that "licensing authorities sometimes have to make difficult decisions relating to the trade-off between risks and benefits of new medicines. These decisions are taken on a case-by-case basis and depend critically on the likely use of the medicine and the existence of acceptable clinical alternatives. Clearly, such decisions cannot always be determined totally by objective criteria, and some information on patients or members of the general public, who may be potential patients and who make the trade-offs between benefits and risks, may be of value and influencial in, ultimately, making the appropriate regulatory decision. For health authorities, who may be involved in determining which medicines are reimbursed and which are admitted to a formulary, health-related quality of life may be of increasing importance."

## The Opportunities

There is undoubtedly a need in the evaluation of new medicines for the determination of hard clinical endpoints as well as an agreement as to what change will represent a clinically significant difference. The degree of the difference that is considered clinically significant is a judgment often made by the researchers based on their knowledge of prognosis with and without treatment. However, in the absence of quality of life data, it is often not clear whether the difference in a clinical measure, such as forced expiratory volume in 1 s ($FEV_1$) as measured in chronic obstructive lung disease, is really significant to the patients concerned and, if so, whether it is relevant as a prognostic indicator or as a determinant of current quality of life. The situation is further confounded if the

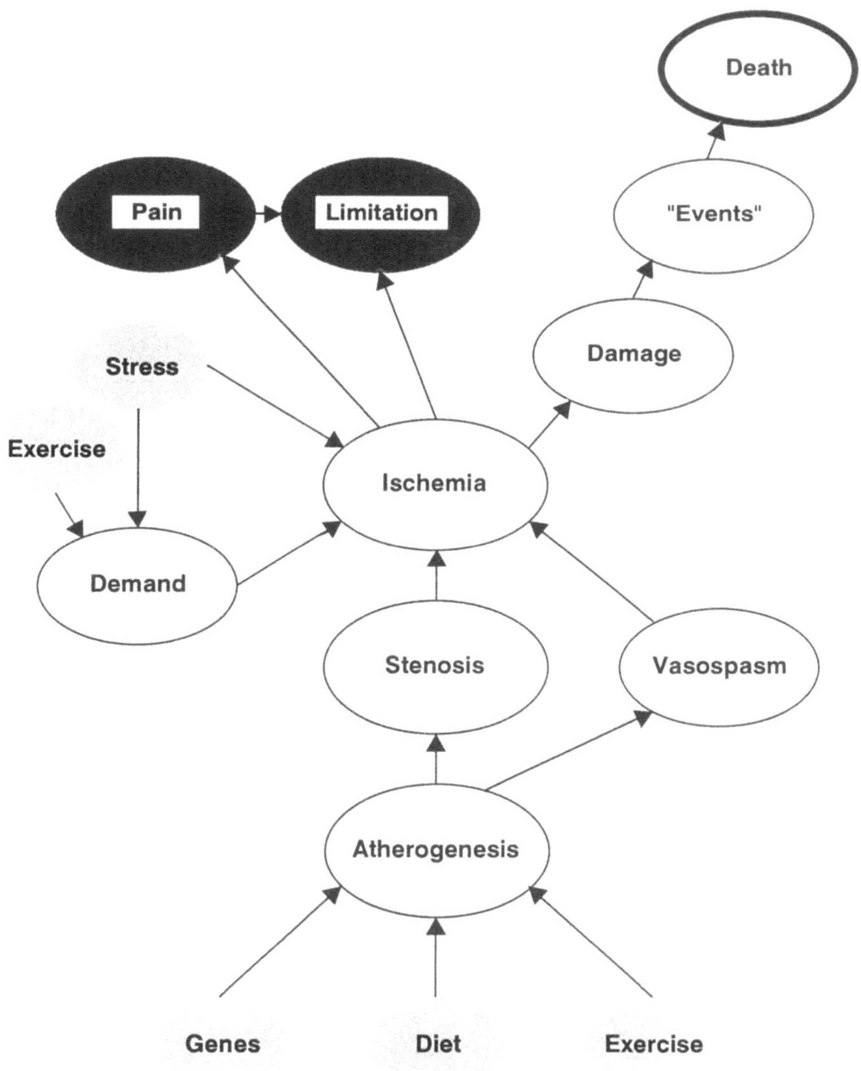


**Fig. 4.** Cardiovascular disease – a medical model. (From [3])

treatment itself has side effects that affect the patient's health status. There is, therefore, a heavy onus on those involved in developing and advocating the use of quality of life measures to ensure that these measures have been subjected to the rigorous assessment of validity and reliability [2].

There are undoubtedly a number of disease areas where the inclusion of health-related quality of life data would be of utmost value in determining outcome. Leighton Read [3] has suggested that, in any area where quality of life is being considered, an important step is to develop a medical model of the disease to be investigated which should, subsequently, be compared with the socioeconomic model. A recent paper [3] provided a medical model for cardiovascular diseases and how this could be considered in terms of socioeconomic issues.

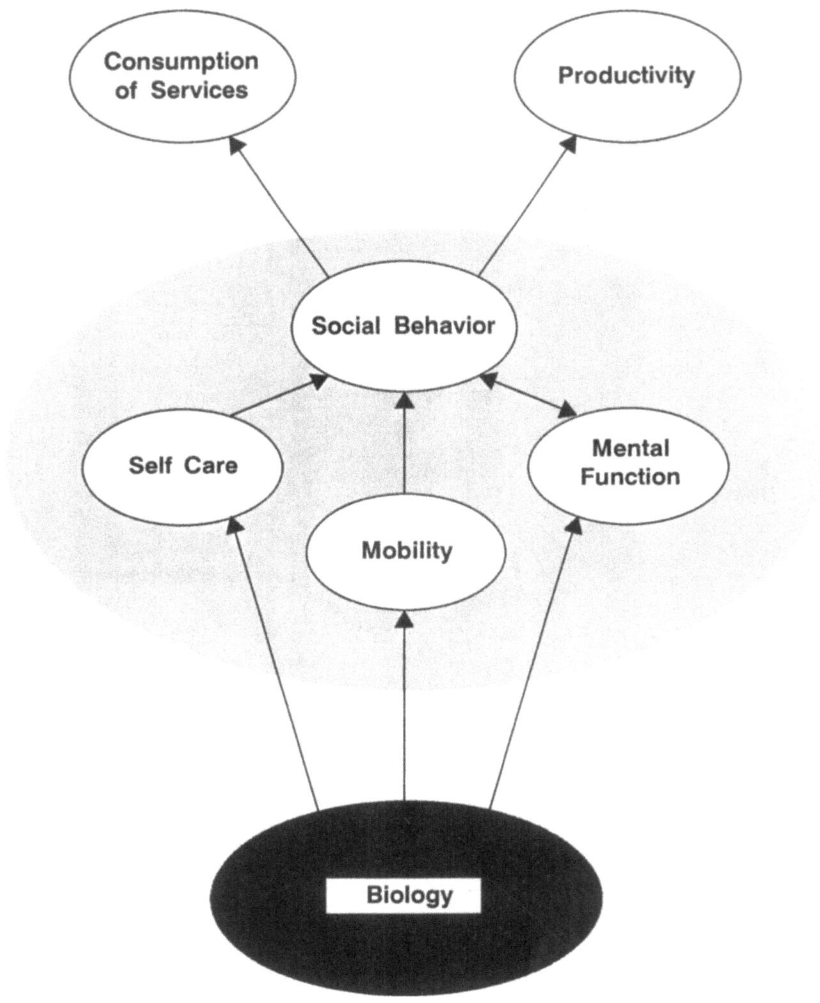


**Fig. 5.** Cardiovascular disease – a socioeconomic model. (From [3])

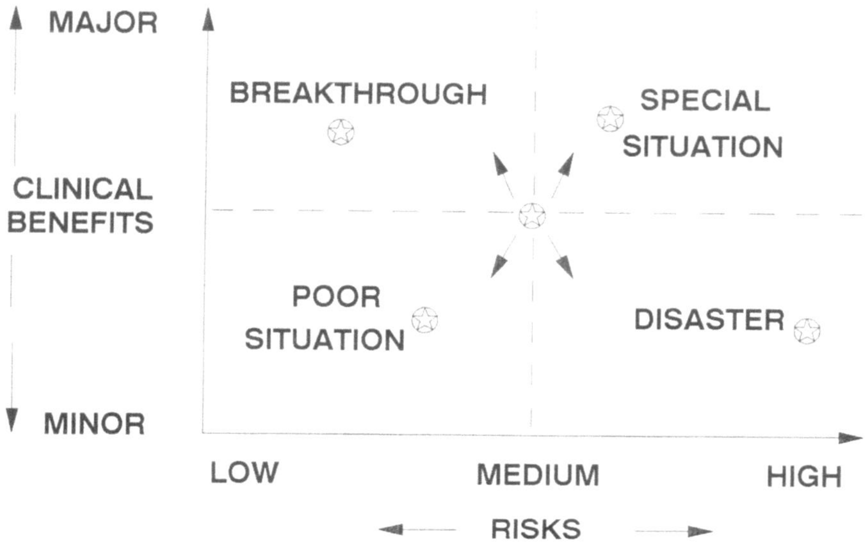


**Fig. 6.** The clinical benefit/risk ratio

A major opportunity provided by health-related quality of life assessment might well allow the repositioning of a new or established medicine in terms of the benefit/risk ratio. With information on clinical benefits and a knowledge of risks from a particular treatment, it should be possible, ideally, to place any medicine within one of the four quadrants (Fig. 6). In general terms, a medicine with major clinical benefits, but low risks, would indicate a breakthrough drug while a medicine with minor clinical benefits, but high risks, would indicate a disaster. Low benefits and low risks might be a poor situation for any medicine, while, in special circumstances, high risks might be tolerated for major clinical benefits in certain life-threatening diseases.

The position of any medicine in Fig. 6 could well be altered by measuring and then combining the clinical benefits with quality of life measurements and economic outcomes (Fig. 7). The measurement of such additional benefits could move a medicine from the lower part of the graph to the higher quadrants.

## The Principles

In considering health-related quality of life studies, the plan should be as follows:

1. Define what one means by health-related quality of life.
2. Develop a conceptual framework initially producing a medical model of the disease and, subsequently, a socioeconomic model.
3. Review the generic and specific instruments available rather than developing a new instrument, unless one is prepared to go through the various issues and procedures required for validating a new instrument.

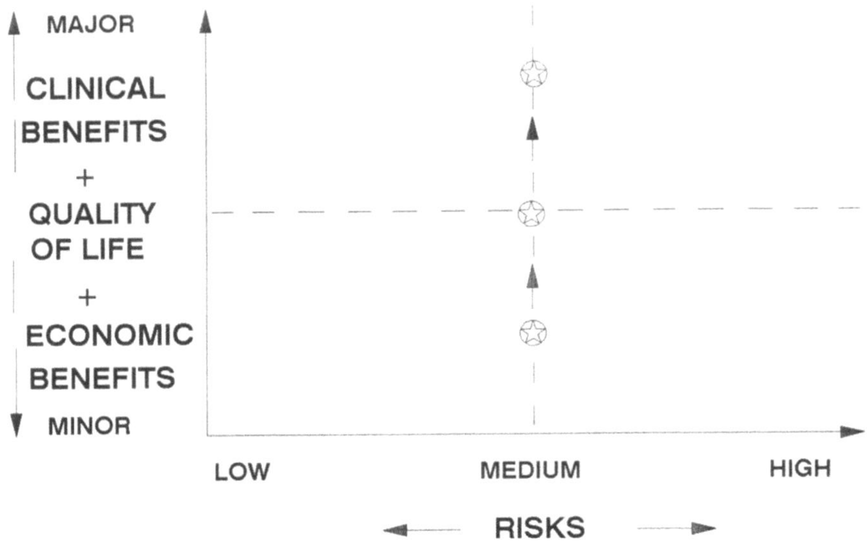


**Fig. 7.** The combined benefit/risk ratio

4. Having selected the appropriate instrument, assess its potential value in the disease area to be examined.
5. Complete a pilot study to identify the applicability and suitability of using such an instrument in the study proposed before a full-scale evaluation is carried out.

Spilker [4] has shown in a recent book that the quality of life field is a rapidly changing and developing medical area. The standards developed over the next few years will probably have a major influence on this area for a very long period. While it may be considered premature to define the golden rules of this field, there is no doubt that serious consideration should be given to the move from solely traditional endpoints to innovative outcomes in estimating the benefits of medicines.

## References

1. Ware JE, Brook RH, Davies-Avery A, Lohv KN (1981) Choosing measures of health studies for individuals and general population. Am J Public Health 71:620–625
2. Buxton MJ, Drummond MR (1990) Quality of life measurement in the development of medicines. Pharmaceut J 3 Mar:260–262
3. Read JL (1988) From medical to socioeconomic evaluation of drug therapy. In: van Eimeren W, Horisberger B (eds) Socioeconomic evaluation of drug therapy. Springer, Berlin Heidelberg New York Tokyo, pp 72–81
4. Spilker B (1990) Quality of life assessment in clinical trials. Raven, New York

# 17. Expanding Measures of Benefit in Socioeconomic Studies

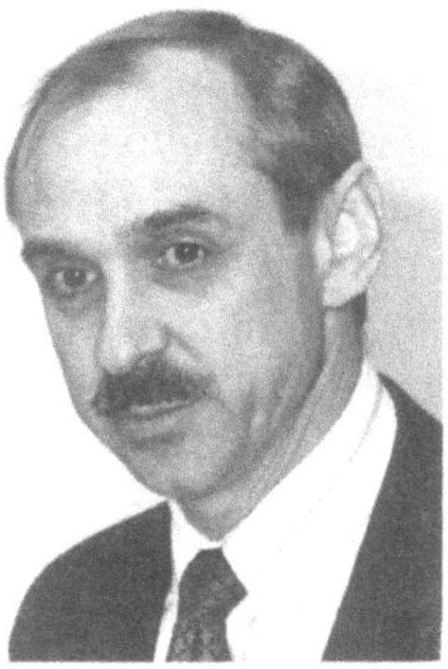

B. R. LUCE

## Introduction

The purpose of socioeconomic studies of pharmaceutical interventions is to estimate analytically the value of those interventions. That valuation process should include all relevant costs and consequences, including side effects, risks, and benefits over all relevant time periods. Often, however, important consequences are not adequately considered by an analysis, which may result in misleading or the misinterpretation of results. Despite increasing interest [6] and methodological advances in the measurement of quality of life in drug studies, many otherwise methodologically sound socioeconomic studies do not include quality of life components, even when their inclusion could make a difference in the interpretation of value.

## Increase Volume of Socioeconomic Studies

As any reader of the health economic literature can attest, there has been an increasing number of socioeconomic studies in the indexed health care literature. In a recent review of that literature, it was shown just how long this trend has been going on [5]. From 1966 to 1988 the number of cost/benefit analysis (CBA) and cost/effectiveness analysis (CEA) articles per year increased from several to over 150. Virtually all of the increase is due to articles published in medical journals rather than other health-related journals. Thus, the clinical community is clearly interested in economic issues. Much of the increase in CBA/CEA articles is found in the United States literature, although non-US (mainly European) CBA/CEA literature has been increasing as well. In the last half of the 1980s we note that socioeconomic studies of drugs may be increasing at a rate much higher than studies of other medical and surgical interventions. Most likely, this is due to the number of studies funded by the pharmaceutical industry. The number of published drug studies doubled during the period 1984–1987 (14 articles per year) compared to the previous 4-year period (7 articles per year) and doubled again in 1988 (31 studies). My impression from anecdotal evidence and first-hand experience is that the dramatic increase noted in 1988 is not an aberrant figure, but a sign of numerous studies to come, since, as noted, many of the studies are funded by the drug industry. Although the literature review referred to above was limited to health economic studies, it is our impression that there are many quality of life studies sponsored by industry as well. Those studies are just beginning to appear in the scientific literature. The question, for present purposes, is whether economic studies of drugs are adequately accounting for potential side effects and longer-term risks of the drugs they purport to be evaluating.

## The Methodology of Cost/Effectiveness Analysis

There have been a number of widely-read articles and texts which describe the methodological issues associated with socioeconomic analyses [2, 5, 7, 8]. An excellent depiction of the analytical formula to be used in a cost/effectiveness study is described by Weinstein [9], who depicts the cost/effectiveness ratio as:

$$\frac{C}{E} = \frac{\triangle C_{Rx} + \triangle C_{SE} - \triangle C_{Morb}}{\triangle Y - \triangle Y_{SE} + \triangle Y_{Morb} + \triangle Y_{Symp}}$$

where:
$C$ = Net increase/decrease in health care costs;
$C_{Rx}$ = Direct costs of treatment, including drugs, physician visits, routine tests;
$C_{SE}$ = Costs induced by side effects;
$C_{Morb}$ = Savings associated with the prevention of morbid events;
$E$ = Net increase/decrease in quality-adjusted life years;
$Y$ = Net change in life expectancy due to treatment;
$Y_{SE}$ = Negative quality adjustment associated with the side effects and complications of treatment;
$Y_{Morb}$ = Positive quality adjustment associated with the prevention of morbid events;
$Y_{Symp}$ = Positive quality adjustment associated with the relief from symptoms.

Thus, theoretically at least, quality of life is incorporated into a complete socioeconomic analysis of a drug (or any other medical) intervention. The question is whether, in fact, it is routinely being included in actual practice. Our review of the literature indicates that it is not. The follow-up question is whether including quality of life makes a difference, and the best answer probably is that it depends. Two recent studies illustrate the issue.

The first example is a study which compared the costs and life-saving effectiveness of traditional antiarrhythmic drug therapy and the totally implantable defibrillator [4]. Using a decision-analytic clinical model, the authors estimated that implanting a defibrillator for patients at high risk for sudden death cost society approximately $ 17000 per year of life saved in 1986. They further found that including quality of life changes for survivors in the model made no difference in the study results, primarily because of the extremely high death rate of the study population. Relatively small changes in quality of life were swamped by the effect of mortality in the analytic model. However, the authors did not examine the significance of the quality of life effect which the competing therapies may have had on survivors, potentially an important issue given the toxicity of antiarrhythmic drugs and the pain and anxiety that accompany electrical shocks to the heart.

The second example also concerns heart disease; this time we look at blood pressure medication. To set the stage, I first refer to an article by Croog et al. [1], which appeared in the *New England Journal of Medicine* in 1986. The authors reported statistically significant differences in quality of life for several antihypertensive drugs across a number of psychometric dimensions, including sleep dysfunction, general well-being, work performance, life satisfaction, and sexual dysfunction. In particular, the study concluded that captopril had a significantly higher positive quality of life profile than did propranolol. More recently, a study of the cost/effectiveness of some of those same antihypertensive drugs appeared in the medical literature [3]. This study used a coronary heart disease epidemiologic risk model to simulate a population aging from 35 to 64 years old and calculated the cost per year of life saved for the various drugs of interest. The authors reported that propranolol was six to seven times more cost effective than captopril. In particular, propanolol was reported to cost $ 11 000 per year of life saved, while captopril cost $ 72 000 per year of life saved. The cost/effectiveness ratio of the other drugs that were also studied, hydrochlorothiazide, nifedipine, and prazosin hydrochloride, fell in between. The researchers chose not to include the measurements of quality of life in the base case of the model. However, in a sensitivity analysis, the authors reported that if quality of life made a 1% difference in overall efficacy of propranolol, then the cost/effectiveness of propranolol would be three times higher ($ 33 000 v. $ 11 000). If quality of life made a 2% difference in overall efficacy, then the side effects of propranolol would actually outweigh the life-saving effect of its efficacy due to lowering blood pressure, in effect reversing the conclusions regarding the relative cost/effectiveness of propranolol and captopril (assuming captopril was not compromising quality of life as well). Therefore, the sensitivity analysis in the above example indicated that, in assessing the socioeconomic value of these particular antihypertensive drugs, the results are extremely sensitive to the value which the analyst ascribes to the effect of the drugs on patient's quality of life. This would seem to make some intuitive sense, since today both clinicians and patients are acutely aware of the burden which the side effects of antihypertensive medications can have on the ability of patients to function normally in society. In this context the term "function" includes the various domains of function, e.g., physical, social, cognitive, sexual, etc. Medications are, in fact, prescribed in part due to their side effect profile. Trying to assess value for money, for instance in a cost/effectiveness ratio, would seem to require the inclusion of the quality of life impact these medications may have.

The problem is that we are better at the theory than at the practice. Although researchers are adept at measuring quality of life along a number of psychometric dimensions, these measurements are not easily translatable to utility scales, which, if done, would permit more comprehensive cost/effectiveness comparisons. Additional methodological research needs to be done along these lines.

This research agenda would consist of several elements. First, quality of life measurements of patients on antihypertensive medications need to be taken for the various drug regimens using the traditional psychometric scales noted above. Second, patient preferences, or utilities, need to be assessed for the various health states described by the psychometric scales. Third, the patient utility values need to be mapped to the psychometric scales. This would permit researchers to estimate the quality of life trade-off to life, since both endpoints would be expressed in the same units. A simple example may help to illustrate the value of such an effort.

Assume that drug A is more efficacious than drug B in terms of gains in life expectancy due to blood pressure control. In fact, over a 40-year period drug A results in a net gain of 0.5 year of life. However, drug A compromises quality of life more than drug B in terms of general feelings of well-being and physical, social, and sexual activity levels. Through various methodological techniques (e.g., time trade-off or standard gamble), we discover that patients value the collective decrement in quality of life to be approximately 0.025 of a life year for each year they take the medication. That is, patients would be willing to trade off a little over 9 days per year ($365 \times 0.25 = 9.15$) to be free of these side effects. This is equivalent to one full year of life over a 40-year period ($9.15 \times 40 = 366$). Thus, we conclude that, on average, patients would prefer drug B over drug A. For the purposes of simplicity, we omitted the economic dimension, which, if included, would permit a calculation of net cost per year of life saved.

## Conclusions

Today, society is asking for more than the safety and efficacy profile of medications as well as of other medical interventions. Society also is interested in providing care efficiently and in protecting the quality as well as the quantity of its citizen's lives.

The medical literature is increasingly including studies which report both the relative cost/effectiveness of competing interventions and the relative impact alternative therapies have on patients' quality of life. These expanded measures of benefit are enriching the literature and, therefore, clinical and health policy decision making.

Nevertheless, more research is needed to be able to express these concepts adequately so that decision makers can make more sense of them.

## References

1. Croog SH, Levine S, Testa MA et al. (1986) The effects of antihypertensive therapy on the quality of life. New Engl J Med 314:1657–1664
2. Drummond MF, Stoddart GL, Torrance GW (1987) Methods for the economic evaluation of health care programmes. Oxford University Press, Oxford

3. Edelson JT, Weinstein MC, Tosteson ANA et al. (1990) Long-term cost-effectiveness of various initial monotherapies for mild to moderate hypertension. JAMA 263:407–413
4. Kupperman M, Luce BR, McGovern B et al. (1990) An analysis of the cost-effectiveness of the implantable cardiac defibrillator. Circulation 81:91–100
5. Luce BR, Elixhauser A (1990) Standards for socioeconomic evaluation of health care products and services. Springer, Berlin Heidelberg New York Tokyo
6. Luce BR, Weschler JM, Underwood C (1989) The use of quality-of-life measures in the private sector. In: Mosteller F, Falotico-Taylor J (ed) Quality of life and technology assessment. National Academy Press, Washington DC, pp. 55–64
7. Stason WB, Weinstein MC (1977) Public health rounds at the Harvard School of Public Health. New Engl J Med 296:732–739
8. Warner KE, Luce BR (1982) Cost-benefit and cost-effectiveness analysis in health care: principles, practice and potential. Health Administration Press, University of Michigan
9. Weinstein MC (1980) Estrogen use in postmonopausal women: Costs, risks, and benefits. New Engl J Med 303:308–316

# Part VI

## Assessing the Risk/Benefit Relationship

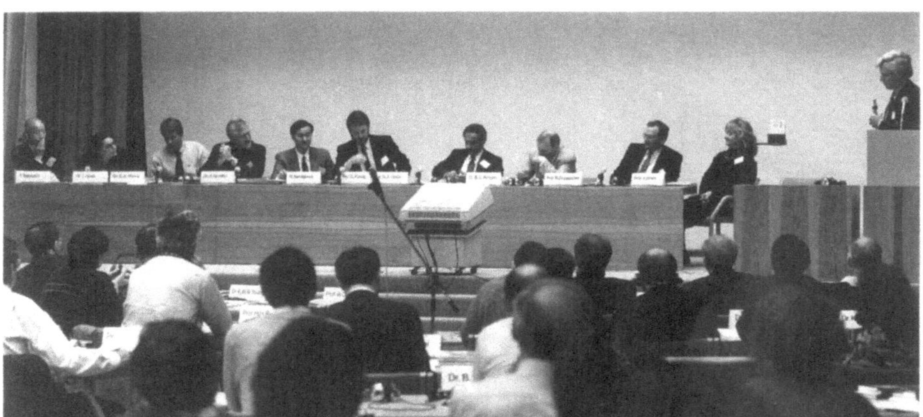

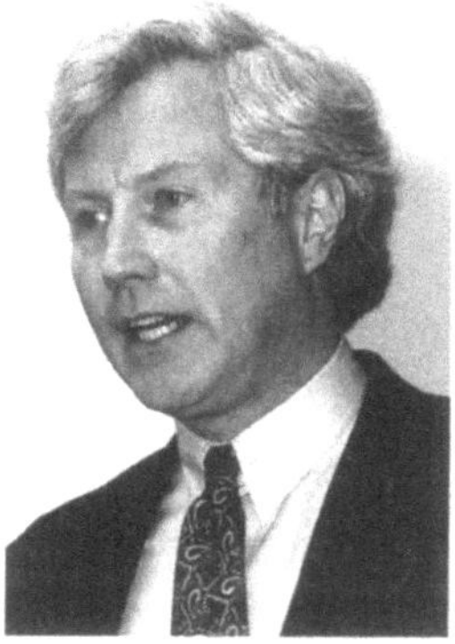

# 18. Challenges in Benefit/Risk Appraisal

W. W. Lowrance

The essential issue for any drug is: How much side-effect risk should be judged acceptable, for how much therapeutic benefit? Manufacturers must take benefit/risk considerations into account as they develop drugs and bring them into market, and iteratively, then, as they refine and shepherd the drugs through their commercial lifespans. Regulators must do the same as they control the admission of drugs into the market and guide refinements (such as reformulation, setting of indications and restrictions, provision of information to users, and so on). Obviously, physicians and other health-care providers and payers must also do so. All of these authorities must consider technical, personal, and social factors, and should think and act throughout in the interest of the ultimate public consumers of the drugs. Because I believe that continuity should be fostered among RAD-AR efforts, and because what I presented at the 1988 Wolfsberg conference [1] is still valid, I will briefly state my core concerns as I have articulated them before.

## Assessment, Appraisal, Response

Dealing with any risk, whether for pharmaceuticals, aircraft, electricity generation, or lunch, involves the following three separable modes of analysis and action [1]:

- *Risk assessment:* description of the likelihood and severity of threat
- *Risk appraisal:* evaluation of the personal or societal burden from the risk, the costs required for protection, and the payback expected from risk-reduction investment
- *Risk response:* prescription of what to do about the risk

Risk assessment is empirical and technical. Risk appraisal and response are much more social and personal; they involve value judgments and ethical considerations. Appraisal and response must be based on sound assessment. What is very special for pharmaceuticals (as compared with television sets or skis, for instance) is that, obviously, drugs are intended for the sole purpose of reducing risk of illness, either to prevent an illness altogether, or to reduce the harm incurred by it. The benefit of a pharmaceutical is the reduction of risk impending from some health threat. So, evaluation in this domain weighs target illness risk against drug side effect risk. The goal is net health risk reduction.

## The Pharmaceutical Comparative Matrix

Ideally, for any drug we would like to have information to fill in the matrix of Fig. 1 [1]. Notice that the "null alternative" is no treatment; this may occur either because a decision is made not to use the drug in question, or because the drug is unavailable practically (e.g., not existing on the market, not recognized as an option, not procurable locally, or not affordable). This comparative matrix constitutes the portfolio or dossier on drugs, and indeed on all other medical technologies and techniques. Although we do not possess all of this information, at least in reliable form, on all drugs, we should aspire to it.

| | Therapeutic efficacy | Risk to patient | Costs (various) | Cost-effectiveness | Benefits (various) | Patient preference and ethics | Societal ethics |
|---|---|---|---|---|---|---|---|
| The drug of concern | | | | | | | |
| No treatment | | | | | | | |
| Alternative drugs | | | | | | | |
| Non-drug alternative | | | | | | | |

**Fig. 1.** The pharmaceutical comparative matrix. (From [1])

## Evaluative Subsets

An even wider perspective must be developed, as depicted in Fig. 2 [1]. Drugs are a risk-reduction subset within the larger set of medicine (which includes health screening, dental and visual prophylaxis, and a wide variety of other activities). Medicine itself is a subset within the much larger health care domain (which includes lifestyle regimens, health statistics, and other activities that are broader than classical medical care). And health care is a subset within the overall domain of health risk confrontation (which includes fire protection, disaster preparedness, and other activities beyond health care). Thus, for any drug the questions are: Is it the best drug for the application compared with other drugs or with nondrug therapy, such as surgery? In a larger framework, does the

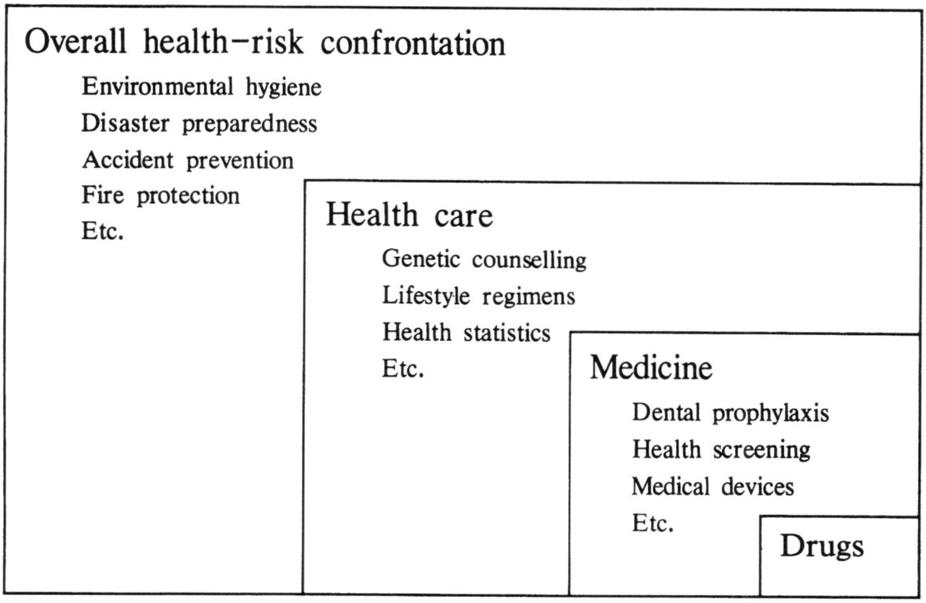


**Fig. 2.** Evaluative subsets. (From [1])

application, such as therapy, promise a higher payback to consumers or society compared with other health care investments, such as prophylaxis? Then, in the grand framework, how does the drug compare with other protective regimens, such as workplace safeguards? The first two of these questions tend to be raised in medical domains, the latter two in longer-term policy and economic domains. All guide the evolution of pharmaceutical development and application.

## The Idea of the Brighton Conference Experiment

Regulators, jointly with manufacturers, approve particular acceptable risk ceilings, and appropriate benefit/risk balances, all the time. But how do they do it? Can empirical studies not be done, at least to make the process more explicit? At a symposium on "The Perception, Measurement and Management of Therapeutic Risk", held at Brighton, England, in 1987, pairs of experts from rheumatology, cardiology, general practice, and surgery were asked "to assess the risks of two diseases and indicate on the logarithmic scale of safety units (previously described by Professor Heilmann and Dr. Urquhart) the number corresponding to the level of treatment-induced mortality that they would consider to be an acceptable risk" [2]. The experts tentatively conjectured, for example, that for a drug effective against congestive heart failure, because of the crucial therapeutic benefit and lack of alternatives, a relatively high risk of fatal side effects (on the order of 1 out of 10–100 patients) should be judged acceptable. Similarly, for a drug for gout, they thought that only a much lower risk of side effects (on the order of 1 out of 10–100 000 patients) should be judged acceptable. This was a very preliminary experiment. Because of imprecision in disease definitions, some ambiguity from the way the issues were presented, and other factors, the doctors were not very comfortable with the poll outcomes. Also, the only side effect risk considered was fatality, not illnesses. The publication deserves to be read for methodological description and for commentary.

Shouldn't much more of this kind of inquiry be pursued, both with people other than physicians and with M.D.s? Shouldn't people who suffer from or represent those who suffer from arthritis, for example, be given the opportunity to conduct such an exercise in parallel with groups of physicians of diverse backgrounds, and then attempts be made to discuss reasons for any differences of judgment, perhaps iterate the exercise, and then negotiate toward harmonization? The outcome, it seems to me, could be immensely helpful to manufacturers, regulators, health care providers, and the public.

## Issues for the Future

The following set of issues should be addressed by regulators and industry representatives. They focus principally on personal and social benefit/risk value judgments, not on scientific uncertainties or on costs.

1. *Opening, "fishing" questions.* At macro, societal levels (e.g., drug companies, regulators), how are benefit/risk judgments made for specific drugs, for classes of drugs, and for specific illnesses? Generally, how is it determined what level of side effect risk is unacceptable for a drug? Is that unacceptable risk level coupled to the benefit level? How is the concept of benefit/risk ratio used? Who makes the judgments and the improvements?
2. *Criteria of judgment.* In the pharmaceutical business (broadly defined), which benefit/risk criteria are applied and are they explicit? Do medical leaders, patient advocate groups, regulators, and manufacturers generally agree on the criteria and considerations?
3. *Established nature of criteria.* Are these judgments made systematically, or ad hoc, case-by-case, and inconsistently? For important, routine medical applications, are benefit/risk criteria and expectations well enough established that everyone can know in advance against what benefit/risk standards a drug will be evaluated? Is historical precedent the only guide?
4. *Consultation with publics.* With respect to classes of drugs or illnesses, how are consumers (or their representatives) consulted as to their benefit/risk appraisal? How multidirectional and robust is the consultation, and could improvements be made to it?
5. *Individuals' judgment making.* With respect to a drug they are personally contemplating taking, how do individual consumers make their benefit/risk judgments? Do we know how these judgments are made? Could improvements be made in this area?
6. *Regulators versus vendors.* On benefit/risk judgments, do regulators and manufacturers tend to agree (a) most of the time; (b) some of the time; or (c) rarely? For what reasons do they disagree?

7. *Universality*. How country- or culture-specific are drug benefit/risk judgments, e.g., once a drug is approved for marketing in one leading country, how likely is it that the drug will be approved in other countries? What are the consequences, and how might they be dealt with?

These issues are central challenges to all of us concerned about more sensitively appraising the benefits and risks of pharmaceuticals in context, thereby enhancing the health of the public.

## References

1. Lowrance WW (1989) A broad framework for confronting health risks. In: Horisberger B, Dinkel R (eds) The perception and management of drug safety risks. Springer, Berlin Heidelberg New York Tokyo, pp. 9–18
2. Burley D, Inman WHW (eds) (1988) Therapeutic risk. Wiley, Chichester

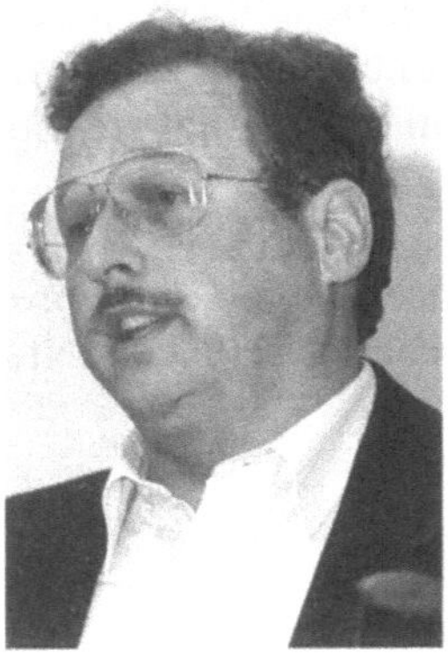

# 19. Analysis and Synthesis of Adverse Drug Reaction Evidence

R. BRUPPACHER

From the viewpoint of the manufacturer, analysis and synthesis of adverse drug reaction (ADR) information is needed on four levels with increasing scope and complexity.

## 1. Adverse Drug Reaction Case Evaluation

The unit of observation of every ADR problem is one case of a drug-attributed adverse event. Spontaneous and single ADR reports are still the most important element for detecting a new adverse drug effect. However, as nobody would accept a therapeutic effect merely on the observation of one or several cases, ADR reports as such can only provide an indication of a possible risk. One well-documented case may trigger actions, even though assessment of a causal relationship in an individual case always remains speculative, however sophisticated it may be. Algorithms can certainly help reproducibility, but will not really improve accuracy over good clinical judgment. Much attention has been given to this type of case assessment; this level of evidence evaluation is closest to the usual work of physicians, and is certainly the best developed method. However, conclusions about the potential harm to other patients cannot really be derived, even though experienced clinicians and clinical pharmacologists may be able to estimate the order or magnitude of a possible risk. The amount of human judgment in such estimates is high in proportion to the level of reproducible, scientific input and this results in great scope for disagreement.

## 2. Issue Assessment

Just as one swallow does not make a summer, one case does not usually make an issue. At the level of issue (ADR problem) assessment, we have to integrate data and evidence from different sources. This in itself necessitates good definitions and a standardized terminology since it is necessary to define what actually belongs to the issue and what does not. Whereas individual case assessment is mainly a question of the quality of the documentation, the major characteristic of a true issue is consistency of information from different sources. An issue concerns a risk, and in order to arrive at frequency estimates data are needed concerning the exposure, i.e., the use of the product.

Validation of an individual case report requires careful documentation. At the issue level we are faced with the need for a rapid validation of the evidence coming from the different sources: animal work, clinical trials, studies, and spontaneous reports. Nothing is more uncomfortable than a worrisome signal that cannot be verified. Indeed, most of today's drug monitoring activities are not so much characterized by a lack of signals as by difficulties in validating them. The current endeavors to increase spontaneous reporting can only be successful if they actually lead to interpretable, high-quality reports. If we cannot understand a message on the radio because of too much static, it is not very helpful to turn up the volume; we need better reception and perhaps also a more informative station. In the same way, a simple increase in the volume of spontaneous reports will not necessarily improve the signal/noise ratio. Turning to other channels (e.g., ARDs, prescription event monitoring, registries, or record linkage studies) may be much more useful.

The rapid introduction of a new drug into a very large market, as planned in the coming European Internal Market, may bring some dangers to the exposed population because a delay between problem identification and decision or action will leave a wider population exposed. On the other hand, rapidly increasing exposure provides also the opportunity of a rapid validation of signals, if appropriate surveillance measures are in place. Important issues may arise some time after marketing, and continuous surveillance will have a better chance of detecting these. The record linkage projects may be especially helpful for rapid validation. In addition to medical specialists and clinical pharmacologists, the collaboration of an epidemiologist is essential at the level of issue assessment.

## 3. Safety Profile Level

It is surprising how much decisions on the fate of a drug are determined by specific issues or even individual case reports. Basically, what counts for the patient is the evaluation of overall risk related to the benefit that a therapy can offer him. Decisions should be determined by the bottom line, and it is therefore necessary to incorporate the specific safety problems into a comprehensive profile characterizing the drug.

This profile may vary significantly for different situations, different populations, and the different characteristics considered. Also, there is a serious problem in weighing different aspects, e.g., what is the importance of a peptic ulcer compared with liver damage? On the bottom line it is the drug's effect on the survival, health, quality of life, or comfort level of the patient that really matters. While we are not doing too well on the level of issue evaluation, we also have to admit that we often do a miserable job on the profile level. Very few decisions have actually been based on a comprehensive analysis and synthesis of a drug profile.

Social and economic factors also need to be considered and this further complicates decision making and increases the difficulty in reaching a consensus.

## 4. Comparative Benefit/Risk Profile

However useful it may be to measure all the positive and negative consequences of a specific medicine and relate them to its therapeutic utility, it still is not enough to enable rational decision making. As important as the cost/benefit ratio (or better, the cost/benefit difference) of a drug is, its comparative utility to other alternative treatments for the same disease may be more decisive. However, few comparative data are usually available. Published evidence is accumulated slowly and selectively and is often prejudiced. Editorial policies do not really safeguard against biases in publication, but often increase them. The fact that clinical trial information on ADRs is usually confidential and that access to many ADR data bases is also quite limited represents a major obstacle for comprehensive, comparative assessment. Many current comparisons between drugs are not very useful; they are based on scanty and selective information, and there is often a hidden agenda behind such comparisons. Incidently, these hidden agendas exist not only in the industry, but sometimes also for so-called independent experts.

## Making Risk Understood: A Joint Responsibility

If we review our ways of dealing with drug risk issues, we realize that we still have a long way to go and a lot to learn if we are to make our risk assessment more rational. The common goal is better therapy for our patients. It is a public goal and cannot be pursued in secrecy and isolation. Open information and constructive dialogue are necessary. We have to work together to create better and more accessible data bases, especially for validating suspected adverse effects. We should join forces to develop more expertise and more openness to new ways of detecting, documenting, evaluating, and reporting adverse drug effects. Legislation always tends to reinforce already functioning systems in the case of drug surveillance, particularly spontaneous reporting. Risk assessment, however, is also a matter of denominators, and probably one of the most serious gaps in our knowledge concerns actual drug usage, where the best information of market research is again not publicly accessible. Open information, on the other hand, can be misused and misunderstood; information on ADR problems may create unfounded scares. To make open information more useful than harmful, we must also provide instruments for the rapid validation of signals. This calls for the broadest possible data bases and for the use of all available instruments. It can only be achieved with the collaboration of all partners involved.

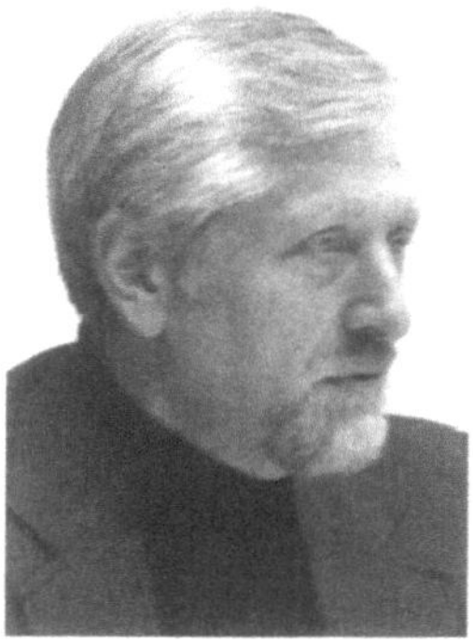

# 20. The Complexities of Assessment

A. J. GORDON

In order to appreciate the complexities faced in using and understanding the common expression *risk/benefit (R/B) relationship,* it is important to stress that the term is flawed from a methodologic perspective. *Benefit* is usually derived from surrogate measurements of efficacy, is assessed prospectively, and involves discrete, often narrow endpoints. On the other hand, *risk* (the chance of harm) is a multidimensional concept usually investigated and measured retrospectively. Furthermore, although we usually think of the R/B relationship in terms of applicability to and perception by a patient, many other constituencies involved in the development and use of medicines (e.g., physicians, companies, regulators) have different perceptions of both benefit and risk for themselves and on behalf of patients. Also, considering that there is considerable misuse or inappropriate use of drugs by both physicians and patients, the true R/B relationship, however measured, becomes distorted; in other words, many risks, minor as well as serious, may be avoidable [1].

The introduction of more science into the area of medication compliance is also affecting our application of R/B concepts. Recent data suggest that patients self-titrate for safety and toleration, the least compliant with prescribed regimens are those with the most adverse experiences [2]. It must also be appreciated that, when considering estimates of risk for application to any R/B assessment, far too little attention has been given to the uncertainty involved [3].

Finally, as we attempt to define and apply R/B assessments across different cultures and within varying regulatory environments, it is important that the terminology and conceptual framework for the various components of both benefit and risk be standardized as much as possible.

## References

1. Venning GR (1987) Rare and serious adverse reactions. Med Toxicol Adverse Drug Exp 2(4): 235-241

2. Petri H, Leufkens H, Naus J, Silkens R, van Hessen P, Urquhart J (1990) Rapid method for estimating the risk of acutely controversial side effects of prescription drugs. J Clin Epidemiol 43(5): 433–439
3 Finkel AM (1990) Confronting uncertainty in risk management. Center for Risk Management, Resources for the Future, Washington DC

# 21. A Review of the Regulatory Process in Japan

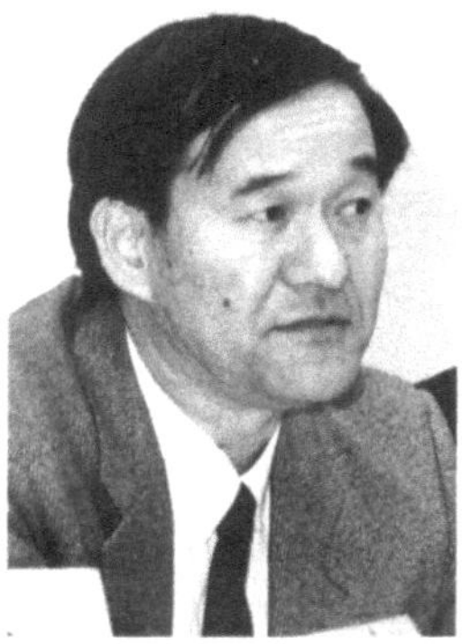

H. NAKAGAWA

In Japan, all the preclinical (mainly animal) and clinical data on drugs are evaluated for their clinical efficacy and safety when an application is made to the Minister of Health and Welfare for their license and marketing. After the approval has been given, the drugs are treated differently depending on whether or not they are new. In cases where the drugs are new (e.g., containing new chemical entities), they have to undergo re-examination 6 years (in principle) after the first approval on the basis of postmarketing information on efficacy and safety. Drugs which are not new undergo re-evaluation every 6 years in order to check their efficacy and safety, although the priority of re-evaluation is given to each drug or group of drugs depending on its clinical importance. All drugs have to undergo ad hoc re-evaluation in the special cases where certain problems regarding their safety or efficacy arise.

In the processes of first application for approval, re-examination, or re-evaluation, only information on clinical efficacy and safety is assessed. Drug usefulness is compared and judged with other drugs of comparable application for use, etc. The economic or marketing aspects are not taken into consideration in these assessments.

In addition to being used in periodical assessments of re-examination and re-evaluation, the Adverse Drug Reaction (ADR) Information System is important in the assessment of the risk of drugs in the postmarketing phase. ADR information is collected in two ways:

1. Voluntary information is collected from selected medical facilities (2178 hospitals in March 1990)
2. Information on any serious ADRs and other ADRs not included in the description on the package insert is reported from private firms as a statutory requirement of the Pharmaceutical Affairs Law

All scientific evaluation in these assessment processes is made by the experts in the Central Pharmaceutical Affairs Council, which is an advisory body to the Minister of Health and Welfare.

At present, a research group from the Ministry of Health and Welfare is looking into formulating standards for the degree of seriousness of ADRs.

Investigations on the degree of seriousness of ADRs related to blood disorders, hepatic dysfunction, renal dysfunction, and hypersensitivity have already been completed and investigations are scheduled for other ADRs. Once these are completed, the pharmaceutical company will make judgments according to these standards, in addition to the attending physician's decision.

## Postmarketing Surveillance for Re-examination

The method of executing postmarketing surveillance (PMS) for the re-examination system begins with the selection of the hospital which will be requested to carry out the survey. The system representative then brings the survey sheets to the physician at that hospital and asks him to carry out a survey on the usage of the drug. One doctor will gather information on 10–20 cases.

Conducting PMS for the re-examination system is unique to Japan; the same is not carried out in Europe or in the United States. In the United States, PMS studies are conducted on specific drugs, but not for all drugs.

PMS has now been carried out for over 100 items under the re-examination system and the results have been presented to the Ministry of Health and Welfare, but an issue has arisen over whether all the information expected was obtained. The reason for this is believed to lie in the fact that the methods of carrying out PMS have been left up to the pharmaceutical companies. There are also several problems to be resolved such as the limited acceptance of the system by medical facilities, the inadequate understanding by physicians, and the defectiveness of survey measures by the re-examination system representatives.

Moreover, carrying out PMS for the re-examination system costs a lot of money and is a heavy burden to the pharmaceutical companies. This surveillance is said to cost between 400 million and 500 million yen for one pharmaceutical. The number of personnel required to put together the data for the surveillance and to make reports has increased greatly, too.

## Good Postmarketing Surveillance Practice

In part due to this state of affairs, the Good Postmarketing Surveillance Practice (GPMSP) has been formulated, with a proposal advanced to ensure the reliability of the PMS results. In addition, a research group from the Ministry of Health and Welfare is conducting a study on methods of carrying out surveillance and improvements in methods can be expected.

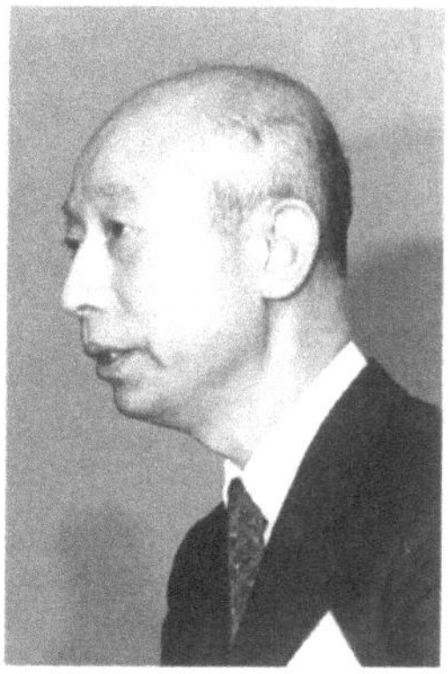

# 22. Postmarketing Surveillance in Japan: An Industry View

Y. Takeuchi

Pharmaceutical companies in Japan carry out several types of postmarketing surveillance. These types of surveillance have been determined under the Japanese Pharmaceutical Affairs Law and pharmaceutical companies make their reports to the Ministry of Health and Welfare. The types of surveillance include:

1. Reported cases of adverse drug reactions (ADRs), which are a collection of spontaneous reports from doctors, primarily in the hospitals.
2. Postmarketing surveillance under the re-examination system, which collects 10 000 cases of ADRs for a 6-year period after a new drug is marketed. It is a cohort survey without control group.
3. Re-evaluation, which evaluates efficacy and safety based on postmarketing literature.

## Collecting and Evaluating ADRs

Once the responsible representative of a pharmaceutical company receives ADR information from a doctor, he reports to the department concerned on a simple survey sheet. The department in charge of the matter then requests and collects the necessary information about the case on more detailed survey sheets. As for regulatory reporting on cases, serious ADRs that are already known as well as serious or less serious ADRs which are unknown must be reported by pharmaceutical companies to the Ministry of Health and Welfare.

Within the pharmaceutical companies, judging whether the collected cases of ADRs are serious or not is very important. A major difference between Japanese pharmaceutical companies and those in the United States and Europe is that clinical doctors are not usually employed by Japanese companies. Consequently, the judgment at a Japanese pharmaceutical company on whether a case is serious becomes based primarily on the opinion of the physician attending the patient at the time the ADR arises. This opinion may vary with the physician, since there are no standards for determining whether an ADR case is serious. To address this, when a pharmaceutical company makes judgments, it often seeks the advice of physicians (specialists) outside the company.

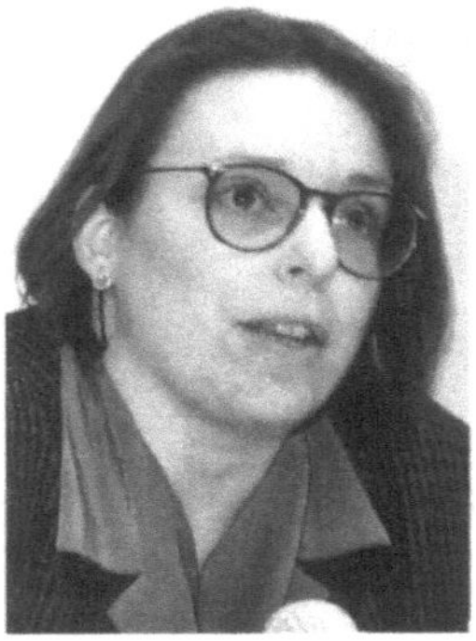

# 23. Distortions in Risk Assessment

J. HAAS

Failure to adjust correctly for severity will invariably distort the assessment of risk in pharmacoepidemiologic studies. Drugs are not prescribed to patients at random. The decision to prescribe a given agent to a given patient is based on assessment of a complex of factors which the prescriber may not articulate. Drugs with certain real or perceived characteristics will be prescribed to patients with certain real or perceived characteristics. This process has been described by Urquhart as channelling. Patients who are perceived as sicker will be prescribed drugs perceived as stronger; patients with previous drug intolerance will be prescribed agents believed to be better tolerated. Moreover, the outcome of the patient's illness is determined primarily by the underlying disease and only secondarily by treatment.

This intrinsic determinant of health outcome may be called the "sick patient effect" by analogy with the "healthy worker effect," which is established as a fundamental source of bias in occupational epidemiology research. Failure to appropriately adjust for the effects of channelling and the sick person effect will distort risk assessment based on pharmacoepidemiologic studies.

Randomization of drug assignment in clinical trials has become standard practice because there proved to be no way to avoid the introduction of bias, either subtle or blatant, when physicians are permitted to assign specific therapy to specific patients. Random assignment of drug therapy is essential to avoid the influence of recognized or unrecognized prognostic factors on patient safety and efficacy.

Much information about safety, however, comes not from clinical trials but from postmarketing experience, as increasing numbers of patients are exposed to the commercially available drug. The world of the randomized clinical trial is left behind: physicians decide which patients will be treated with the newly marketed drug. Stable and well-controlled patients are not likely to be selected for treatment with a new medication. Therapeutic failure, whether due to lack of efficacy or tolerance, is likely to be the reason for switching a patient to a new therapeutic modality. This process can sometimes be well documented using available data sources. Initially, most patients who are prescribed a substance will be switched from a previous drug, possibly of the same class. This phenomenon will mean that in the first years after a drug becomes available, the recipients will be a special cohort of difficult-to-manage patients within a given therapeutic indication.

For these special patients, selected by their physicians to receive a new therapy, the natural course of their disease is likely to be different from that of other patients with the same diagnosis. The underlying disease will be the major determinant of the disease outcome. The prognosis of these patients will be determined, largely, by the severity of their disease.

Therapy will modify the course of the underlying disease, but it will not remove the influence of underlying prognostic factors. If the basic determinants of disease outcome are not identified and not removed by appropriate adjustment, then it will be impossible to separate the effects of therapy from the effects of the underlying disease. This brings us to the sick patient and healthy worker effects mentioned above.

The healthy worker effect is a term used to describe the phenomenon whereby workers, even in the face of occupational hazards and poor working conditions, have overall health patterns which are better than those of the general population. This is particularly true of cardiovascular and respiratory mortality. Once recognized, the reason becomes obvious: there is a strong selection bias for good health in employed populations. In particular, workers able to hold a job requiring physical labor in dirty, demanding conditions are likely to be selected for the absence of health problems. Their underlying vigor may make it difficult, in occupational epidemiology studies, to identify deleterious influences of the work environment on a worker's health. The sick patient effect is the mirror image of the healthy worker effect. Here the underlying disease is a major determinant of patient outcome and will make it difficult to identify the influence of therapy.

Although this effect of intrinsic patient prognostic factors on the findings of pharmacoepidemiologic studies may seem obvious, it is, in fact, often ignored or adjusted for inadequately. An example of such inadequate adjustment occurred in studies of an asthma death risk and the use of the $\beta_2$ agonist fenoterol [1,2,3]. The investigators recognized the potential for bias resulting from the channelling of the new drug to sicker patients, but they chose to address this by adjusting for severity using ad hoc measures which they labeled "measures of chronic severity." A closer look at their findings showed that the patients labeled severe had a better prognosis than those not considered severe. This was the result of using measures of treatment intensity as measures of disease severity. Since asthma is a disease in which treatment does modify prognosis, the adjustments produced paradoxical results making interpretation of the studies impossible. Spurious associations have probably been created.

Thus, channelling of therapy and the sick person effect are virtually unavoidable problems in pharmacoepidemiologic studies. These factors must be addressed with the same care as the primary factors under study. If ignored, apparent drug-outcome associations will be created which are of no significance to the risk/benefit profile of the drug. The effort to confirm this, however, may result in a costly diversion of energy and resources.

## References

1. Crane J, Pearce NE, Flatt A et al. (1989) Prescribed fenoterol and death from asthma in New Zealand 1981–1983: case control study. Lancet I: 917–922
2. Pearce N, Grainger J, Atkinson M, Crane J, Burgess C et al. (1990) Case control study of prescribed fenoterol and death from asthma in New Zealand, 1977–1981. Thorax 15: 170–175
3. Poole C, Lanes SF, Walker AM (1990) Fenoterol and fatal asthma. Lancet 335: 920

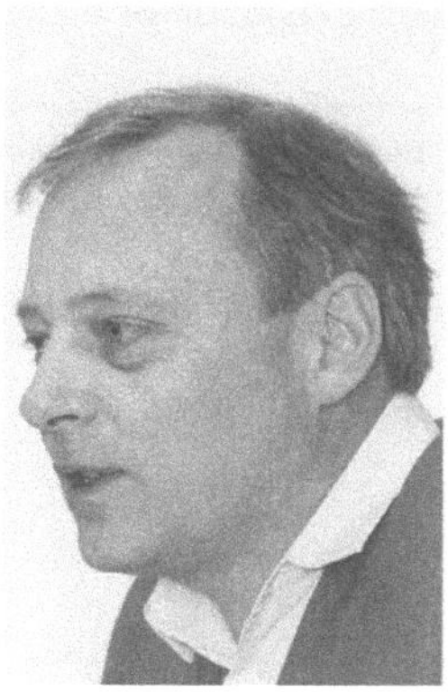

# 24. Weighing Risk/Benefit Assessment: Views of a Swedish "Regulator"

B.-E. Wiholm

The process of weighing drug-induced risks against disease-induced risk is a complicated multistep procedure. Although the basic principle was laid out more than 2000 years ago by Hippocrates – *primum est non nocere* – the interpretation and implementation of this principle has varied over time and has become more complicated in the present situation with the advent of modern pharmacotherapy.

We have come a long way from the period when foxglove leaves were dosed up till the patient showed signs of intoxication and then lowered somewhat. Dose finding is, however, still a major problem, both in drug development and in clinical practice. In fact, incorrect dosing is still the most common mechanism for drug-induced morbidity, both causing hospital admission and during hospital treatment. If dose-related adverse effects of cytostatic and immuno-suppressive medicines are included, the so-called type A reactions are also responsible for the majority of drug-induced mortality. In spite of this, most drug withdrawals because of safety issues have been caused by the appearance of rare, but dramatic and serious, idiosyncratic (type B) reactions. The interpretation and evaluation as well as the relevant preventive measures of drug-induced risks are heavily dependent on the nature of the problem at issue. Therefore, the evaluation of new potential adverse effects of medicines is a multifaceted and complicated procedure which includes at least the following steps:

- Detection and hypothesis generation
- Verification or refutation of the hypothesis
- Quantification to estimate the incidence
- Exploration of underlying mechanisms
- Identification of possible high-risk populations and the search for markers of increased susceptibility
- Evaluation of the clinical impact of the reaction on the individual and the population
- Identification of possible preventive strategies, including regulation of the use of the medicines as a last resort
- Information to the prescribers, the patients, and the relevant receivers in the medical community

**Table 1.** Major obstacles to scientifically solid decisions of risk/benefit evaluation of medicines

| |
|---|
| Lack of valid background data on the natural occurrence of events and diseases in populations and subpopulations, as well as lack of valid data on the natural history of many diseases |
| Uncertainties of the mechanisms of new events and their frequency of drug-induced occurrence |
| Lack of valid data on disease-related risks for comparison |
| Lack of valid expression of risk for idiosyncratic reactions, where risk is not independent of time |
| Time constraints and pressure |

These steps, however, only take the risk side into account and only the risk of the medicine under study. Before regulatory action is taken, the risk associated with available alternative therapies should ideally be evaluated and compared with the risk at issue. Moreover, the benefits of the actual and alternative therapies should be evaluated and weighed in the final evaluation of the situation.

To do these analyses in a proper way calls for an experienced body of multidisciplinary experts who have all relevant background data at hand. There are, however, several obstacles to scientifically solid decisions, some of which are depicted in Table 1. The last point in Table 1 is especially influential and cumbersome if a crisis is at hand or perceived by some party involved.

Given these uncertainties and the fact that most diseases can be treated using a number of medicines and other therapeutic measures, the standpoint of the regulator, whose responsibility primarily is to protect the public, most often must be to withhold rather than to free a medicine. This may lead to temporary or, in the worst case, permanent restrictions in the use of a medicine, even if it is not proven beyond doubt to be guilty or if all the risks of alternative therapies are not known.

Today, many medicines are approved for the market on the basis of data which actually offer no proof of equal efficacy or safety, but rather show an inability to demonstrate any difference from an already existing medicine. Thus, the argument is unfounded that taking a medicine off the market without 100% proof of guilt of its causing a serious problem deprives most patients of a medicine which to them is uniquely valuable. Actually, the evidence for such statements is, in my opinion, just as anecdotal as spontaneous ADR reports, or even more so. In fact, such cases presented with rechallenge seem even rarer than spontaneous ADR reports with a positive re-exposure.

To improve the weighing between risks and benefits of medicines, we need to develop further both the evaluation process and the instruments used therein, as well as the validity and availability of the necessary background information. Some principles for the advancement of the risk/benefit evaluation process are suggested in Table 2. The first principle in Table 2 is focused on the problem of comparing risks and benefits when they are perceived to be qualitatively

**Table 2.** Some principles suggested to improve the risk/benefit evaluation process

1. Risks and benefits should as far as possible be expressed in comparable units of measure
2. Risk should preferably be expressed in absolute terms, i.e., excess risk
3. The risk/benefit comparison could be made in relative terms as a relative risk, i.e., the risk of dying from disease as compared to the risk of dying from the available treatments

different, e.g., the benefit of being relieved of a headache against the risk of dying from agranulocytosis or acute gastrointestinal bleeding. It will improve the possibility to make valid comparisons if benefits are expressed as the reduction of risk from disease per unit time. For example:

- Reduction of risk of dying from disease per unit time as compared to the risk of dying from the treatment per unit time of exposure.
- Reduction of quality of life from disease per unit time as compared to reduction of quality of life from treatment per unit time.

(NB The risk of idiosyncratic adverse reactions are seldom independent of time, which introduces a problem of measuring the relevant period at risk; the traditional measure "person time of exposure" often is not applicable).

The second principle in Table 2 is intended to improve our measurements and expressions of risk. Excess risk is an estimate of how many extra cases of the disease or symptom are caused by use of the medicine instead of how much the risk is increased by the medicine as compared to a nonmedicated state. For instance, a low relative risk (e.g., 2 extra cases) of inducing a common problem, e.g., gastric ulcer (natural occurrence about 1/1000 patient-years), may be much more important to public health than a high relative risk (e.g., 20 extra cases) of inducing a rare disease, i.e., agranulocytosis (total occurrence about 9/1 000 000 patient-years).

The third principle in Table 2 points out the importance of comparing the risks of disease and treatment. To this should be added the comparison of risks inflicted by alternative treatments or no treatment at all.

To implement these principles some actions can be suggested (Table 3). When, for example, a new medicine is developed that would work in reducing

**Table 3.** Actions suggested to accomplish the principles for improved risk/benefit evaluation

1. Create a program devoted to the collection of descriptive epidemiologic data on specific subpopulations
2. Create a program of record linkage systems designed for these purposes
3. Create a program of case control surveillance of rare diseases which could be used to quantify the risk of new drugs
4. Create an international foundation for the sponsoring of important pharmacoepidemiologic studies

the loss of quality of life by alleviating problems of mictural incapacity, which up to now have required surgery, the background morbidity in the population of potential users of the medicine should be investigated thoroughly.

Present record linkage systems have the disadvantage that they were created for the reimbursement of medical treatment and sick leave. In the near future important changes in the approval process and probably also in the postmarketing surveillance of new medicines are going to take place. With the simultaneous introduction within the European Community of new chemical entities, much more emphasis has to be placed on a structured follow-up on effects that cannot be detected in the clinical trials program. To ensure early detection of potential problems, the spontaneous reporting systems already available will most probably be sufficiently effective if they can be coordinated and open to all parties involved. The quantification of rare but serious reactions, however, still presents a problem.

Even though these diseases and reactions are rare, they have been responsible for the majority of drug withdrawals where safety has been at issue. Such a program should include biology, the study of mechanisms behind idiosyncratic reactions, with the aim of defining risk groups and markers of the pharmacogenetic phenotypes who are at increased risk.

A major obstacle to the rapid evaluation and quantification of serious but rare adverse reactions has been the lack of funding for the large-scale studies needed. To overcome this obstacle it seems rational to create an international foundation with multisource sponsoring which could take on the responsibility for sponsoring studies that are important not only to a single company or country, but to public health in the international community. Such a foundation could preferably be arranged under the auspices of CIOMS or some other independent international organization.

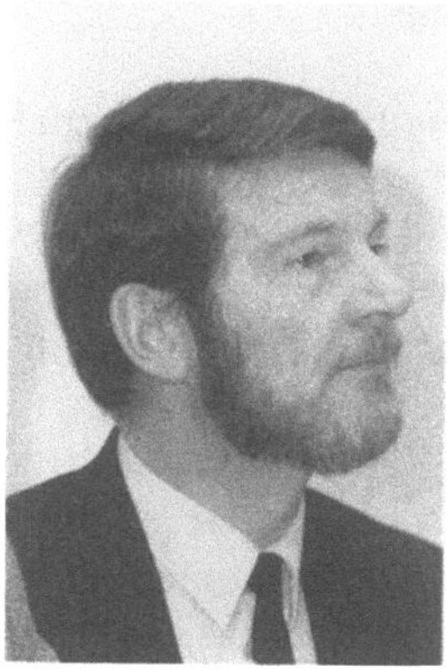

# 25. Scientific Evaluations and Personal Judgments

G. KREUTZ

For any pharmaceutical intended for patients, the applicant for marketing authorization has to document and substantiate to the authority granting the licence pharmaceutical quality, therapeutic efficacy, and medical safety. During the administrative approval procedure, these three qualifications are well examined on the basis of scientific knowledge and established standards. But the extent to which these attributes are predefined varies considerably. Requirements to be fulfilled and definitions to be applied are more developed, for example, with respect to pharmaceutical quality and toxicology and less developed with respect to all other constituents of medical safety. And scientific methods to verify therapeutic efficacy in many indications are worked out well and applied more or less uniformly while, for example, ways to define contraindications and especially evaluate potential adverse drug reactions are much less agreed upon.

## Benefit and Risk: Probabilities and Their Estimates

We must recognize that the evaluation of benefit and the evaluation of risk involve different approaches; as a method to critically examine the effects of pharmaceuticals, each of these evaluations, although it follows accepted rules, is based on different grounds. The prerequisite for therapeutic benefit to patients is therapeutic efficacy as measured by accepted endpoints. Predictability, whether a specific patient will experience efficacy of the pharmaceutical, depends greatly on the proportion of patients who have experienced efficacy in a controlled clinical trial. Because this proportion usually is high, it is highly probable that the patient will experience efficacy, that something good will happen to him or her.

With respect to risks we have to take into account a different situation. The probability that somebody will experience a harmful adverse drug reaction is low in most cases and for most types of reactions. The lower the probability, the more difficult it is to present valid figures which give an estimate close to the true value. On the other hand, the uncertainty about any given figures is high which means that any calculated confidence interval covers a wide range.

## Benefit and Risk: Comparison Without Standardized Scale

The comparison of benefit and risk is an expert evaluation based on personal judgment. There is at this time no scientific method used or even validated using any kind of calculation that could lead to a result which could be used in decision making. Any such method would have to weigh adverse drug reactions according to their type or severity. These weights should be variable depending on therapeutic class or indication. It would be, for example, necessary to specify different weights for agranulocytosis and for blurred vision as adverse drug reactions, and different weights would be assigned to each single adverse drug reaction like agranulocytosis if it occurs related to use of an antirheumatic or a cytostatic pharmaceutical. This would be an altogether tremendous task and the judgment would be very difficult to agree upon.

## Benefit and Risk: Population and Individual Patient

We have to differentiate between evaluation of benefit and risk for a patient population and for an individual patient within a population. The benefit and risk relation should be interpreted differently for each of these cases because of the differences already described.

Altogether, what we sometimes call "assessment" is much less a decision based on defined methods, although this may be the impression conveyed by the use of this word. It is, rather, an evaluation based on personal judgment that can be followed only after all the relevant arguments have been made.

# 26. Discussion

One of the problems with the use of benefit/risk ratios is that people generally unfamiliar with the assessment of benefits and risks ascribe a precision and a certainty to these ratios that simply do not exist. In reality, benefit/risk assessment is applied ethics. It is important to make clear to everyone that these ratios are based ultimately on personal judgments, even though scientific methods often are used in the estimation process. It also is important to understand that risk and benefit are multidimensional entities; for example, benefit is not the same as efficacy, which is a surrogate measure, and risk cannot be equated with the level of safety as measured in clinical trials.

Each constituency affected by the use or development of drugs thus thinks about the benefit/risk relationship from its own perspective. Manufacturers, physicians, and regulatory authorities understandably assess this relationship in terms of their own needs, not on behalf of patients. It is natural that, in developing and marketing a drug, a manufacturer would ask: "What are the benefits and risks for me as a manufacturer?" Yet this means that the risks for and the benefits to the patient who is directly impacted by the drug may not be adequately considered in overall benefit/risk assessments. The only way the patient is able to introduce his or her own benefit/risk judgment into this process is through self-initiated modification of a drug dose or frequency.

The panelists urged that greater attention be given to the specification and analysis of actual patient drug use patterns, about which little is known. This matter will have to be addressed primarily by the pharmaceutical companies or other nongovernmental bodies, however, since only in major crises will regulatory authorities give this matter the attention it requires. These authorities are responsible, through the drug approval process and the enforcement of laws, for ensuring that drugs are safe and effective. For better or worse, their mission is not to monitor comprehensively the public's drug use patterns. Even when the people who are charged with postmarketing surveillance within a regulatory authority are different from those people who approve the drugs, there still are internal conflicts regarding the interpretation and application of the minimal drug use data that exist. Moreover, the range of government authority control tends to be limited to the proper, not the improper, use of drugs. Yet it is often important to consider what the safety margin of a drug is in the likely event of its being used improperly, as in a patient-initiated overdose of a psychoactive or nonsteroidal antiinflammatory drug.

Facts are a scarce and precious commodity. While panelists favored the expansion and linkage of drug use data bases, they also cautioned that such data should not be equated or confused with facts. To sort out the effects of a medication from the patient's underlying disease is extremely complicated and difficult, and is at the core of the problem faced by pharmacoepidemiologists in drawing conclusions from drug use data. Such information cannot be used in isolation, but must be used in conjunction with patient information. To illustrate, postmarketing data on risks and benefits are normally generated according to the way the drug is prescribed, not the way it is taken. Moreover, ADR data are collected in a milieu of improper prescribing practices and patient noncompliance; hence, drug use data do not indicate what the incidence of harm would be if patients took all their medicines according to the prescribed frequency and dose. It is hoped that the emerging field of population pharmacokinetics will be able to improve the reliability of drug use studies in the future.

The perspective of the government regulatory authorities is quite different from that of the patients. The former's concern is to safeguard the public in general through the drug approval and withdrawal process and is reflected in their attention to rare idiosyncratic events, severe or even fatal reactions, and broad issues of disease and health. The patients, on the other hand, worry about such personal symptomatic discomforts as dizziness, nausea, and incontinence, reactions which are of immediate concern but cannot be measured easily, if at all. Patients generally tend not to take seriously longer-term severe reactions; in a study for a new antihypertensive drug, for example, over 90 % of the patients for whom the drug was prescribed on a continuing basis purchased the drug only once.

One might characterize the importance of a particular ADR as the product of its severity times its frequency. If an ADR is frequent but minor, it is usually recognized by the regulatory authorities at the time the drug is initially approved and can be communicated to the patients. Patients, in turn, self-censor themselves. If an ADR bothers them enough, they take care of that problem. At the other end of the spectrum are rare but severe ADRs. In these cases, while regulatory authorities are very interested in knowing about important life-threatening, unknown, unlabeled ADRs, once they are assured that these reactions are quite rare, they generally limit their intervention to requiring an appropriate warning in the labeling of the drug. Further involvement by these authorities is unlikely to influence either the patients' willingness to use the drug or the physicians' therapeutic choices.

In the history of drug withdrawals, one of the biggest problems has been the failure to anticipate the actual pattern of use in the population. Both physicians and patients act differently in coping with actual problems than in idealized settings. Indeed, many withdrawals involve the failure to anticipate accurately how people act in real-life situations. Regulatory authorities as well as pharmaceutical manufacturers have an obligation to give much greater attention to anticipating problems that might arise in the use of drugs as they make their risk/benefit assessments.

The panelists emphasized the difficulty in deciding upon inappropriate thresholds of risk for a given clinical indication or drug category. With respect to case assessment, the notion of overall risk has no meaning. Rather, there is a risk for a specific patient in a specific situation. Just as there exists a case assessment of an ADR that has occurred, so too there exists an assessment of a specific indication for a specific drug in a specific patient. As for assessments of specific ADR issues, the panelists thought they are quite well done, although not as well done as on the individual level. But even for these ADR issue assessments it is very difficult to establish the overall bottom line, the overall risk profile, of a drug. As a result, epidemiologists tend to limit themselves to consequences (for example, mortality) rather than diagnoses of specific risks.

Given the current competitive environment within the pharmaceutical industry and the difficulties associated with generating valid data on drug risks, government regulatory authorities lack comparative risk data on the drugs with which they work. Therefore, in the absence of risk standards and absolute risk levels, these authorities must exercise considerable judgment in the drug approval process. All parties need to understand that there are no absolutes in this process; no rigid criteria are applied, either at the clinical trial stage or at the postmarketing surveillance stage. Within the FDA and other regulatory agencies, approval remains somewhat dependent upon who the reviewer is, which drug class is being considered, which diseases are the target of the drug, etc.

Nevertheless, a few operating principles have emerged in these agencies. For example, if a thorough investigation of a drug shows the risk of a particular reaction to be very small, it is simply acknowledged as such in the labeling and no restriction is placed on the use of the product. Increasingly, also, government authorities believe that it is necessary and appropriate to consider all causes, not to single out one body system or one particular reaction. The FDA, for example, in contrast to most other national regulatory agencies, did not move to take phenylbutazon off the market; even though the FDA recognized that the drug had a greater propensity to cause immunologic reactions than did other nonsteroidals, it did not feel that the available data on overall risk differentiated it sufficiently from these other drugs. Most regulatory authorities deal with risk uncertainty by collecting more data. If definable concern exists at the time a drug is being considered for approval, a clinical trial or targeted epidemiologic study often is conducted before a decision is made.

Yet more data and more analysis are not enough; value judgments must still be used in the drug review and approval process. One consideration is whether there are alternative therapies on the market; if not, regulatory authorities may alter the intensity with which a potential problem is pursued. Other considerations are whether the population to be exposed to the drug is the same one studied in the trials; whether the disease being treated is severe; and whether preliminary signals that appear raise "red flags." It is important in making these value judgments that the regulatory authorities try to anticipate problems on the basis of their broad experience with other drugs.

The panelists expressed interest in instituting routine 3-year or 5-year reviews both by the pharmaceutical manufacturer and by the government regulatory agency of each new drug approval to ensure that it is given a second look based on accumulated experience. Routinizing the review process in this manner would lessen the appearance of a crisis when a regulatory agency invites a company to discuss one of its drugs. In Japan, for example, there is a 6-year review after the initial approval in the case of new drugs, although a few drugs may be reviewed conditionally after 4 years; a review system also is in place for drugs other than new ones. In general, whether 3, 5, or 6 years is a reasonable review period for a drug depends very much on the frequency of the use of the drug, the indications of the drug, and whether sufficient information can be obtained during the review period to conduct a thorough reassessment.

Pharmaceutical company representatives expressed the concern that such periodic postapproval drug reviews might not be coordinated across countries. It is crucial that there be broad acceptance of the standard information that should be provided to the various national regulatory authorities and that there be some uniformity of review periods among the developed countries. In fact, standardization of the information required across countries by their respective regulatory authorities is a concern at all stages in the drug development, marketing, and postmarketing process. Although the plans for an integrated European Community by 1993 could lessen these concerns, it is unlikely they will be resolved without the continued efforts of the full spectrum of drug safety constituencies.

Several concluding comments brought the discussion back to the topics addressed earlier. If more and better ADR information cannot be generated, then drug and ADR epidemiology, evaluation, and interpretation will decline in quality. Animal studies may be able to help provide the required information, provided there is more emphasis on the quality than on the quantity of evaluation. As to the information obtained through clinical practice, the first person who generally recognizes the presence of an ADR is the patient, who usually then seeks the advice of a physician. Legal barriers or industry incentives should not prevent the physician from being able to inform the patient of signs to look for rather than confusing or frightening the patient later with the ultimate diagnosis. The physician also must be better able to recognize ADRs early in their development. Postgraduate education for the physician is very important, as is the provision of graphic information to the physician by the industry. Lastly, more people experienced in the recognition and interpretation of ADRs are needed not only on the faculty of medical schools, but also in community medical advisory centers and the media.

# Part VII

# Expectations in Drug Safety Communication

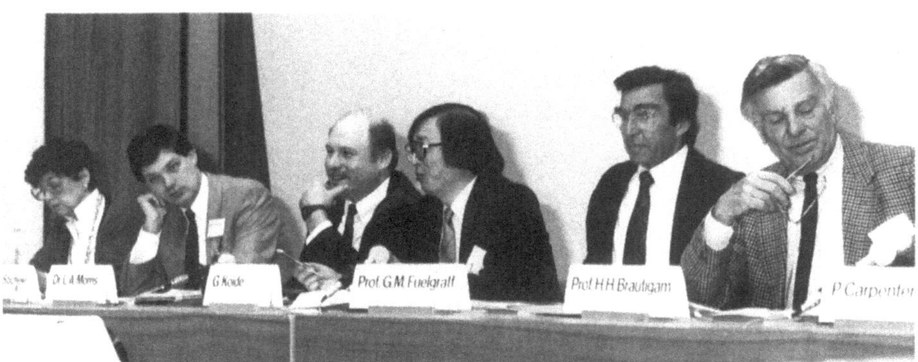

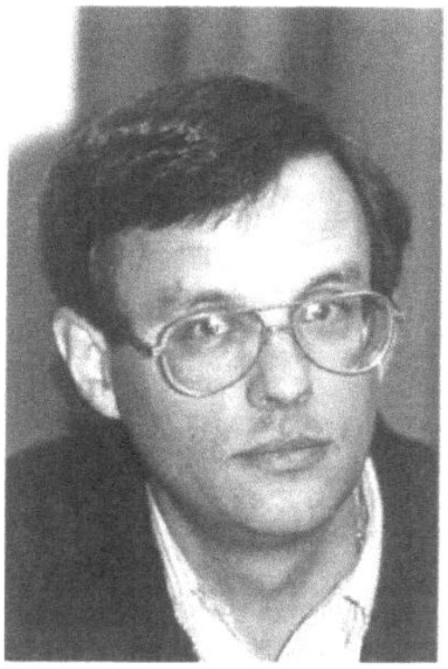

# 27. The Challenge of Communicating Drug Safety Information

P. CARPENTER

Our task becomes more difficult as we make the important transition to the stage of communicating information, a field where there is a need for more experience and knowledge; a field where we currently rely much more on art than on science. It is a very difficult challenge to move from the arena of knowledge collection and analysis, which has come to be based on "objective" science, to the arena of knowledge communication, which heretofore has been based on the creative arts. That challenge is to link the creative arts to the objective sciences, and to do so on the basis of philosophical standards. We provide this information so the participants in the decisionmaking process, particularly the patient, can make an informed choice. Three ethical principles that lead us to recognize the importance of informed choice are nonmaleficence, beneficence, and autonomy. The first principle is an area where medicine has distinguished itself for generations. In recent years, with the application of science, we have become increasingly capable of providing benefits. Now one of our most important challenges is to ensure the right of individuals to make their own choices. It is important that we recognize the need of patients to believe that they have some reasonable command oven their own lives. To paraphrase Robert S. Morison [4], if we fail to do that, they are simply going to give up supporting what they perceive as the elements in society that systematically deny them the ability to control their own fates. We see this increasingly in our society as many people turn to other forms of medicine such as homeopathy, herbal medicines, and over-the-counter medications. I suggest that one of the motivations with respect to prescription medicines is that far too frequently the individual feels a complete lack of self-determination.

As stated by Diana B. Dutton [2], all medical advances involve risk: nothing ventured, nothing gained. But that does not mean that all risks are worth taking, or that we all would make the same choices. Risks to individuals and society as a whole are the prices we pay for medical progress. Some hazards are known, or can be discovered with more extensive testing, but new and untried therapies will always entail unpredictable risks. Only the people who bear those risks can legitimately decide that they are worth taking. It is for this reason, as we discussed in 1988 at Wolfsberg, that we developed the concept of pharmaceutical informed choice. Simply stated, this means that the patient's right to decide can be effectively exercised only if the patient possesses enough information to permit an intelligent choice. To achieve this, the physician and the pharmacist should be provided with adequate information about a pharmaceutical product and its alternatives so they can improve their presentation to the prospective user and increase that person's understanding of the options.

In addition, whenever we present pharmaceutical product information directly to patients, our objective should be to inform regarding benefits and risks, rather than to promote use of the product. To paraphrase Sir Walter Bodmer, improving the public understanding of science and in this case the public understanding of the risks and benefits of drugs is an investment in the future, not a luxury to be indulged in, if and when resources allow [1].

Hopefully, the ethical foundation that we have discussed, (the principles of nonmaleficence, beneficence, and autonomy) combined with objective science regarding knowledge acquisition and analysis, the very creative capabilities of our industry, and the concepts of pharmaceutical software and informed choice will lead us in a very new direction.

As a noted physicist, Richard P. Feynman, has said, "Our responsibility is to do what we can, learn what we can, improve the solutions, and pass them on" [3]. That is our challenge today.

## References

1. Bodmer, W (1985) Report of the committee on public understanding of science. Royal Society, London.
2. Dutton DB, Preston TA, Pfund NE. (1988) Worse than disease: pitfalls of medical progress. Cambridge University Press, Cambridge
3. Feynman, RP (1988) What do you care what other people think?: further adventures of a curious character. WW Norton, New York
4. Morison, RS (1969) Science and social attitudes. Science 165: 150–6

# 28. The Media Perspective

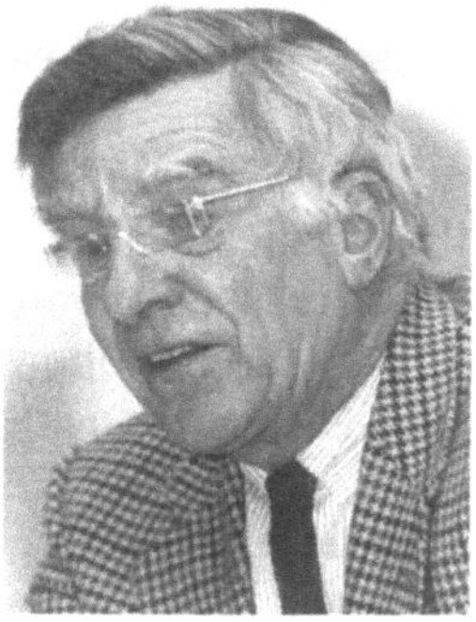

H. H. BRÄUTIGAM

Whether we like it or not, we need to face the fact that there is a new scenario in drug safety and risk communication, and that new players are appearing on the health care scene. Among these new players are the media in their role as communicators to and on behalf of the public. Although the media have embraced the role of watchdog for health matters, the quality of information provided by the media is, at present, rather poor. The reason for this is twofold: pharmaceutical companies are not trained in communicating with journalists and journalists lack basic knowledge of biostatics and pharmacoepidemiology. Both of these gaps must be filled if we are to see an improvement in drug safety information.

Let me give you an example of one series of events that underlined how unwilling those involved in the health care process are to communicate openly with each other. Some years ago, while I was chairman of the obstetrics and gynecology department of a West German teaching hospital, a situation arose in which a number of patients developed blood poisoning shortly after giving birth. The staff immediately started to question the patients' relatives and to study the medication that the patients had received to try and pinpoint the cause. Finally, we were able to come up with a set of facts: all the women who were suffering from blood poisoning were previously healthy rhesus-negative women who had given birth to rhesus-positive babies. All of the women had been injected with anti-rhesus immunoglobulin to prevent rhesus incompatibility in future pregnancies.

We suspected an adverse drug reaction, but had no proof. In the course of the following days, we informed the pharmaceutical manufacturer involved, the regulatory authority, and the government. The manufacturer denied any responsibility and asked the hospital to contain the problem, not to inform the media, and to return all the ampules for examination. The regulatory authority suggested, after 8 weeks, that the ampules should go to a state institute for examination. In the meantime, the hospital had already decided to take action by sending a few ampules to an independent foreign serum institute. The results of the tests arrived within a few days, they showed that toxins had been discovered in two out of the three ampules.

The consequences for all those involved were catastrophic: one patient died, compensation took 10 years to sort out, the managing director of the pharmaceutical company went to prison, and the regulatory authority lost credibility in the eyes of the public.

I would like to suggest a few ways in which the current situation could be improved. To communicate risk and benefit data to the public, Madison Avenue-style advertising people are not appropriate. Information should only come from trained staff in the pharmaceutical industry. Industry should follow three simple rules in communicating with the media: straightforwardness, objectivity, and reliability.

Straightforwardness in the industry's dealings with the media is a priority, since the public often gleans more information about medical problems from the media than from their doctors. Pharmaceutical companies provide doctors with information on new developments and treatments, but doctors often cannot or do not want to find the time to spend on patient information, and, consequently, the patient is the receiver of poor quality information. To counteract this, the results of pharmacoepidemiological studies, particularly where they concern the relation between risk and benefit, should be made accessible in an understandable manner to the public. It is the consumer's right to receive proper information which he or she can use to make a choice.

In order to make a sound choice on which course of action to follow, the information that is at the consumer's disposal should be objective. A number of options are open to the consumer, who must choose not only between certain drugs, taking their risk/benefit relationship into consideration, but also between drug or nondrug therapy. Again, this is the patient's decision, and not that of the physician or counsellor. The concept of an available range of options is accepted in the area of surgical treatment, and written informed consent is mandatory. This range of options should also be presented in the case of drug treatment, and informed consent of a patient could also be required for treatment.

Reliability is the last principle. The consumer should be able to have confidence in the data at his or her disposal. These data should present both the positive and negative aspects of drug studies and postmarketing surveillance. If this is not the case, the result in the long run is a loss of confidence, which is extremely damaging to all parties concerned.

To improve the quality of information, industry should arrange seminars and workshops with journalists from the nonscientific media and begin to establish contacts during the "good times" which may be of help in the cases of "bad times". Seminars should focus on pharmacoepidemiology and the perception of risk. With honest and open communication, one can ensure the adequacy of newspaper reports.

Target-oriented product information should be separated from general information which could be provided by a risk/benefit industry foundation. The public have a highly developed interest in drugs and already make use of the available literature on this subject, such as the Swedish FASS directory. There is room for more, similar literature. Patient package inserts are necessary, but since they are only available after the drug has been prescribed, their existence cannot influence the decision making process. Nevertheless, they should be looked at with a view to demystifying the expert language and replacing it with something that can be understood by the average individual.

The new issue in developed countries is defensive medicine, and we will have to deal with it practically.

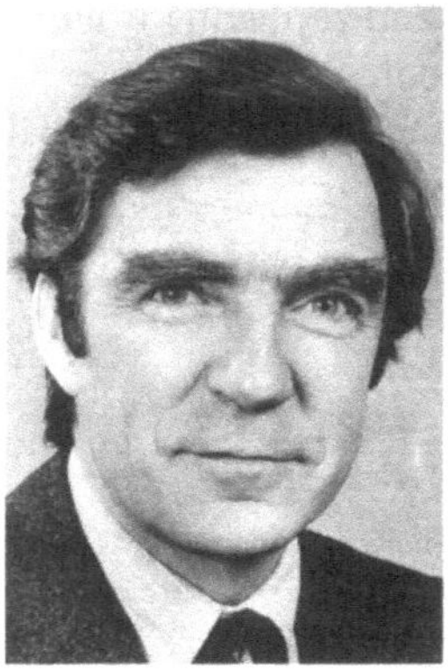

# 29. The Culture of Weighing

G. M. Fülgraff

Pharmaceutical companies are the primary source of information on their products within the information and communication triangle (Fig. 1), and should fulfill their role and responsibility here, even though some of the information pathways and communication means are under the tutelage of regulatory authorities. In continental Europe, tradition and legislation provide an established and regulated information pathway from the manufacturers to the drug users in the form of mandatory patient package inserts (PPI). Since drugs are dispensed only in original packages, every drug user is in possession of the mandatory PPI.

The safe use of drugs depends largely on the form and substance of the manufacturers's information to prescribing physicians and to drug-using patients, since drugs are integrated wholes of hardware and software, the latter being decisive for overall safety. Hence, benefit/risk assessment and communication cannot strictly be separated from each other, because any assessment

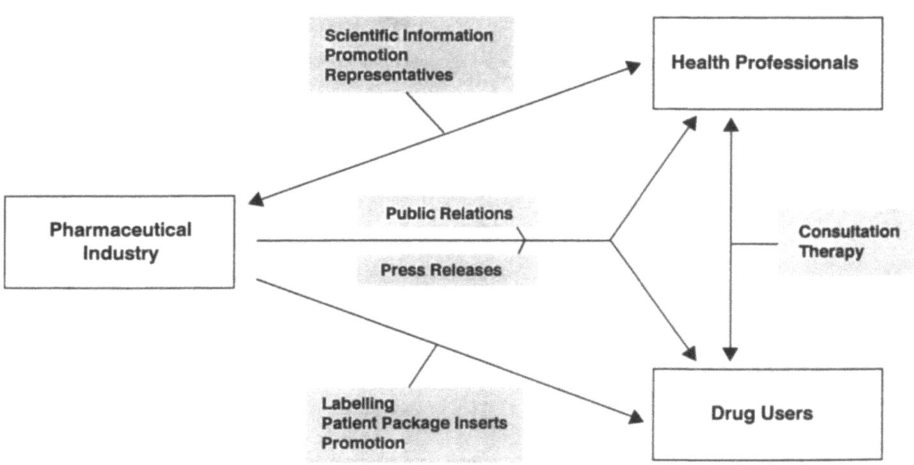


**Fig. 1.** Sources of information on pharmaceutical products

takes into account a given form and substance of information, particularly the way claims and risks are expressed.

Communication about drugs is applicable when it is embedded in an outflow of a culture of weighing. A culture of weighing encompasses two meanings:

1. That statements provide the necessary particulars on benefits and risks, allowing judgments which may, to a certain degree, differ when undertaken by different individuals.
2. That both risk and benefit are expressed as being essentially probabilistic and, in addition, often controversial and disputed.

The fact is, however, that risk is usually described as controversial and probabilistic, whereas the benefit is expressed in factual terms.

To illustrate the practical consequences, we will look at a disease characterized by green pimples on the face and a drug product marketed under the brand name Pimplex with the claim "makes green pimples disappear" and the adverse drug reactions (ADR) warning "may, in rare cases, cause swollen red nose." Regarding the effects of the application of Pimplex, there are four possible outcomes:

1. Unchanged green pimples: worthless Pimplex
2. Green pimples disappeared: wonderful Pimplex
3. Green pimples disappeared and swollen red nose: dangerous Pimplex
4. Green pimples still present and swollen red nose: disastrous Pimplex

The above-mentioned usual information in claims and ADR warnings refers only to the outcomes outlined in points [2] and [3], and does not refer to the outcomes mentioned in points [1] and [4]. Ideally, Pimplex should only be marketed when individuals who would have outcome [2] could be identified in advance, but we are, in most therapeutic situations, far from that point. This lack of targeting the drug should be compensated for by informing doctors and patients of the four possible outcomes and, if possible, their rough probabilities. For a typical drug product to lower blood pressure which is recommended for the treatment of borderline or slightly elevated blood pressure, the claim should consequently read: "This product will probably lower your blod pressure, but whether this will be of benefit for you in terms of a longer and better life or in terms of preventing typical complications of high blood pressure is a matter of controversy."

One should perhaps not ask too much at once. But there are, nevertheless, minimum requirements for communication within a culture of weighing, such as congruence of knowledge and behavior and consistency of all information on a drug through the manifold channels which are used by a company, from scientific information to promotion, from representatives to pharmapolicy, and from the registration department to marketing. Marketing of drugs in a culture of weighing meets the challenge to clearly distinguish between:

- What is known and what is assumed
- What is a generally accepted benefit and what is still controversial or disputed
- A lack of risks and a lack of knowledge of risks

These distinctions allow the addressees to make their judgments by comparing the chance of therapeutic efficacy and the chance of harm. The marketing items and messages should be revised to fit into the culture of weighing.

The principle of weighing must also dominate communication and discussion about drug products in general. All of the constituencies involved in the safe use of drugs should jointly destroy the phantom of drugs as the last resort of an intact world, and give up *expressis verbis* the illusion that the development and the use of modern therapeutics could reasonably be guided by such a principle as "above all, do no harm." We should, instead, make joint efforts to raise the public awareness that there is a good chance that drugs will relieve or improve a situation, but that they are also linked with a chance of harm.

In conferences devoted to the improvement of drug safety by more appropriate means and contents of communication, it is not surprising that the principles of a culture of weighing meet with broad approval. This is due, at least in part, to the selection of the people attracted to the subject. It is, however, far from the truth that all information given on drugs is imbued with the principle. To improve the situation we should regularly ask ourselves two questions:

- Do I know all channels by which my institution communicates, and are they all in line with the culture of weighing so that I can fully agree with them?
- Whom would I primarily have to influence within my institution to better approach the principle and to attain congruence and consistency?

It must be realised, however, that consent to principles is one thing and application in daily practice is another. The devil is in the nuts and bolts. Authenticity and trust are reached neither by asking for principles nor by mere acclamation of them, but by patient, steady, and sustained efforts to communicate within a scope defined by the principles.

It could be an attractive task within the framework of RAD-AR to elaborate and then propose to the pharmaceutical world an internationally acceptable set of principles for good communication practices (GCP) according to the culture of weighing. GCP would exclude such practices as warranting 100% efficacy as well as "no harm." Such promises cannot be considered innovative marketing, but simply unethical.

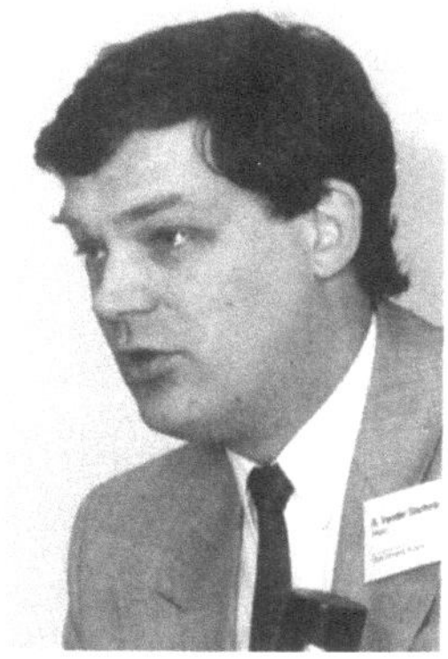

# 30. Patient Package Inserts: Carriers of Consensus Information

R. VANDER STICHELE

In the information network surrounding the individual patient, there are many oral information sources, each playing its role. The health professionals, i.e., physicians and pharmacists, are the information sources preferred by the patient [1, 2]. Field studies, however, have demonstrated that information from these sources is limited, especially with regard to risk communication [3, 4]. Traditionally, there has been very little cooperation between physicians and pharmacists in bringing information about medications to the patient [5, 6] (Fig. 1). A social network of relatives and friends surrounds the patient. Patients consult this network when in trouble, e.g., when deciding whether to seek

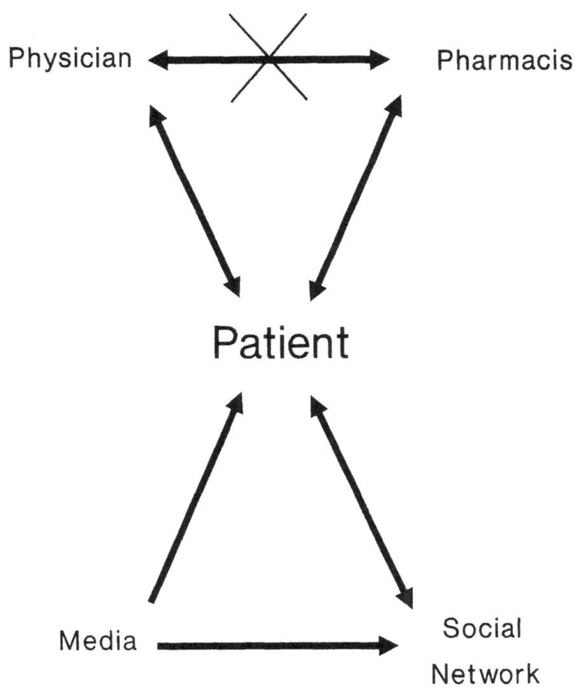


**Fig. 1.** Patient interaction with information sources

professional help or to start (or continue) taking medication. The media influence the patient directly, and through the social network. Some of the information provided by these sources is repetitive, some is conflicting, and some diverges from accepted knowledge.

## Written Medication Information

One way of providing a clear reference to accepted medical knowledge is written medication information, in the form of books, leaflets, or inserts. In the United States the Physicians' Desk Reference is a bestseller among the general public. Specialized information services, professional associations of physicians and pharmacists, pharmaceutical companies, and consumer organizations provide leaflets, mostly for classes of medications. These leaflets are provided on a voluntary basis and originate from a single source. Although their communicative quality may be obvious, the distribution of these leaflets to the patients in need of information is problematic [3].

In some countries of Western Europe there is a longstanding tradition of original drug dispensing with an information insert enclosed in each individual retail package. The concept of patient package inserts (PPI) brings together three important notions:

1. The linkage of the chemical substance (the medication) and the information that goes with it (the insert) into one branded product (the package) in the course of retail distribution
2. The notion of intended, and legally enforced, readability
3. The notion of consensus medication information

## The Patient Package Insert as a Source of Consensus Information

The PPI can be regarded as a direct communication between the individual patient and experts in medication information [7]. The experts in the medical professions, the regulatory authorities, and the pharmaceutical industry seek consensus. The result of this consensus-seeking process is the product summary or data sheet (Fig. 2).

From the data sheet a concise piece of paper, the PPI, is derived. It is present in every package, as an extra channel of information, not to replace, but to supplement and facilitate other communication. The PPI is like a safety net, in case the physician or the pharmacist did not have the time or the inclination to give essential information to the patient.

## Risk Communication on a Time Axis

The encounters of the patient with medication information sources can be plotted on a time axis: first, the physician control visits; second, the pharmacist refill visits. An important moment comes when the patient returns home with

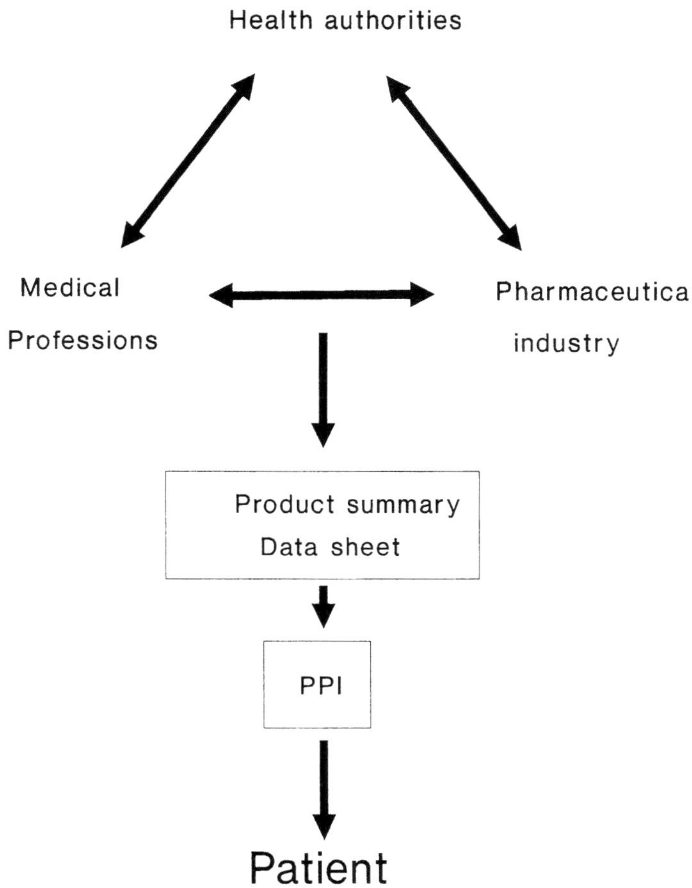


**Fig. 2.** The patient package insert as a source of consensus information

the dispensed medication and decides on his or her own whether he or she is going to take the medication. Research conducted in Belgium (a country with PPIs in every medication package) indicates that most patients then read the insert [8] (Fig. 3).

The insert may also be important later on the time axis when a problem arises that might be caused by the medication. The time of onset of side effects is unpredictable. However, an appropriate and swift reaction is often crucial. With some side effects, e.g., allergic reactions, the patient should stop the medication and then consult the physician. With other side effects, the patient should continue medication, because abrupt halting might be hazardous. For some side effects the physician should be informed with the shortest possible delay, for others only at the next scheduled routine visit. It is obvious that some important decisions in the therapeutic process are left to the patient.

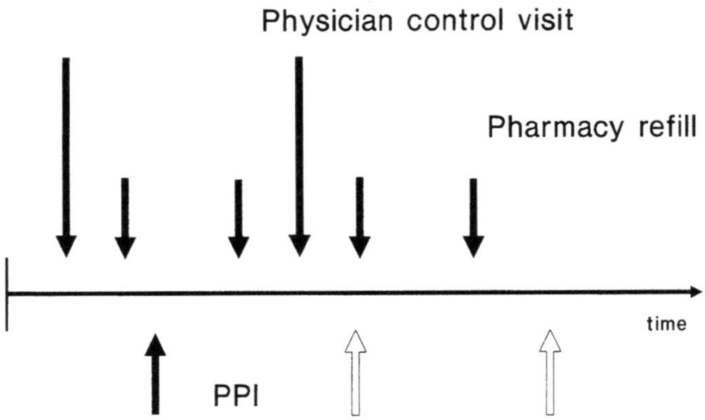


**Fig. 3.** Patient encounters with information sources over time

## Self-Efficacy of the Patient

Our therapeutic interventions rely strongly on the inevitable procedure of self-administration of medication by the patient. The patient has the possibility to refuse treatment and must be motivated to continue treatment. Last, but not least, in dealing with side effects, the patient must make autonomous decisions [9]. At these moments, a well-written instructional package insert can be valuable.

When PPIs were first proposed in the late 1970s in the United States, there was much opposition, especially from physicians and pharmacists. They feared the PPI would suggest side effects, frighten the patient, damage his relationship with the health professional, and jeopardize compliance. A full decade later, those early fears have not been confirmed.

## Conclusion

PPIs are soon to become part of branded products in the European Community [10]. This new medium is certainly not the ultimate communication tool, and it is still in a somewhat experimental phase. In the future, PPIs within original drug dispensing distribution systems will probably play a key role in communicating risk to the individual patient. Physicians and pharmacists will have to learn how to interact with this new medium in order to ensure good communication with the patient and proper utilization of medication.

## References

1. Morris LA, Grossman R, Barkdoll GL, Gordon E, Soviero C (1984) A survey of patient sources of prescription drug information. Am J Public Health 74: 1161–1162
2. Baldwin HJ, Cosler LE, Schulz RM (1987) Opinion leadership in medication information. Commun Q 35: 84–102

3. Morris LA (1982) A survey of patients' receipt of prescription drug information. Med Care 20: 596–605
4. Scherwitz L, Hennrikus D, Yysim S, Lester J, Vallbona C (1985) Physician communication to patients regarding medications. Pat Educ Couns 7: 121–136
5. Norwood GJ, Seibert JJ, Gagnon JP (1976) Attitudes of rural consumers and physicians toward expanded roles for pharmacists. J Am Pharm Assoc 16: 551–554
6. Woroniecki CL, McKercher PL, Flagler DG, Berchou R, Cook JA (1982) Effect of pharmacist counseling on drug information recall. Am J Hosp Pharm 39: 1907–1910
7. Herxheimer A, Davies C (1982) Drug information for patients: bringing together the messages from prescriber, pharmacist and manufacturer. J Roy Coll Gen Pract 32: 93–97
8. Vander Stichele R, Bogaert MG (1989) Patient package inserts: the Belgian experience with a mandatory program. Drug Inf J 23: 673–677
9. Leventhal H, Cameron L (1987) Behavioral theories and the problem of compliance. Pat Educ Couns 10: 117–138
10. Sauer F (1989) EEC regulatory initiatives on drug information. In: Bogaert M, Vander Stichele R, Kaufman JM, Lefebvre R (eds) Patient package insert as a source of drug information. Excerpta Medica, Amsterdam

# 31. The Patients' View

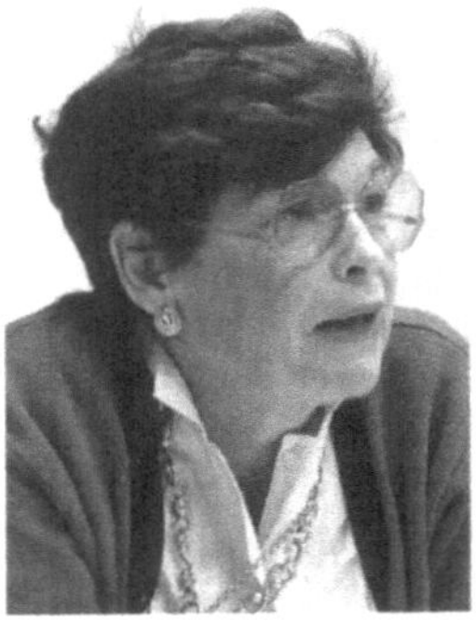

K. Whitehorn

Medicines are taken for illness; so it comes as a surprise to discover that, in Britain at any rate, the majority of drugs are bought by healthy people. The biggest users are women over 50 who are in the upper socioeconomic groups, so on all these counts I am typical of the UK drug user. What these figures really tell us, though, is that taking pills and medicines is part of our normal way of life, and not just something we resort to in extreme emergency.

Given that the taking of drugs is such a normal activity, it is surprising that patients' expectations of them should be so extremely wide of the mark. My purpose in this chapter is to try and show how wide is the gulf between what medical professionals and drug companies think their ministrations will do, and what the patients expect them to do, and the even wider gulf between the way in which the professionals assume the patients will follow their treatments, and what the patients actually do.

Patients' expectations are, I am afraid, totally unrealistic. We expect, for a start, that everything sold over the counter is quite safe, or it would, of course, need a prescription. This begs entirely the question of what happens if you take an overdose. One sad phenomenon doctors often find is that some hysterical youngster has staged a "suicide" with paracetamol, not really meaning actually to die, the classic "cry for help" in which the young person subconsciously makes sure that help will arrive in plenty of time. The suicide is found, rushed to hospital, treated, and surrounded by upset friends and relations, i.e., just the effect intended; but then, all too often, death follows some days later, from liver damage.

Along with the assumption that everything sold across the counter is safe goes a presumption that anything "natural" is safe. Natural is about the most imprecise word in the English language. The philosopher Professor Whitehead used to discourage its use by peering coldly over his spectacles at anyone who used it, and saying, "Which of the one hundred and twenty meanings of that word are you intending in this instance?"

Patients' use of the word is woolly in the extreme. Some people regard it as the opposite of "drugs". "Oh, I don't take *drugs,*" one woman said, "only aspirin." This goes along with an uninformed distrust of drugs; Calhan's 1986 study [1] found that women in lower socioeconomic groups (4 and 5) particularly are in a state of total confusion about what is or is not a drug: "Disprin is safe – not like aspirin; that's very dangerous." Others assume that anything that comes from herbs, or arrives in homeopathic bottles, or is in any way linked with alternative medicine may well be ineffective, but at least can do no harm.

Many of you will remember the scare recently over L-triptophane, a "natural" drug which suddenly started producing appalling side effects in a few people in the United States. It now seems likely that there was one contaminated consignment, rather than inherent trouble with the stuff; but the possibility of contamination is not one that crosses the mind of a patient buying a "natural" remedy. One man known to The Patients Association had kidney problems and an associated condition of high blood pressure, for which he was given some medication; he took it, but felt he ought to do something more about his blood pressure. He was found to be swallowing enormous doses of the veterinary garlic he gave to his racing greyhounds for their high blood pressure. I shudder to think what he must have smelled like.

Another area in which patients' expectations present or should present the health professionals with a big headache is the assumption that a doctor will remember what else his patients are taking. The doctor does not, of course, remember, partly because he perhaps simply does not know which laxatives, painkillers, and other oddments the patient may be buying over the counter, but also because he does not remember what he, or maybe another member of the practice, or even the hospital prescribed earlier.

Patients' expectations of the doctor are perhaps the most unrealistic of all. Even now, in Britain, patients tend to look at the doctor with a reverence which turns them to jelly in his presence. They expect him to be God, that he will tell them all they need to know; what they don't realize is that they would not take in most of it even if he did. Studies have shown that a patient takes in a maximum of four pieces of information at a consultation; Ley and Spelman's work [2] suggests that patients' recall of instructions is even less than their recall of information.

Patients assume the doctor will warn them of any possible side effects. On the whole he does not do so, at least partly because any good doctor knows the therapeutic benefit to be derived from saying in ringing tones, "This stuff is going to make you *better.*" Many doctors, too, think it unnecessary to alarm the patient; I am not so sure. One Dick Francis thriller begins with a city gentleman going off his head in the forecourt of a bank. This was based on a real incident, when Dick's wife, Mary, found her old and ailing mother apparently becoming senile in her sheltered bungalow; the old lady was well on the way to being taken off to a mental home when the doctor revealed that what was wrong with her was simply the side effect of some medication she had been prescribed. In that case all was well – that time.

If the doctor does not explain, many patients think the pharmacist will. Some of them do, but far too many of them do not. In theory, the pharmacist counsels the patient carefully over the counter; in practice he is often in the back dispensary reading a newspaper. Often, even if he has doubts, he is inclined to leave the responsibility with the doctor. One patient had some nose drops prescribed for a throat condition and thought this was stupid. When she queried the pharmacist, he just said, "I daresay the doctor knows what he's doing" when he should have explained *why* the nose drops would benefit the throat, i.e., because the throat was being affected by matter from the nose. On another occasion a pharmacist did have doubts, but dispensed the drug anyway. Later he was asked, "Why didn't you ring the doctor and check?", to which he retorted, "Have you ever tried ringing a doctor? You don't get past the receptionist." And many pharmacists actually make matters worse by plastering "To be taken as directed" labels over the manufacturer's instructions and even removing the patient packet insert. We have had many examples of both. About the only instruction that seems routinely to appear on bottles of pills is "Keep away from children. Avoid alcohol." One woman wrote to *The Times* to say that she felt she would have a better chance of doing the second if she could only manage to do the first.

Nonetheless, where a pharmacist is inclined to be helpful, he can be a good source of information: because he is not intimidating, patients feel they can ask questions. The doctor may be God, but the pharmacist is not – God doesn't try to sell you hot water bottles.

Where do patients learn about drugs? It is often assumed they read the patient packet inserts but, in Britain at any rate, they do not (only the Tampax ones get read by schoolboys eager for precise anatomical information). Some 60% of writers of inserts do not try them out on a test population before printing them in thousands, and far too many of them can be misunderstood. If they were written with short words in short sentences, patients might glean more from them; but there is an unfortunate parallel with domestic appliances. For example, when you think you have a lot of instructions for your microwave, what you often have are the same instructions in seventeen languages, not well written in any of them; you will have probably lost the bit of paper by the time you need to look up anything. The man who pinned up the despairing notice on a machine "As a last resort, read the instructions" knew what he was up against.

Patients may have learned a little in schools, but not much: the greatest quantity of what is taught in schools is thankfully forgotten as soon as school is over. On the whole, patients pick up what they know from folklore, from what their mothers said, and from what they remember once having been told. A young general practitioner in Britain tried to find out what his patients really wanted, and eventually established with the aid of a few studies that they wanted to know what was wrong with them, why they had got it, and whether they would get better. In meeting these expectations, he feared Aunt Nelly was much better than a doctor. "You've got a chill," she would say. "You got it from going out without your scarf." And, of course, we know that most patients recover from most ills spontaneously anyway. The tide of inaccurate shared information in which most patients swim should not be underestimated: people look at each other's pills – "Oh, I know that one, I had it for my stomach" – never mind that the area being treated has nothing to do with the stomach this time.

I have stressed the unreality of our expectations and the inadequacy of our knowledge, but that does not mean that patients are not increasingly eager to be informed, to make their own choices, and to help decide whether this is the treatment for them or not. I would only emphasize that if one wants to get more information across to patients, one should remember that a good many of them, and those are the most vulnerable, may have a vocabulary of about 600 words and an attention span of 3 minutes at the most. It is no good giving them sound information if they cannot take it in. "The nutritional value of food not eaten is nil," say the dieticians; this is also true of information not taken in. But patients can understand, if they are addressed in the right way, and the right way was defined by a wise old editor on a popular newspaper who said of his readers what we might well say of patients: "Never overestimate their knowledge nor underestimate their intelligence."

## References

1. Calhan M (1987) Health and illness: the lay perspective. Tavistock, London
2. Ley P, Spelman MS (1967) Communicating with the patient. Staples, London

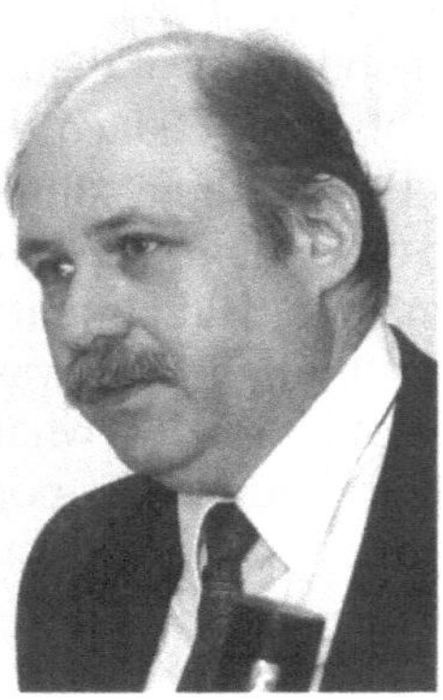

# 32. Patient Motivation*

L. A. MORRIS, E. TABAK, and N. OLINS

Educating patients about the medications prescribed for their treatment is essential. From 30% to 50% of patients taking medication fail to adhere sufficiently to the prescribed regimen, risking therapeutic failure due to inadequate dosage or toxicity from overdosing. Adverse drug reactions may also cause morbidity, hospitalization, and mortality. Elderly patients are especially susceptible to undertreatment or adverse drug reactions because of the large number of therapeutic agents they take and the serious illnesses they experience that require treatment.

Numerous programs have been developed to provide elderly patients with information about their medicines. However, the most successful of these programs require a mixture of both low-cost print information and high-cost interpersonal counseling with health care providers. Maximizing the educational impact of print media is an important cost-reducing, patient education strategy.

There are numerous programs designed to provide prescription drug information to patients. The National Council on Patient Information and Education lists 190 institutions with patient education programs [2]. Most of these programs provide information that health professionals believe patients need to know about their medications. A communications program designed by "experts" assures that essential information is disclosed to patients taking prescription medication.

However, "expert" systems do not assure that the provided information will be desired by patients. Although health professionals are likely to know the informational content that needs to be transferred to patients to encourage safe use, they cannot assure that patients will be motivated to read the information carefully, understand it, or remember the material when they need to utilize the information.

Therefore, in addition to understanding the content of prescription drug information that needs to be transferred to patients, designers of a patient

* The views expressed are solely those of the authors and do not reflect the policy of the Food and Drug Administration or the American Association of Retired Persons Pharmacy Service.

education system also need to be aware of patients' motivations to read, understand, and remember the provided information. If patients' motivations are clearly understood, materials can be created that more clearly focus their content on patients' needs and provide instructions that can help patients achieve their personal goals.

Unfortunately, there are multiple reasons underlying patients' motivation, and patients may vary in terms of why they may or may not be interested in drug information. For example, some patients may want to know drug information because of their desire to take care of themselves, while others may want to know more about their medication so they can communicate more clearly with their physician. Assessing patients' motivation to learn about their medication requires measurement of multiple motivations.

## Food and Drug Administration – American Association of Retired Persons Pharmacy Study

A benefit segmentation study is being performed to measure the reasons patients may be interested in learning about their medications. Benefit segmentation analyses seek to group people into homogeneous but distinctive patterns by virtue of the expected benefit from using a product or service. In this case we are seeking to group patients into patterns based upon why they are interested in learning about their antihypertensive medication. Once these groupings are formed and differential motivations understood, materials can be developed which are targeted to the different groups.

The study is being performed jointly by the Food and Drug Administration (FDA) and the American Association of Retired Persons (AARP) Pharmacy Service and data collection is currently underway. Members (patrons) of the AARP mail order pharmacy receiving thiazide medication for hypertension are mailed a response card soliciting their participation in the study. Those agreeing to participate are sent a 110-item questionnaire that measures patient knowledge, motivations, attitudes, and demographic information.

### *Questionnaire Design*

A literature search was conducted to review motivations for drug information seeking. Questions were simplified, adapted, and grouped into a logical order to form a questionnaire.

One major line of questions involved information about hypertension medication. Items included measures of both self-perceived and actual knowledge. The knowledge areas probed included when and how to take the medication as well as information relating to precautions and side effects of the drug. Additionally, subjects' sources of information about their medications were assessed, based upon earlier findings by Morris, Grossman, Barkdoll, and Gordon [6]. These authors found four distinct patterns of drug information seeking behavior (i.e., physician, pharmacist, self-reliant, and noninformation seeking).

Another set of characteristics evaluated were subjects' attitudes and beliefs about both having hypertension and taking medication to control hypertension. A set of questions was developed from the health belief model [1] to assess perceived severity of high blood pressure and susceptibility to problems from having high blood pressure, as well as perceived benefits and barriers to taking the medications.

Rosenstock, Strecher, and Becker [7] subsequently posited the addition of self-efficacy to the health belief model as a separate independent variable. Consequently, we added items designed to examine subjects' beliefs about their personal abilities in relation to their high blood pressure. Self-efficacy was evaluated both in terms of knowledge levels (whether subjects understood how to take their medication) and skill level (how confident subjects were of their ability to carry out the medication schedule).

Information-seeking orientation and preference for active participation in medical care were measured with a scale developed by Krantz et al. [3].

Motivational factors were assessed in two ways. One set of items was designed to analyze various motives and disincentives for learning. This was an original scale based upon focus group data and a broad literature review [5]. The other set of questions assessed subjects' involvement levels with learning about medication. Involvement along various dimensions has been tested as a set of antecedents to the consumer decision making process [4]. There were four categories of questions here, representing components of attributions to learning about the medications, pleasure value (emotional responses to learning), social value (importance of others' judgments), the importance of negative consequence to the subject (significance of the risks of not learning about the medication), and the subjective risk of a mis-choice (probability of risks if patients do not learn about the medication). Questions were asked that assess these values in the two contexts, learning about medication and taking medications.

The attitudinal, motivational, and self-perceived knowledge items were constructed using four-point response scales. The factual knowledge items use a simple agree-disagree dichotomy (rather than true-false), with an option for "don't know." Additionally, demographic and other subject background characteristics are assessed for potential cross-tabulations with the responses. These include indicators of social support, perceived health status, concurrent risk factors, and a self-report compliance measure.

### *Use of the Data*

Once data have been gathered, they will be analyzed to define groupings based upon patients' motivations. Involvement levels as well as reasons for learning about the medication will also be combined to serve as the basis for assigning patients to different groups. Other data solicited in the questionnaire will be used to describe and discriminate between these groups, so we can learn more about the different patient education segments. Demographic and psychographic (attitude items) will be used to describe the segments.

If reliable segments can be defined, the next step will be to design and test the materials for their effectiveness. We aim to discover whether targeted materials are more effective than mass-directed information in terms of improving patients' knowledge about their medication.

## References


1. Becker MH (1974) The health belief model and personal health behavior. Slack, Thorofare NJ
2. Bullman RW, Rowland F (1985) Directory of prescription drug information and education programs and resources. Washington DC NCPIE
3. Krantz DS, Baum A, Wideman MV (1980) Assessment of preferences for self-treatment and information in health care. J Personality and Social Psychology 39 (5):977–990
4. Laurent G, Kapferer JN (1985) Measuring consumer involvement profiles. J Mark Res 22:41–53
5. Morris LA (1990) Communicating therapeutic risks. Springer, Berlin, Heidelberg, New York, Tokyo
6. Morris LA, Grossman R, Barkdoll G, Gordon E (1987) A segmentational analysis of prescription drug information seeking. Med Care 25 (10):953–964
7. Rosenstock IM, Strecher VJ, Becker MH (1988) Social learning theory and the health belief model. Health Educ Q 15 (2):175–183

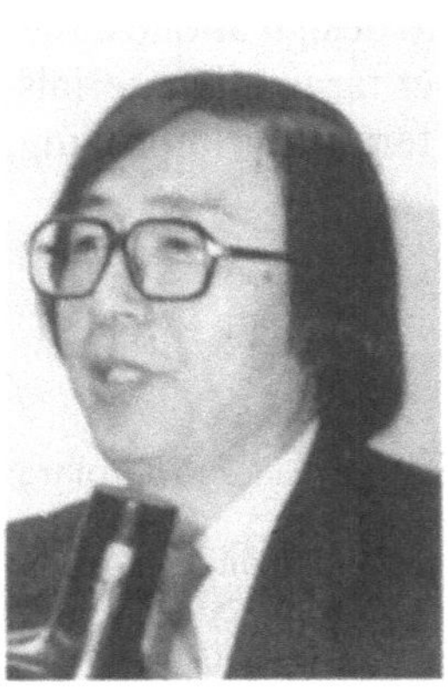

# 33. Japan's Other Drug Market: Exports via Tourists

G. Koide

About 2 years ago, many Americans rushed into pharmacies near Tokyo International Airport and bought packs of a drug called Dextran Sodium Sulfate (DSS), which was originally developed in order to prevent deposition of atheromatous plaques around the artery walls. Most paid about $ 650 for DSS because it was believed it might be effective in fighting AIDS. The case is a typical example of people's attitudes and behavior toward drugs based on information and misinformation. In this chapter, I shall discuss this aspect, using other examples to illustrate how the media can help the public to better understand the benefits and risks of drugs. These examples concern the "gray market" of drug sales from Japan to other countries.

## What Drugs Do Asian People Carry Home From Japan?

According to statistics published by the Japan Pharmaceutical Manufacturers Association, Japanese drug imports in 1988 totalled 1614 million and exports totalled 742 million [1]. The imports, therefore, accounted for 2.2 times as much as the exports. Japanese products go to the United States, Europe, and Asia, as shown in Fig. 1. The recent tendency has been toward a steady increase of exports to Asian countries (+4.3 % in 1988/1987), and a decrease to all others (−24.6 % to the United States and −13.2 % to Europe). The share of exports to Asia has increased to 30.5 %. Figure 2 shows that antibiotics, nutrients, and vitamins are the three main classes of drugs exported to Asian countries.

However, these statistics show only one side of drug traffic. Besides official overground marketing, there is an underground flow of drugs to Asian countries. It is an everyday occurrence for drugs to be purchased at tax-free pharmacies and carried home from Japan. Who carries them? They are carried out of Japan primarily by tourists and workers from Asian countries such as China, Taiwan, Korea, Hong Kong, India, and Pakistan.

Table 1 shows the top five drugs sold at the tax-free pharmacy in Tokyo. All may be sold without prescriptions. Ruru is one of the popular cold remedies. It is taken three times a day (after each meal) at a dose of three tablets for adults, two

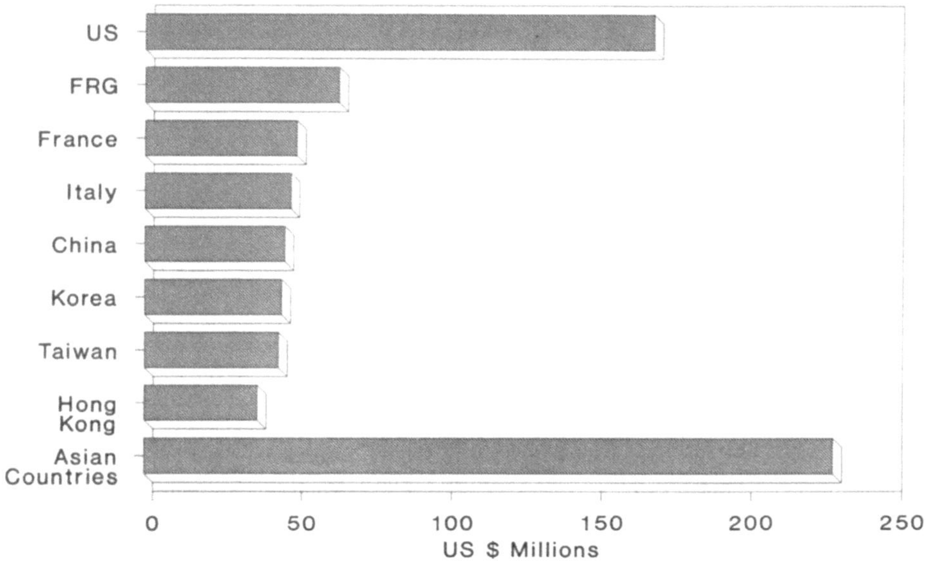


**Fig. 1.** The export of drugs from Japan (1988)

tablets for children aged 11–15, and one tablet for children aged 6–11. An adult dose of nine tablets a day contains clemastine fumarate (1.34 mg), lysozyme hydrochloride (60 mg), acetaminophen (900 mg), dihydrocodeine phosphate (24 mg), noscapine (36 mg), DL-methylephedrine hydrochloride (60 mg), potassium

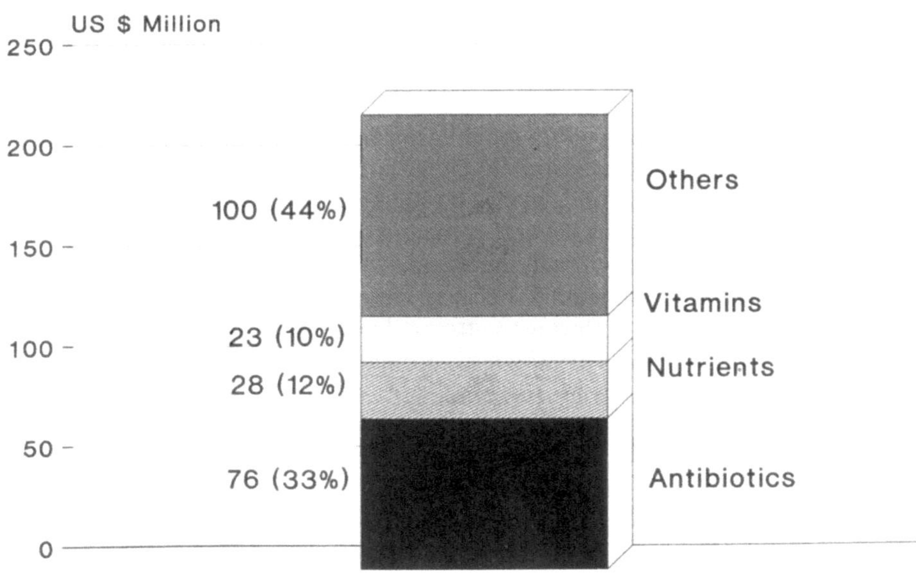


**Fig. 2.** The export to Asian countries (1988)

**Table 1.** Top five drugs sold at the tax-free pharmacy in Tokyo

| Name | Composition | Effects |
|---|---|---|
| Ruru | Clemastine fumarate<br>Lysozyme hydrochloride<br>Acetaminophen<br>Dihydrocodeine phosphate<br>Noscapine<br>DL-Methylephedrine hydrochloride<br>Potassium guaiacolsulfonate<br>Caffeine<br>Benfotiamine | Cold/sneeze remedy, anti-fever, etc. |
| Seirogan | Creosote<br>Philodendron bark<br>Geranium herb<br>Glycyrrhiza<br>Citrus peel | Diarrhea, food or water intoxication, etc. |
| Alinamin | Fursultiamine<br>Vitamin $B_6$, $B_{12}$, $B_2$ | Vitamin preparation |
| Combantrin | Pyrantel | Anthelmintic |
| Trocy | Tioconazole | Antifungal |

guaiacolsulfonate (240 mg), caffeine (75 mg), and benfotiamine (24 mg). Similar kinds of cold remedies are sold under such commercial names as Benza, Pabron, Contac, Zikinin, and so on. Why do people prefer Ruru to others? They can memorize and pronounce it easily because it has the shortest name of all, only two syllables. They buy Ruru for this simple reason, and it is now used in Asian countries as aspirin is used in Europe and the United States.

Seirogan, with a comparatively long history of about 100 years, is taken for diarrhea, vomiting, food or water intoxication, etc. It is also taken three times a day (after each meal) with a dose of three tablets for adults, two tablets for children aged 8–15, and one tablet for children aged 5–8. Nine tablets, one daily dose for adults, contain creosote (375 mg), philodendron bark (300 mg), geranium herb (300 mg), glycyrrhiza (150 mg), and citrus peel (300 mg). Seirogan is manufactured by several companies and is not a brand name, but people wish to purchase, above all, the brand of seirogan which carries the bugle trademark. The bugle trademark became famous because Japanese soldiers used that brand as a cure-all during the Russo-Japanese war in 1904–1905, which Japan won. During the days of Japanese colonial expansion, seirogan became a popular drug in Asian countries. Its name, written at first in Chinese characters, meant a tablet to conquer Russia, and though more peaceful letters are now attached to it, a bugle still remains in the memory of Asian people as the symbol of an effective drug to fight powers and diseases. It is noteworthy that people buy a drug not just for its effect, but for such other reasons.

Alinamin is a vitamin preparation which is taken by adults in a dose of four tablets a day. This daily dose contains fursultiamine (100 mg), and vitamin $B_6$ (10 mg), $B_{12}$ (20 μg), and $B_2$ (10 mg). Television commercial films have helped

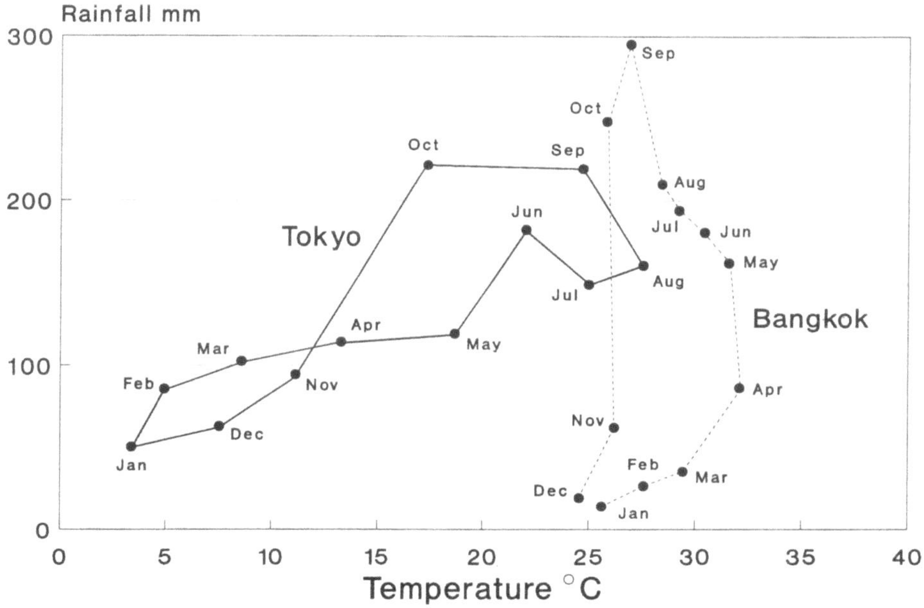


**Fig. 3.** Temperature – rainfall relation

Alinamin prevail over other vitamin agents. The other two drugs in Table 1 are not so familiar to people outside Asian countries. Combantrin is an anthelmintic, and Trocy is an antifungal cream.

The list in Table 1 testifies to the peculiar situation of Asian countries, where 60 % of the world population is concentrated, and which belong to the tropical and subtropical zones in the so-called monsoon belt. Bangkok, Thailand, is a good example. Compared with the temperature–rainfall pattern in Tokyo, that of Bangkok is quite different, as shown in Fig. 3. Bangkok's temperature is remarkably high throughout the year and the rainfall is intensive, especially in summer [2]. The higher temperature and humidity, together with an unsanitary social environment, especially in the countryside, create a hotbed for various fungal diseases, e.g., athlete's foot, which occurs when fungi like Trichophyton invade the skin between the toes. It begins with itching and blisters, then the skin cracks, making it vulnerable to secondary infection bacteria [3]. In addition, a lifestyle in which people live in rural environments and eat rare foods inevitably causes the spread of parasitic worms. That, in turn, leads to the demand for anthelmintic pills.

It is an accepted practice for tourists to import drugs. When they return to their countries, a customs declaration is not even necessary if passengers bring in fewer than six small bottles of each drug. The reason why these tourists are anxious to buy drugs in Tokyo is that they believe Japanese drugs to be pure and effective. In Tokyo, there are several pharmacies in the Shinjuku and Ikebukuro areas which specialize in selling to tourists from Asian countries. The most typical one is "Treasure Island", a big tax-free souvenir shop in Ikebukuro. It is usually crowded with people seeking drugs and cosmetics as well as famous Japanese electrical goods. According to the owner, each customer spends about $ 100 and 30 %–50 % of the sales come from the pharmacy, though the pharmacy occupies only one-fifth of the shop.

It is surprising that people take drugs so freely, without giving any thought to risk. If drugs hide risky side effects, the easy-going attitudes and behavior toward them may cause abuse; and the misuse of drugs may have serious consequences. Indomethacin, for example, is a commonly used drug, dispensed without prescription to treat lumbago in the countryside in Thailand. It is an anodyne and anti-inflammation capsule for rheumatism with occasional adverse effects such as leukopenia, a condition in which the number of white blood cells decreases [4].

A further example is provided by a muscle-building agent containing an anabolic steroid which is often given to boys by poor parents who wish their sons to become famous kick-boxers and to get rich. People in Thailand enjoy kick-boxing, or Thai boxing, which is a national and professional sport, and many youngsters admire and respect a champion. It was Ben Johnson's use of an anabolic steroid that invalidated his gold medal at the Olympic Games in 1988. Neither pharmacists nor parents know the side effects of these drugs.

The problem is that these drugs flow into the Third World through both overground and underground routes [5, 6]. Even if the overground route were to be prohibited, the other would remain. It is probable that antibiotics stream into Asian countries illegally through private traffic. Abuse of antibiotics can result in a serious increase of antibiotic-resistant diseases, above all, sexually transmitted diseases [7].

## Why Was DSS Carried Home From Japan?

The problems illustrated by my examples are not limited to Asia. The behavior adopted by people who want to get drugs is universal. I would like to return to the example of Americans bringing DSS home from Japan. In 1988, many Americans were eager to buy DSS because a scientific paper suggested that DSS might be effective in treating AIDS patients. DSS had not been approved by the Food and Drug Administration (FDA) in the United States because the FDA had found no evidence that DSS was effective in treating AIDS patients. Without scientific proof that a drug is safe and effective, the FDA does not permit it to be marketed in the United States.

At a meeting in San Francisco, homosexuals exchanged information about the reported effectiveness of DSS against AIDS and its availability on the Japanese market. New York AIDS organizations provided information by telephone on how DSS could be obtained. Demonstrators sat in the corridor of a Japanese company to demand that DSS be made available, despite the FDA's legal prohibition. Clearly, the public believed that DSS might be a cure for AIDS [8]. Friends and relatives of the AIDS patients, tourists, and even brokers came to Japan and bought as much DSS as possible for shipping to the United States. Cartons of DSS, often labeled "fragile china", were sent by air to New York, San

Francisco, and Los Angeles. Dealers doubled the price once it entered the United States.

Both the Asian and American examples illustrate how quickly information and misinformation about drugs are disseminated worldwide, regardless of natural borders or great distance. Furthermore, they suggest that on understanding a variety of aspects of a situation – including social, behavioral, and cultural factors – is inevitably necessary for risk and benefit assessment of drugs.

## Why Are the Mass Media Important for Risk and Benefit Assessment of Drugs?

As the average life expectancy lengthens, health and health care become increasingly the objects of public concern. People tend to consume a lot of drugs, believing them to be good for health; in reality, drugs can have disastrous consequences because of unexpected adverse effects. It is one of the professional responsibilities of the mass media to provide people with accurate, relevant, and multidimensional information quickly, thereby checking the spread of misinformation and preventing abuse of drugs and resulting disasters. Another aspect of the professional responsibility of the mass media is to find the hidden problems and inform the general public.

Past experience with the adverse effects of drugs such as subacute myeloopticoneuropathy (SMON) caused by chinoform shows that the mass media have played an important role in identifying problems, giving a warning, helping individual patients decide what to do, encouraging responsible organizations to take action, and, finally, assisting the unfortunate patients. In general, a hidden problem becomes an open problem once the media report it to the public. In other words, there is often no perceived problem *unless* the media provide the information to the public. It is only the public who is able to put the pressure on responsible organizations to prevent the proliferation of adverse effects of drugs.

Of course, risk and benefit assessment should be determined after prudent and unbiased consideration. Accordingly, the public should have unlimited and uncontrolled information to facilitate their consideration of acceptable risks. In this connection, the mass media have an important role and responsibility in ensuring the public has adequate, unbiased information on risks and benefits.

## Conclusion

DSS was carried home from Japan by Americans who believed it might give relief to AIDS patients. Various drugs, possibly including antibiotics, are carried home by Asian people who expect them to bring good fortune. The dependence on drugs for maintaining health will become stronger both in advanced and developing countries towards the twenty-first century. Misinformation about drugs inevitably increases abuse and misuse. Consequently, the probability of drug disasters will increase unless some steps are taken to adequately inform the public. The mass media are responsible for providing people with information as fast as possible and helping them consider the risks and benefits of drugs.

*Acknowledgement.* I am grateful to those who helped me write this article. Special thanks for invaluable help are due to Professor Gen Ohi, University of Tokyo; Professor Akio Akagi, Keio University; Professor Ichiro Kai, Teikyo University; Dr. Takao Kano, Tokyo Hygienic Laboratory; Dr. David Taylor, Ciba-Geigy; and Arihumi Kishimoto, NHK Publishing Co.

## References

1. Japan Pharmaceutical Manufacturers Association (1989) Data book. pp. 30–31
2. Sasa M et al. (1978) Diseases in Asia (in Japanese), Shinjukushobo: pp. 4–14
3. Dixon B (1986) Health and the human body. Perseus Press: pp. 174–175
4. Mizushima H et al. (1989) Drugs – 1989. Nankodo
5. Silverman M et al. (1982) The prescription for death – the drugging of the third world. University of California
6. Melrose D (1982) Bitter pills. OXFAM
7. Ashford WA et al. (1976) Penicillinase-producing neisseria gonorrhea. Lancet II:657–659
8. NHK-TV news, July 21, 1988

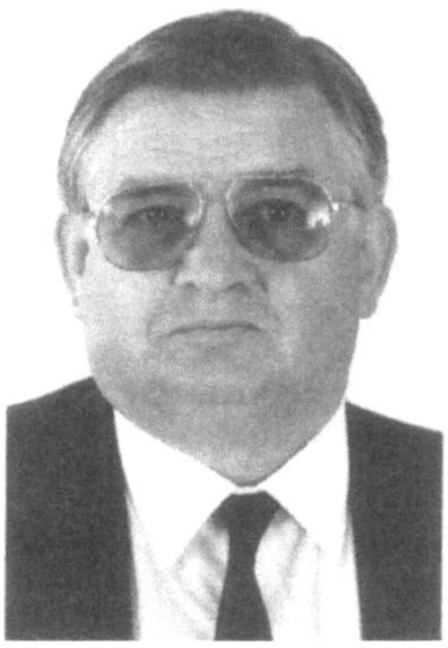

# 34. Controlling Drug Safety: Making Cautious Changes*

R. D. MANN

What principles or broad policy issues should be occupying our attention as we consider the subject of drug safety some 29 years after the thalidomide disaster of the early 1960s? In the United Kingdom, the Medicines Act of 1964 was a direct outcome of the thalidomide disaster and this Act introduced an integrated drug regulatory process in which the safety, efficacy and quality of a medicine are considered together as a comprehensive scientific whole. So we do not have a long experience in the modern process of drug registration and regulation, and we should accept the need for humility in discussing principles to lead us into the future. We need to be careful in changing the processes and procedures that we use in controlling drug safety, but changes will necessary. The principles that should be kept in mind in making these changes include the following:

1. The concept of informed consent should be replaced by that of *informed choice*. Informed consent is a paternalistic and passive concept of a legal nature. It implies that the decision regarding benefit and risk is made by the professional adviser, and the patient consents to this decision on the basis of the information given. Informed choice is a more active process and requires that the medical adviser educates the patient so that he or she can make a selection from all of the choices available. The changed emphasis is on greater communication and on being as open with the patient as that person's wishes and education will permit. It is the patient who has to live with the choice, and the choice should be left to the patient to the greatest extent possible.

2. *Patient information* should be provided on a scale which greatly exceeds that which has been traditional. The forthcoming EEC Directive on this subject is to be welcomed, but it is necessary to ensure that comprehensive drug safety information is made available to patients and their medical advisers. There are difficulties with this as such information can be misinterpreted, but these difficulties can be explained in documentation covering the published data. It is the job of the adviser to explain, but the data should be in the public domain so

* The views expressed in this article are, of course, those of the author and are not necessarily those of other members of the Consultant and Pharmacoepidemiology Groups of RAD-AR UK.

that when questions arise in the mind of the patient, he or she can seek answers and make choices based upon realistic expectations.

3. As drug safety cannot be guaranted, *no-fault compensation schemes* should be developed to care for those who suffer drug-related injuries. With many drugs the risks of rare but serious adverse reactions must be accepted unless the risks of the disease being treated are preferred. New hazards, reminding us of the practolol incident, will arise despite our methods of integrated drug regulation. And, in a manner which has been fully reviewed elsewhere [1], the community, which benefits from the efficacy of medicines, should accept the ethical necessity of caring for the victims of these iatrogenic events.

4. Careful consideration should be given to *altering the current methods used in marketing pharmaceuticals.* It should be recognized that the pharmaceutical industry has provided almost the whole of the contemporary pharmacopoeia, but its profits depend, to an unreasonable extent, on marketing methods which lead to over-prescribing. Drug safety is likely to be improved if the techniques of commodity advertising are excluded so that medicines are promoted only on the basis of the Summary of Product Characteristics for each drug and the papers which have appeared in refereed journals about it. The profits of the pharmaceutical industry should be preserved and the investment of that industry in new drug research supported. Drugs should be used less, they should cost more so that they provide a proper financial return to their developers and, at the same time, carry the premiums of no-fault compensation schemes with them.

5. The *continuing medical education of prescribers* should be strengthened so that doctors use drugs only under conditions in which their benefit to risk ratio is most advantageous in the individual patient. Some doctors are, it would seem, in need of far greater educational support than has, in the past, been provided, and a great deal of the safety of drugs in the future will depend on the quality and availability of the continuing education provided to those who prescribe them.

6. Care needs to be taken over the way in which *changes in the drug regulatory process* are undertaken. The changes currently proposed in the EEC are driven, to an undesirable extent, by political and economic needs and ambitions. It is essential that changes should be made in response to scientific and not political imperatives, and that they should be made cautiously and on the basis of valid experience and experiments.

7. Finally, it is needful to develop *the means of adverse reactions monitoring and postmarketing surveillance.* These means, in their infancy in many of the countries of Europe, are truly essential if unexpected problems with drug safety are to be detected and dealt with at the earliest possible moment. There is a great need to train pharmacoepidemiologists and to construct multipurpose data bases and it is an important principle that these needs should receive attention.

It is clear that the RAD-AR initiative, in bringing together academics, regulators, and members of the regulated pharmaceutical industry, can contribute to the implementation of the principles discussed above and advanced by other contributors to this symposium.

## References

1. Mann RD, Havard J (1989) No fault compensation in medicine. Royal Society of Medicine Services, London

# 35. Discussion

The general discussion began with an observation that the patients' first acquaintance with a pharmaceutical company and its products is through package inserts. Because physicians often have inadequate time or interest to help patients understand what is written on these inserts or to teach the patients how to use drugs properly, it was suggested that the pharmaceutical companies work with the media to ensure that the patients are informed and able to ask their physicians the right questions. This communication strategy also enables the patients to assume greater responsibility for their decisions.

One panelist took the view that a market-driven strategy for communicating with patients is more appropriate than a science-driven or ethics-driven strategy, because in reality the market is the patient, not the pharmaceutical company. In order to communicate with the patients, it is important to know what they understand. The industry, the government regulatory authorities, the health professions, and other constituencies often actually communicate only a small amount of the information they intend – and expect – to deliver to the patients, and yet there is very little evaluation of their drug communication materials and techniques.

Several points were also raised regarding physicians' and patients' knowledge of drug information. Physicians should be trained to explain in common words what a drug is and how it should be used; they also should be fully informed about over-the-counter (OTC) drugs. For their part, patients should be knowledgeable about the symptoms treated by an OTC drug, and also should have the opportunity to become familiar with the risks, benefits, and use of a drug before it is prescribed for use.

Final comments focused on the importance of pharmaceutical company outreach initiatives to establish long-term communication channels as a means to improve media understanding and coverage of drug safety issues, as well as on the realities of establishing internationally consistent standards among national regulatory authorities.

# *Part VIII*

# *Experiences in Drug Safety Communication Through Traditional Channels*

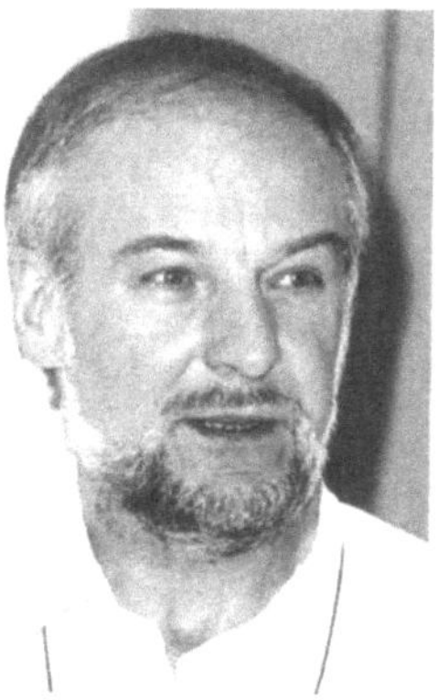

# 36. Principles, Experiences, and Desired Actions

G. LEWANDOWSKI

## Importance of Product Information

A drug is a substance plus information, as has been stated repeatedly. Without sufficient knowledge of its properties, benefits, and risks, a drug cannot be handled properly, so appropriate information is an essential and indispensable promotional tool. As a consequence, product information must be considered a cardinal element in the development, promotion, marketing, and usage of drugs and its importance is still growing for a number of reasons, including:
- A growing amount of knowledge generated
- A growing number of drugs at our disposal
- A growing sophistication of modern therapies
- An increasing scientific and professional interest in how drugs work
- An increasing political and economic interest in the safety and cost/effectiveness of drugs
- Modernization of promotional efforts on the part of the pharmaceutical industry
- Corresponding evolution of international drug regulation

## Traditional Channels

This analysis focuses on traditional information channels, such as
- Printed scientific and professional information and advertisements
- Scientific and professional communication, meetings, and media
- Package inserts for physicians and patients (these have a long tradition, e.g., in continental Europe, and EC pharmaceutical regulation will expand this kind of patient information)
- Communication through medical representatives
- Drug formularies and compendia
- Regulatory communication

Drug information and communication through traditional channels have been overwhelmingly professional and directed mainly, but not exclusively, at the medical profession. Only a minor part of them has been targeted at lay audiences. Drug information and communication are mainly scientific and professional in character, but promotional elements are frequent in material generated by pharmaceutical manufacturers.

## Sources of Information

The manufacturer is generally considered to be the main source of drug information. This is in line with his primordial responsibility for the overall quality of the product (in the sense of total or overall drug quality comprising the essential drug evaluation QESUNC criteria, i.e., Pharmaceutical Quality, Efficacy, Safety, Usefulness, Need, Cost/Effectiveness; compare [2]: p. 22) which he has developed and introduced into the market and is further motivated by his commercial interest in its viability and longevity. But other sources, e.g., scientists, health professionals, health authorities, regulators, and critics, to mention only the most important ones, should not be neglected.

## From Information to Communication

Pharmaceutical product information is not and has never been the one-sided and one-way sending of identical messages from producer to user. The complexity of therapeutic knowledge, the variety of professions and disciplines involved in its generation and development, and the diversity of interests at stake have increasingly made pharmaceutical product communication an open process with multiple players communicating to various addresses through various channels [3]. To a large extent such communication forms part of the often heterogeneous scientific and medical debate.

## Communication of Benefits and Risks

Today all the elements that make up the social value of a drug must be considered, i.e., pharmaceutical quality, efficacy, safety, usefulness, medical need, and cost/effectiveness of the pharmaceutical concerned. They are mostly dependent on each other and can only be considered, debated, and judged in context. This is why drug safety communication cannot be confined to safety aspects in the narrower sense of communication on damage and harm, hazard, and risk. It has to comprise the other components mentioned as well. Drug safety communication deprived of benefit considerations is meaningless.

## Sharing of Power

Pharmaceutical product communication, like all communication, is more than information, even more than education, and goes beyond the mere transfer and exchange of knowledge. Like all other public communication, besides the intellectual component linked to the crucial issue of how to be truthful and understandable, product communication also contains elements of a social and political power struggle and is to an often considerable extent part of this struggle. One might consider professional assessment, transparency of decision making, and public participation as basic elements of modern benefit/risk communication (cf. [3] pp. 14–23). In the area of pharmaceuticals, the issue at stake is who provides the best cure and under which conditions – a traditional source of political conflict. In today's safety communication the issue of acceptable risk stands out in the foreground, and not every scientific answer is accepted as adequate. In modern democratic society, in the face of such controversy, appropriate communication has not just to inform, but to help clear positions, facilitate dialogue, work for consensus, and overcome mistrust. This is easier said than done, but there is no alternative as daily experience in the public debate of technical risks should teach us. We will have to learn to live in a world of more and still more heterogeneous and incongruous information and conflicting demands.

## Entertainment

Communication embraces at least one more element which is often not fully understood, accepted, and acknowledged in pharmaceutical product communication: the element of entertainment. People experienced in advertising and the media and politicians will easily understand, however. Politics and medicine are highly entertaining for many people, and pharmaceutical communication cannot always escape the impact of this predilection. Public regulatory hearings, drug liability trials, scientific conferences, and television appearances of prominent actors offer the most impressive material, and a considerable impact on the final outcome of the issue has to be assumed. Diverting elements are always present in communication. It is, however, difficult to deny that drug communication aiming at ensuring and improving a rational use of drugs, at facilitating and supporting scientifically and medically justified therapies and at helping the physician and the patient to make well-informed decisions should first and foremost strive for the transfer of truthful and reliable knowledge and resist the temptation to entertain. There are, however, exceptions: first, when the entertaining character of a piece of communication helps the better understanding of the message; and second, when the entertaining component is clearly understood and accepted by the community, as regularly happens in advertising.[1] Entertainment is not easily tolerated on traditional channels.

---

[1] This remark should not be misinterpreted as a justification of lack of judgment or bad taste, or in contempt of advertising. Good advertisements, apart from promotional effects, can even be valuable cultural contributions. The interesting esthetic aspects of communication cannot be elaborated here.

## Emotions

There are important emotional aspects in drug safety communication. Emotions are seldom discussed in technical papers and not mentioned in regulations and guidelines, yet they are strong in drug safety issues and, not surprisingly, their impact has often been enormous. Our technical systems do not foresee emotional solutions; they try to exclude feelings. Yet the presence of these emotional aspects is real and demands understanding, concern, and response. We will have to learn to accept other people's emotions and to become aware of our own. This is a most difficult task and one of the noble challenges in our work. We should sometimes stop wrestling with technical systems and devote more time and effort to our neighbor.

## Proposals for Change

In such vast, intricate, and contradictory surroundings it may seem an extremely ambitious venture to suggest principles and put forward ideas for further actions, the task getting still more complicated when we imagine ourselves living in a pluralistic internationalized society undergoing rapid and deep changes in informational behavior and becoming increasingly multicultural. We will not be able to propose sweeping solutions. Modest but resolute steps directed towards practical improvement are necessary and should be tried. If we agree, first, that the main purpose of pharmaceutical product communication is to achieve optimal therapy, i.e., optimize benefit and reduce risk; second, that this communication must, in addition, enable patients and physicians to take autonomous and informed decisions; and third, that this communication takes place in an ongoing multidisciplinary and interactive process affected by divergent responsibilities, goals, and interests and is subject to a set of rules – legal, technical, and other – then we could attempt to subscribe to the following few simple principles:

1. Product communication must be relevant and truthful
2. Communication should be understandable and related to relevant and demonstrable facts
3. Distortion and misunderstanding should be avoided
4. New findings should be communicated without delay
5. Promotional statements should be clearly distinguishable and not be mixed up with factual information
6. Drug safety communication must relate to and respect the context of comparative benefit/risk assessment
7. Stay open to authentic dialogue
8. Keep in mind that you are responsible for human beings

Although all this has often been said before and is frequently repeated, I think it makes sense to say it once more and make it daily practice. When communicating on drugs, very often complexity of the subject matter, uncertain knowledge, or complicated legal or technical rules are not the greatest obstacles to effective and credible communication, but rather our own shortcomings in dealing with the truth and refraining from hyperbole. Exaggerated claims and other mistakes in communication have played a notoriously negative role in major historical drug issues (compare [1]). Without conscious and prolonged efforts to overcome these, there is little hope of marked improvement. A critical look at the development of this issue over more than 20 years, namely, since the thalidomide catastrophe, seems to support this point: regulation and guidelines have multiplied, product communication has become more complicated and research more sophisticated, but the old mistakes are made all over again, and the public credibility of the whole system remains as poor as ever. We need more than technical improvement; we need a profound change of mentalities, maybe a different culture of public communication.

Efforts are needed from all actors and parties concerned, from scientists and doctors, from regulators, from industry and critics, from politicians and the media, and last, but not least, from the consumer himself. As long as the other party is declared guilty right away and held solely responsible, decisive improvement will be very difficult to achieve.

## Particular Responsibilities

Pharmaceutical manufacturers and drug regulatory authorities, however, each have a particular responsibility for appropriate product communication: both are in parallel held responsible for the overall quality of the product [2], especially its favorable benefit/risk ratio in general usage, throughout its whole life cycle. In this respect, their responsibility for drug safety is virtually unlimited, and therefore their mistakes are judged more severely by the public, who, by contrast, seems to accept a considerably less balanced attitude on the part of other actors, e.g., issue advocates, and prominent journalists, without detriment to their credibility.

## Actions

Being convinced that a profound change in attitudes and prolonged multiple efforts are required, I find it very difficult to propose a necessarily limited number of appropriate and promising actions. Considered carefully, preparing a revolution, designing specific strategies, selecting suitable triggering events, and developing decisive tactics are not so simple either. Success in these matters very much depends on a good organization, reliable comrades, supporters, allies, critics, and public sympathy, and on being always ready to swiftly exploit favorable opportunities. And a patient, legal, and peaceful effort of conviction can be very successful. RAD-AR could be perceived as being just such an effort and should be actively pursued. Maybe an annual drug safety communication award created within its frame and to be awarded by an independent council could send just one additional signal and rally further support. In private, a prominent conference participant jokingly suggested that the award be given annually for the worst example of drug communication. This would make it more effective. The idea should be studied, but competition will be fierce. "Communicatio" means doing things in common.

## References

1. Lewandowski G (1988) What can be learned from drug safety issues? In: Horisberger B, Dinkel R (eds) The perception and management of drug safety risks. Springer, Berlin Heidelberg New York Tokyo, pp. 158–160
2. Luce BR, Elixhauser A (1990) Standards for socioeconomic evaluation of health care products and services. Springer, Berlin Heidelberg New York Tokyo
3. National Research Council (1989) Improving risk communication. National Academy Press, Washington DC

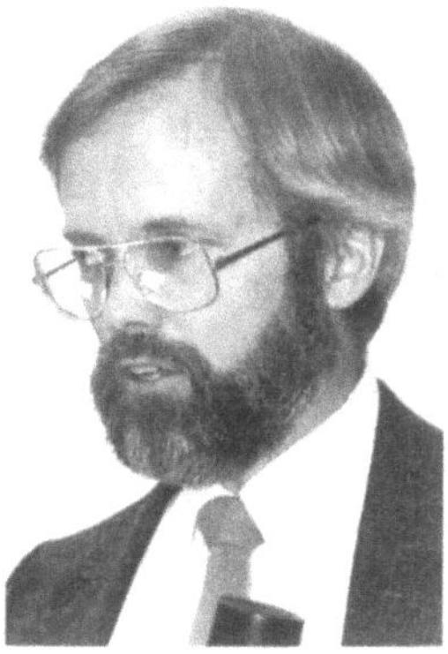

# 37. Physician-Patient Communication and Decision Making

P. ARNTSON

A major goal of our research program is to increase citizens' competencies to make health care decisions concerning their own lives [1]. One of the most important decisions they can make concerns when and how to use prescription drugs. Their ability to make competent drug treatment decisions can be greatly influenced by how physicians and patients discuss the use of drugs. Information about prescriptions is most salient during the consultation when medications are introduced by physicians in order to solve health problems. Furthermore, a high percentage of the population relies on doctors for health information. Yet, before recommending how physicians and patients can most functionally discuss the risks, benefits, and use of prescriptions, we must conduct research that describes the current state of communication and decision making about drugs. This research will then provide a credible data base from which to suggest possible improvements.

For this report, the following questions will generate descriptive answers:

1. Where do patients get most of their information about medicines?
2. What kind of drug information is exchanged during the physician-patient consultations?
3. How do patients perceive the process of information exchange and decision making about drugs?
4. How are the prescribed medications used?
5. Do patients seek additional information about their prescribed drugs?
6. How do physicians perceive the process of information exchange and decision making about drugs?
7. How do the patients' sociodemographic characteristics affect communication before and after the medical consultation?

These questions follow from the six initial questions that generated this project [2]. At this point, we are most interested in describing how physicians and patients talk about prescription drugs, the patients' and doctors' perceptions of the communication, and what happens after the patients have left the doctors' offices.

## Method

### *Subjects*

Thirty-eight general practitioners in the Oxford Regional Health Authority (United Kingdom) agreed to let us videotape a morning or afternoon surgery. The general practitioners were either trainers of general practitioners or were partners in training practices, all of whom had experienced being videotaped quite regularly. The general practitioners did not know that we were looking at how they discussed medications. Between 16 and 38 patients were videotaped with each doctor, an average of 24 patients per doctor.

Of the 905 patients who were videotaped, 301 patients said they had received a new prescription drug. For this report, we will be analyzing the physician-patient consultations for these 301 patients. The average age of the 301 patients was 38 years. There were 180 females and 121 males in the sample. Their average age at leaving school was 16. The mean number of years that they had been with the practice was 12.3. The average number of visits they had had with a doctor over the previous 2 years was 4.6.

### *Research Design*

There were five data collection points in this project. We attempted to gather data beginning with doctor-patient communication about prescription drugs, afterwards by asking the patients what had occurred during the consultations, then by reviewing what the doctors wrote down on the medical record, and 2 weeks later asking patients about their experiences with the drugs. Finally, when all the other data had been collected, we asked the doctors what they thought about their interactions with patients concerning medications.

*Videotape Analysis.* Each videotaped consultation was analyzed for both the content and the form of the interaction. The consultation was also timed. For this report we only analyzed the communication about prescription drugs. The following items on the contents checklist were analyzed in the doctor-patient interaction about prescription medications:

1. The name of the medication
2. The medication's intended benefits
3. The medication's mode of action (i.e., how it works)
4. The medication's possible side effects
5. The medication's possible risks
6. Precautions associated with taking the medication
7. The patients' opinion about the medication
8. The patient's ability to follow the treatment plan

For the first seven content categories, the coders could check whether or not it was discussed and whether the doctor or the patient initiated the discussion. For the last item, the coders checked either yes or no.

These items were a product of many revisions and tests that occurred both during the pilot study with four doctors and 18 patients and during our coders' training sessions. Thirty-four coders were assembled in a senior seminar at Northwestern University, in the United States, during the Winter Quarter 1990. They were trained for 4 weeks in using a contents checklist and an interaction analysis system. Each week during the 10-week quarter a different videotaped consultation was analyzed by all the coders. Twenty of the coders achieved at least an 85 % agreement score for each of the contents checklist items by the 4th week. These 20 coders then analyzed, in rotating pairs, the 301 videotaped consultations in which the patient said a new drug was prescribed. Their coding was spot checked during the remaining 6 weeks of the quarter. The 20 selected coders had, on average, over 90 % agreement on the contents checklist for the remaining six weekly reliability checks. During the Spring Quarter, ten of the trained coders rechecked each of the 301 new-drug consultations, comparing the videotape with the checklist. Any discrepancies were brought to the attention of the research team. In summary, each new drug consultation was coded by at least three coders.

**Patient Questionnaire.** Immediately after the consultation each patient filled out a four-page questionnaire. The questions came from our earlier work with over 3000 patients in England [3], 300 patients in Florida [5], and the pilot test for this study [2]. There were four sections in the questionnaire. In the first section, the patients indicated where they got most of their information about drugs. In the second section, we asked patients to indicate how strongly they agreed or disagreed on a six-point scale to statements concerning their self-efficacy, their health locus of control, their state of health, and the consultation itself. The third section contained questions pertaining to the patients' sociodemographic characteristics. In the fourth section, we asked patients who said that they had received a new prescription drug to indicate how strongly they agreed or disagreed on a six-point scale with statements concerning how the doctor talked to them about their prescribed medications. For the purposes of this report we will focus on the results from the fourth section.

**Medical Record Review.** Two research nurses reviewed the medical record of each patient after the consultation with the doctor. Continuity of care was measured, and information was recorded concerning any drugs that were prescribed, including how the drugs were to be taken.

**Telephone Interviews.** Two weeks after the consultation, every patient who said that he or she had received a new prescription was called. Based on the pilot study, we modified the questions and format. The patients were asked questions about how many pills they had left, whether they were taking the drug as prescribed, why were they doing something different, whether the drug helped, if they had any side effects, if they knew ahead of time about the possibility of side effects, how they knew, if they reported the side effects, if they read about the drug, and if they talked to anyone about the drug. Other questions were also asked, but these are the questions that will be reported on here.

**Doctor Questionnaire.** After all the consultations had been videotaped and the telephone calls were completed, a questionnaire was given to each of the participating general practitioners. The questionnaire contained four sections. In section one, the doctors were asked both to indicate how important (on a scale of 0–10) they thought it was to accomplish 22 consultation tasks and to indicate the approximate percentage (scaled from 0 to 100) of their consultations in which they actually accomplished the tasks. Embedded in this section were the following six tasks concerning prescription drugs:

- To explain all the risks of any medications prescribed
- To explain fully all possible side effects of the medication prescribed
- To find out what patients think about the medications prescribed
- To explain all the benefits of the medications prescribed
- To provide complete instructions for taking the medications prescribed
- To discuss the patients' abilities to follow the treatment plan suggested

In section two, we asked the doctors to rate how desirable (0–10) it would be for their patients to possess 26 specific characteristics. Next we asked them to indicate approximately what percentage of their patients (scaled from 0–100) actually possessed each of these characteristics. Four of these characteristics were specifically related to the patients' taking medications:

- Read about the treatment prescribed before taking it
- Want a full account of the risks of any treatment before taking it
- Fully adhere to the treatment prescribed
- Ask other people about the treatment prescribed before taking it

In section three, we asked the doctors to describe their communication styles. Section four asked for sociodemographic information, years in practice, and type of booking system.

Some of the statements came from an earlier study of doctors' attitudes towards their own communication styles and patients' health competencies [3]. Other statements were developed specifically for this research project and were pilot tested with family practice residents in the United States and general practitioners in England. For our purposes here we will only report on the statements related to prescription drugs.

### *Procedures*

After getting permission from the general practitioners to conduct the study in their offices, the research nurses set up the cameras for a morning or afternoon surgery. Patients were asked for permission to videotape their consultations. If permission was not granted, the camera was turned off. After the consultation, the patients immediately filled out the questionnaire. The research nurses immediately reviewed the medical record. Two weeks later, those patients who said they had received a new prescription were called. Multiple calls were made in order to complete the phone questionnaire. After all the other data had been collected, questionnaires were mailed to the doctors. A follow-up letter and then a telephone call were made if the questionnaires were not returned.

## Results

The results presented here are organized around the first six research questions. The last question concerning how patients' sociodemographic characteristics affect their decision making will be answered in relationship to the other questions.

*1. Where do patients get most of their information about drugs?*

As noted in Table 1, the patients indicated overwhelmingly that the doctor was their primary source of information. Furthermore, 68 patients even refused to indicate a second source of information. Pharmacists were a distant second. Only 43 patients did not choose the doctor as one of their information sources. We found the same pattern of results in the pilot study.

*2. What kind of drug information is exchanged during the consultations?*

The major question in the study and the one to which all the other data are related concerned the drug information exchanged during consultation. Table 2 shows whether the content category was mentioned in the consultation, and if it was, who initiated the discussion. Seldom were the drug risks (2 %) or side effects (23 %) discussed, and there was little mention of what precautions should be taken when using the drug [5]. What we do not know is whether side effects, risks, and particularly precautions should have been discussed.

About half the time the doctor mentioned at least one benefit of taking the drug. Perhaps the doctors who did not talk about benefits assumed the patients knew about the benefits of the drug. The name of the drug and instructions on how to take the drug were mentioned about 80 % of the time. About a quarter of the time the doctor explained to the patient how the drug worked, but less than 8 % of the time did the doctor discuss the patient's ability to follow the treatment plan. Discussing benefits, risks, how to take the drug, how the drug works, and the patient's ability to follow the treatment plan are all consultation behaviors that can increase patients' competencies to use prescription drugs.

**Table 1.** Sources of drug information[a]

| | *n* |
|---|---|
| 1. Doctors | 258 |
| 2. Chemists | 103 |
| 3. Family/friends | 63 |
| 4. Papers/magazines | 36 |
| 5. Labels | 29 |
| 6. Leaflets | 18 |
| 7. Nurses | 8 |
| 8. Other | 19 |
| 9. (Only circled doctor) | 68 |

[a] Patients could circle two choices

**Table 2.** Communication content of consultations

| | Not discussed (%) | Physician started (%) | Patient started (%) |
|---|---|---|---|
| 1. Drug's name | 20.1 | 74.1 | 3.9 |
| 2. Drug's benefits | 49.8 | 48.1 | 0 |
| 3. How drug works | 72.4 | 25.4 | 0 |
| 4. Side effects | 74.9 | 19.8 | 0 |
| 5. Drug's risks | 96.5 | 1.1 | 0.7 |
| 6. Instructions | 15.2 | 82.7 | 0.4 |
| 7. Precautions | 93.3 | 4.9 | 0 |
| 8. Patient's opinion | 64.0 | 14.5 | 19.8 |
| 9. Patient's ability | 92.6 | 7.4 | 0 |

In only 15 % of the consultations did the doctor ask the patient his or her opinion about the prescribed medication. However, in about 20 % of the consultations the patient offered an opinion about the medication, making it unnecessary for the doctor to ask. Overall, this means that the doctor may not have known patient's opinion about the drug 64 % of the time.

It is clear that patients are fairly passive in discussing prescription drugs. At most, patients initiated specific comments about the drugs 4 % of the time in a given category and less than 10 % overall. This is about the same level of patient participation that other studies have found in the United States [5].

Given the importance of discussing benefits and side effects and the fact that there was some variability in these categories, we compared benefits and side effects with other variables. We found that in those consultations where benefits or side effects were discussed, the consultations took on average 1.5 minutes longer than those consultations that did not discuss benefits or side effects. Both findings were statistically significant ($p < 0.05$). The age of the patients was also related to whether or not side effects were discussed. In those consultations where side effects were discussed, the patients were on average 11 years older than the patients in consultations during which side effects were not discussed.

Each prescription drug was coded according to the British National Formulary [4]. Table 3 shows whether or not doctors and patients mentioned side effects for each of the major drug classifications. In this table, we get a better understanding of when doctors think it is important to discuss side effects. For instance, drugs that were prescribed to treat central nervous system problems, cardiovascular system problems, and obstetrics, gynecology, and urinary-tract disorders had side effects discussed by the doctor about one-third of the time. In contrast, the side effects of drugs prescribed to treat infections were discussed less than 10 % of the time. Even within these general classifications, the need to discuss side effects will vary greatly according to the specific type of drug.

**Table 3.** Side effects mentioned by drug category

| | No. of prescriptions ($n$) | Not discussed (%) | Physician started (%) | Patient started (%) |
|---|---|---|---|---|
| 1. Infections | 122 | 89 | 9 | 2 |
| 2. Respiratory disorders | 42 | 76 | 24 | 0 |
| 3. Skin complaints | 38 | 79 | 21 | 0 |
| 4. Central nervous system disorders | 36 | 58 | 36 | 6 |
| 5. Musculoskeletal and joint diseases | 32 | 66 | 28 | 6 |
| 6. Gastrointestinal diseases | 25 | 76 | 16 | 8 |
| 7. Cardiovascular disease | 14 | 57 | 36 | 8 |
| 8. Endocrine disorder | 14 | 86 | 14 | 0 |
| 9. Eye complaints | 9 | 67 | 22 | 11 |
| 10. Obstetrics, gynecology, and urinary-tract disorders | 9 | 67 | 33 | 0 |
| 11. Ear, nose, and throat complaints | 8 | 75 | 25 | 0 |

*3. How do patients perceive the process of information exchange and decision making about drugs?*

In section four of the patient questionnaire, there were five statements concerning how the doctor discussed prescription drugs with the patients (Table 4). The patients were asked to respond on a six-point scale that ranged from very strongly disagree (1) to very strongly agree (6).

Overall, the patients did not see the doctors as asking them to choose a treatment. On average they neither agreed nor disagreed about whether the doctor gave them enough information to make their own decision. The patients

**Table 4.** Patient perception of information exchange and decision making about drugs

| | Mean | Standard Deviation (±) | Median |
|---|---|---|---|
| 1. The doctor asked me to choose a treatment for my health problem | 1.95 | 1.58 | 1 |
| 2. The doctor gave me enough information to make my own decision about which treatment to choose | 3.31 | 2.05 | 3 |
| 3. The doctor fully explained the benefits of the medicine he/she prescribed | 5.10 | 1.43 | 6 |
| 4. The doctor fully explained the risks of the medicine he/she prescribed | 3.63 | 2.11 | 4 |
| 5. The doctor did *not* ask my opinion about taking the medicine he/she prescribed | 3.00 | 1.95 | 2 |

slightly disagreed on average that the doctor did not ask their opinion about the drug. However, the distribution is bimodal for this statement, meaning that most people either strongly disagreed or strongly agreed.

The patients' responses to the questions concerning risks and benefits were more illuminating. Overall, the patients strongly agreed that the doctors fully explained the drug's benefits. They only slightly agreed that the doctor had fully explained the risks. In Table 5, the patients' perceptions of how fully the doctor explained the medication's risks are presented by the general type of drug that was prescribed.

Notice that in those drug categories where at least one-third of the time side effects were actually mentioned (i.e., obstetrics, gynecology, urinary-tract disorders, central nervous system, and cardiovascular systems), the patients' average scores are above the overall mean of 3.63. The mean for infections, where side effects were mentioned less than 10 % of the time, is 3.32. However, the means for respiratory drugs and gastrointestinal system drugs do not correspond with the frequency of side effects that were mentioned.

There is even less correspondence between what the patients said happened in the consultation and what actually was coded in the consultation. Table 6 shows

**Table 5.** Patients' estimates of how fully doctors explained risks[a]

| | (Scale 0–10) Mean | Standard deviation | *n* |
|---|---|---|---|
| 1. Infections | 3.32 | 2.08 | 113 |
| 2. Respiratory disorders | 4.06 | 2.01 | 33 |
| 3. Skin complaints | 3.45 | 2.20 | 31 |
| 4. Central nervous system disorders | 4.29 | 1.99 | 24 |
| 5. Musculoskeletal and joint diseases | 3.70 | 2.12 | 30 |
| 6. Gastrointestinal diseases | 3.06 | 2.29 | 16 |
| 7. Cardiovascular disease | 3.92 | 2.19 | 12 |
| 8. Endocrine disorder | 3.56 | 2.19 | 9 |
| 9. Obstetrics, gynecology, and urinary-tract disorders | 5.22 | 1.39 | 9 |

[a] This is for patients who received only one prescription drug

**Table 6.** The congruency between patients' reports of their doctors' communication and the actual communication

| All Risks (patients, *n* = 229) | Patients | |
|---|---|---|
| | Disagreed (%) | Agreed (%) |
| Not mentioned | 41.9 | 28.4 |
| Mentioned | 8.3 | 21.4 |
| Benefits (patients, *n* = 243) | | |
| Not mentioned | 7.6 | 42.4 |
| Mentioned | 2.9 | 47.1 |

the degree of congruency between the patients' perceptions of what the doctors said and what was actually said.

In the first column for the "All Risks" cross-tabulation are patients who either very strongly disagreed or moderately strongly disagreed that the doctor fully explained the risks. In the second column are patients who either moderately agreed or very strongly agreed that the doctor fully explained the risks. We dropped from the analysis patients who only slightly agreed or disagreed. In row one for the "All Risks" cross-tabulation are all the consultations where side effects, risks, and precautions were not mentioned by anyone. In row two are those consultations where at least one of these aspects was mentioned. A little over 28 % of the patients moderately or strongly agreed that the doctor had fully explained the drug's risks when no one had actually mentioned risks, side effects, or precautions.

For the "Benefits" cross-tabulation, the columns are set up in the same way as the "All Risks" cross-tabulation. The patients either very strongly and moderately strongly disagreed or very strongly and moderately strongly agreed that the doctor fully explained the drug's benefits. For the two rows, either the doctors did or did not mention benefits. Here we see slightly more incongruity between patients agreeing that the doctors mentioned benefits when they did not (42.4 %). These findings fit in with a general pattern of patients overestimating what the doctors were doing. This incongruity points to the importance of analyzing actual communication about prescription drugs in consultations.

### *4. How are the prescribed medications used?*

Out of the 301 patients who said they received new prescriptions, we were only able to contact 244 of them by telephone. Some did not have phones; others could never be reached even after repeated attempts. Fifty-four patients reported that they did not take the drug as prescribed, which is consistent with our estimates obtained by comparing how many pills we calculated patients should have left with the number they reported having left. When asked why they did not follow the original treatment plan, patients gave the kinds of answers presented in Table 7.

**Table 7.** Reasons given by patients for not following original treatment plan

| | *n* |
|---|---|
| Got better | 16 |
| Side effects | 15 |
| Doctor's advice | 5 |
| Forgot | 3 |
| Drug was no help | 3 |
| Other/do not know | 12 |

We also asked the patients if the drug helped as expected. In all, 70 % of the patients said yes, 17 % said no, 10 % said they did not know, and 3 % did not respond. Of the 40 people who said that drugs were not helping them as they expected, 26 of them kept on taking the drug anyway. The question arises of how many of the patients who did not think that the drug was helping them, or did not know if it was, would volunteer that information to their doctors during their next appointments. Unless the doctors ask them specifically about the last visits' prescriptions, both a feedback opportunity to the doctors and an educational opportunity for the patients may be missed.

Fifty-seven people reported they had side effects from their prescription drugs. This means that 42 patients continued taking their medications as prescribed, even though they reported having side effects. When asked if they knew ahead of time about these side effects, 29 said yes and 28 said no. When we compared the ages of these two groups, we found that the people who said they knew ahead of time about the side effects had a mean age of 50, while the people who did not know about the side effects ahead of time had a mean age of 40. This 10-year difference was statistically significant. The fact that the older patients were more likely to know about the side effects ahead of time may be related to the earlier finding that consultations with older patients were more likely to have discussed side effects than consultations with younger patients.

The patients who knew ahead of time about the side effects reported that they had learned from the sources shown in Table 8. Of the 57 patients who had side effects, only 14 of them (24 %) learned about the side effects from their doctors. Since we do not know if the problems they thought were side effects are actually related to the prescription drugs, we must be careful in drawing conclusions. Only one person said that he had learned about the side effect from a chemist. The role of chemists in informing patients about prescription drugs is quite minimal in this study.

We then asked the 57 patients if they had reported the side effects to their doctors. Twelve said yes, and 45 said no. Of these 45, 14 said that they would be seeing the doctor anyway. If these 14 patients actually reported their side effects to the doctor at their next visit, then over 50 % (31 patients) of the side effects would still go unreported unless the doctor specifically asked about side effects from previously prescribed medications. Once again there can be a breakdown

**Table 8.** Patients' source of information about side effects

| Source | *n* |
|---|---|
| General practitioner | 14 |
| Taken drug before | 5 |
| Label on drug container | 4 |
| Leaflet | 1 |
| Medical literature | 1 |
| Chemist | 1 |
| Other/do not know | 3 |

in the feedback loop to the doctors if neither the patients nor the doctors discuss the previous visits' treatment outcomes.

### *5. Do patients seek additional information about their prescription drugs?*

We asked the patients if they read anything about the drug they were prescribed. Their answers are presented in Table 9.

We also asked them if they talked to anyone about the drug (Table 10). Only 11 % of the patients who said they read something about the drug also said they had talked to someone. There is not much overlap in the patients' information-seeking strategies. More to the point, there is very little information seeking occurring about their prescription drugs. Further, relatives and friends seem to be a more important reference group than allied health professionals (e.g., chemists and nurses).

**Table 9.** Sources of additional written information for patients concerning prescribed drugs

| Source | % |
|---|---|
| None | 78.2 |
| Label on bottle | 10.9 |
| Leaflet | 7.9 |
| Medical literature | 2.2 |
| Books/magazines | 0.9 |

**Table 10.** Sources of additional verbal information for patients concerning prescribed drugs

| Source | % |
|---|---|
| None | 77.7 |
| Relatives/friends | 16.2 |
| Chemists | 1.7 |
| Other health workers | 1.7 |
| Nurses | 1.3 |
| Others on the drug | 1.3 |

### *6. How do physicians perceive the process of information exchange and decision making about drugs?*

To date, 33 general practitioners out of 38 have returned their questionnaires. Six questions asked them both to indicate how important they thought it was to accomplish certain drug-related consultation tasks and to indicate the approx-

**Table 11.** Doctors' mean ratings of drug consultation tasks

| Task | How important to accomplish[a] | Percentage actually accomplished |
|---|---|---|
| 1. To explain all the risks of any medications you prescribe | 5.96 | 40.9 |
| 2. To fully explain all possible side effects of the medications you prescribe | 6.00 | 38.5 |
| 3. To find out patients' opinion | 6.94 | 48.8 |
| 4. To explain all the benefits of the medications you prescribe | 6.45 | 47.6 |
| 5. To provide complete instructions for taking medications you prescribe | 8.15 | 61.2 |
| 6. To discuss the patients' abilities to follow the treatment plan you suggest | 7.03 | 49.4 |

[a] Rated on a scale of 0–10

imate percentage of their consultations in which they actually accomplished each task. Table 11 shows both how important it is for the doctors to accomplish these tasks (0–10) and in what percentage of consultations they think that the tasks have actually been accomplished (on a scale of 0–100).

As expected, providing complete instructions was rated the most important to accomplish and the most likely to be accomplished. The task rated least important to accomplish was to explain all the risks of any medications, followed closely by explaining all possible side effects. The doctors also indicated that both tasks are least likely to be accomplished. Both sets of findings corresponded to what the doctors actually did in the consultations. Surprisingly, the doctors did not rate the task of explaining all the benefits of the prescribed medications very high in either importance or accomplishment, even though the benefits were enumerated about 50 % of the time in the consultations. The doctors rated the importance and accomplishment of both finding out what the patients think

**Table 12.** Doctors' mean ratings of their patients' characteristics

| Characteristic | How desirable is this characteristic[a] | Percentage actually possessing this characteristic |
|---|---|---|
| 1. Read about treatment before taking it | 5.94 | 24.8 |
| 2. Want a full account of the risks of any treatment | 5.42 | 27.9 |
| 3. Fully adhere to the treatment prescribed | 7.52 | 45.8 |
| 4. Ask other people about the treatment prescribed before taking it | 3.22 | 35.6 |

[a] Rated on a scale of 0–10

and discussing the patients' abilities higher than explaining the drugs' benefits. Yet the doctors did relatively little of either task in the consultations.

Table 12 shows how the doctors rated the four patient characteristics that are related to taking prescription medications. The doctors indicated both how desirable each characteristic was (0–10), and what percentage of their patients possessed the characteristic (on a scale of 0–100). The doctors were least keen on patients who ask other people about the treatment before taking it. They valued more highly patients who read about the treatment before taking it. Yet the doctors indicated that their patients were a little less likely to read about the treatment than talk to someone about it. In fact, the patients reported that they did little of either information-seeking activity. The doctors were fairly accurate in predicting their patients' lack of information seeking about prescription drugs.

The doctors highly valued patients who fully adhered to the prescribed treatment. Yet, the doctors indicated that fewer than 50% of their patients would fully adhere to the treatment plans. They did not so highly value patients who wanted a full account of the risks of prescribed treatments nor did they think many of their patients actually wanted a full accounting of the risks.

Without relating the doctors' answers to their actual communication behaviors and their patients' responses, we can only draw tentative inferences from these results. Relatively speaking, the doctors did not think that it was very important to explain all the risks, side effects, and benefits for the drugs they prescribed. On average, they estimated that these tasks were accomplished less than 50% of the time. They were fairly accurate on how often benefits were discussed, but overestimated how often side effects and risks were mentioned. They rated as more important finding out what their patients think and discussing their patients' abilities. However, the doctors overestimated how often either of these tasks was accomplished in the consultations.

The doctors found least desirable those patients who asked other people about the drugs. Perhaps this is because doctors felt that the patients would be misinformed. They were not too keen either about patients who wanted a full account of any risks or would read about the drug before taking it. They estimated that fewer than 30% of their patients wanted a full account or read about the drug. Relatively speaking, the doctors were accurate in predicting that their patients would more likely talk to someone than read about the drug. The doctors were much more interested in having patients who would adhere to the treatment than having patients who wanted information from other people, printed materials, or more information from the doctors.

## Discussion

Any conclusions that we might draw from this report must be tentative because we have not fully analyzed all the data or all the possible interrelationships between the variables. Furthermore, we must remember that the consultations were being videotaped and that the general practitioners or their partners were mostly trainers. Yet, the way this data set was collected and who was involved mean that the doctors were on their best behavior and we were recording some of the best general practitioners in the Oxford Regional Health Authority. In a random sample of doctor-patient consultations, there may be even less communication about the risks and benefits of drugs and less importance placed on accomplishing certain drug-related tasks.

There are three tentative conclusions that we can make. First, doctors are the primary source of drug information for this sample of patients. When we asked patients to circle two choices of drug information, doctors were their overwhelming choice. Only about 20 % of the patients indicated that they had read or talked to anyone else about the drugs that were prescribed. However, this presents a dilemma for patients, drug manufacturers, and regulatory agencies who want complete drug information given to patients. Doctors rarely mentioned risks and precautions, and only slightly more often talked about side effects in this study. On average, the doctors indicated that they did not consider it very important to talk about risks and side effects.

Second, there is room for improvement in how doctors communicate about prescription drugs. It is important to say up front that there was no gold standard used to say when risks, side effects, or precautions should have been discussed. Both the specific type of drug and the type of patient will affect what is said. And doctors are reluctant to mention side effects because the side effects may occur based on the doctors' suggestions. They are also sensitive to the fact that some patients may not take medications when doctors have mentioned the medicines' rare risks. Time may also be a reason that some physicians are hesitant to discuss the side effects and benefits of drugs. In this study, the consultations were significantly longer when benefits or side effects were mentioned.

Regardless of the reasons, it was surprisingly that precautions on how to use the drugs were mentioned so seldom and that benefits were only discussed by the doctors in 50 % of the consultations. Talking about precautions may help avoid serious side effects. Mentioning benefits may help in persuading patients to take the medications. Discussing patients' abilities to follow the treatment plans and finding out their opinions about drugs, two infrequently used content categories, may help overcome resistance to using the drugs or can alert the doctors to the need for alternative treatment plans.

Third, there was low patient participation in discussing drugs during consultations. Patients initiated discussion about any one content category less then 5 % of the time. This level of patient involvement corresponds to what other researchers have found in the United States. Another measure of patients' involvement in their own care may be the fact that about 20 % of the telephoned patients talked to someone or read about their prescribed medications. Efforts by the National Council on Patient Information and Education in the United States to foster physician-patient communication seem clearly warranted.

These conclusions are not revolutionary. More sophisticated results must await further analysis of the data we have already collected. Tripling the number of doctors in the study will allow us to test how doctors' individual differences may affect their actual communication in consultations, their patients' perceptions of the consultations, and their patients' use and understanding of prescription drugs.

The final projected outcome of this study, and others like it, is to use the results as a basis for developing educational interventions for primary care physicians. The aim of the interventions would be to help doctors improve the ability of their patients to make competent decisions about using prescription drugs.

## References

1. Arntson PH (1989) Improving citizens' health competencies. Health Commun 1:29–34
2. Arntson PH (1990) Doctor-patient communication and decision-making about prescription drugs. In: Shimizu N, Tanaka Y, Jones J, Taylor D (eds) Improving drug safety: the assessment, management and communication of therapeutic benefits and risks of pharmaceutical products. Pharma International, Tokyo, pp. 180–185
3. Arntson PH, Makoul G, Pendleton D, Schofield T (1989) Patients' perceptions of medical encounters in Great Britain: Variations with health loci of control and sociodemographic factors. Health Commun 1:75–95
4. British Medical Association and Royal Pharmaceutical Society of Great Britain (1989) British national formulary number 18 (September 1989). British Medical Association and the Pharmaceutical Press, London
5. Makoul G (1990) Health locus of control and concern as predictors of health information attention and acquisition. Communication in Health Care Conference, Oxford University

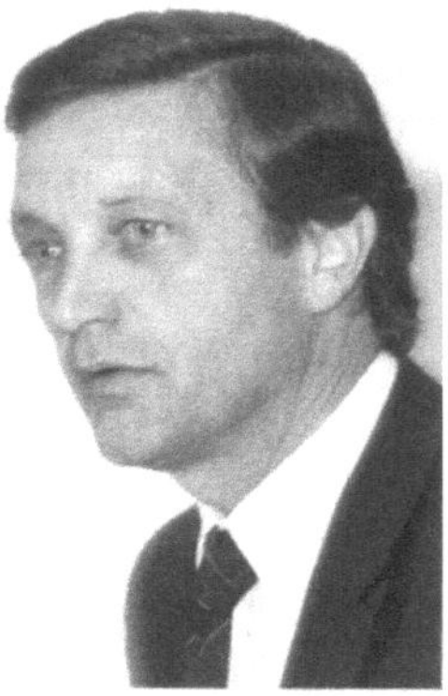

# 38. Problem-Oriented Drug Information Services

F. Follath

The discussion about the various aspects of drug safety is usually focused on newly introduced therapeutic agents. Data on potential benefits and risks are generated in preclinical studies, in clinical trials involving carefully selected patient groups, and, more recently, in postmarketing surveillance studies. Not surprisingly, the main role in this process is played by the pharmaceutical industry and the drug regulatory agencies. The third party, i.e., the prescribing physician, is often neglected. However, adverse drug reactions (ADRs) represent a common problem in everyday medical practice not only with new but also with older drugs having well-known side effect profiles. The type and frequency of ADRs certainly depend on the pharmacological and toxicological properties of chemical compounds, but they are also influenced to a large extent by the mode of the drug's clinical use (Table 1). The wrong drug, a wrong dosage, an unsuitable drug combination, or errors of drug intake represent frequent causes of ADRs in ambulatory or hospitalized patients. Thus, the

**Table 1.** Types of adverse drug reactions

| | | | |
|---|---|---|---|
| **Unexpected ADR (mainly new drugs)** | | | |
| Organ toxicity<br>Teratogenicity<br>carcinogenicity | not predictable (?) | | |
| **ADR due to suboptimal use (old and new drugs)** | | | |
| Wrong drug choice<br>wrong dosage<br>wrong drug combination | predictable and often avoidable | ⇦ | Problem-Oriented Drug Information |
| Erroneous drug intake | | | |

prescribing physicians probably influence the ultimate risk/benefit ratio of drug treatment and the overall incidence of drug-related problems to a greater extent than commonly appreciated.

What could be done to improve the practical use of drugs and reduce the incidence of predictable side-effects? More efforts could be made to teach medical students and practicing physicians about the basic rules of clinical pharmacology and therapeutics, including regular education programs about new therapeutic developments. However, the rapidly growing number of drugs and the complex influences of genetic factors, organ disorders, and interactions on the efficacy and tolerance of pharmacological agents make it increasingly difficult to have up-to-date knowledge of all relevant drug-related problems. Although written, published information is abundantly available, it is difficult to retrieve the appropriate data since the proper sources are often unknown and the search is too time-consuming [2]. Most physicians could therefore benefit from an easily available interactive and comprehensive drug information system. For this reason, we have developed and prospectively evaluated a clinical pharmacology-based drug information service, accessible to hospital and community physicians as well as to pharmacists serving a population of about half a million people in the region of Basel. In this short report I describe the initial experience over a period of 2 years and discuss the potential usefulness of such information systems. The drug information team is located in the Clinical Pharmacology Division of the University Hospital, Basel. Drug- and treatment-related questions are received by telephone and first evaluated by a pharmacist. For all the clinical aspects of therapeutic problems, a physician team member is always consulted. Data on specific drugs are retrieved from computerized data files, standard textbooks, or by direct on-line literature searches. A final written answer is provided to all inquiries following a regular weekly discussion by the entire clinical pharmacology team.

During the past 12-month period (1989), the drug information service answered more than 300 drug-related questions. About half of the demands came from hospital physicians, the remaining in equal proportion from practicing physicians and community pharmacists. The most frequent reasons for addressing the drug information serivce were problems concerning drug treatment in individual patients (72 %) such as side effects, dosage, interactions, and the optimum choice of drugs. The majority of physician inquiries were classified as urgent (67 %) and required a rapid answer. Questions by pharmacists were also of practical importance, but usually less urgent and addressed more general therapeutic principles. The main advantage of our multidisciplinary team, staffed by experienced physicians and pharmacists, was the possibility to evaluate clinical, pharmacokinetic, and pharmaceutical aspects of drug-related questions simultaneously. Furthermore, the direct contact with physicians allowed a more precise assessment of the therapeutic problems and provided comprehensive information about all coadministered drugs and specific characteristics of the patient. Thus, answers considering only a partial aspect of the therapeutic problem could be avoided. The services of the drug information team were generally well received by physicians and pharmacists, who repeatedly asked for further information following the initial contact. Our experience corresponds to those of similar services of clinical pharmacology groups in Sweden [1] and Great Britain [3].

We believe that regionally organized hospital-based drug information services could play an important role in helping physicians to use drugs in a more optimal way and reduce the incidence of ADRs. Multidisciplinary teams consisting of properly trained clinical pharmacologists and pharmacists are able to deal with the various and often complex aspects of drug therapy. Such drug information services could also serve as centers for the collection and evaluation of ADR reports. Drug information centers are currently being organized by all the clinical pharmacology divisions of university hospitals in Switzerland. At a later stage national and international cooperation could further facilitate and improve the activities of such information centers.

## References

1. Alvan G, Ohmann B, Sjöqvist F (1983) Problem-oriented drug information: a clinical pharmacological service. Lancet II:1410–1412
2. Covell DG, Uman GC, Manning PR (1985) Information needs in office practice: are they being met? Ann Intern Med 103:596–599
3. Davies DM, Ashton CH, Rao JG, Rawlins MD, Routledge PA, Savage RL, Thompson JW, Zar MA (1977) Comprehensive clinical drug information service: first year's experience. Br Med J 1:89–90

# *Part IX*

# *Responses Beyond Traditional Communication Channels*

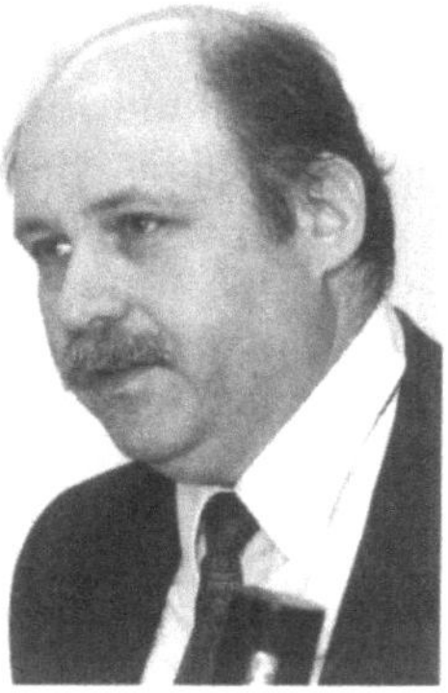

# 39. Manufacturer Standards for Communicating Pharmaceutical Risks and Benefits*

L. A. Morris

When a close friend was completing his medical residency, he once remarked that one of his greatest fears was becoming a "country doc." I was surprised. I envisioned an old greying man taking care of close friends and loved by all. As a career goal, becoming a country doc seemed admirable. However, my friend's vision was quite different. To him, a country doc was not an old man, but someone who had graduated from medical school 4 or 5 years ago. These doctors were well meaning, but simply out-of-date with current standards for medical practice. From a physician's standpoint, staying up-to-date with therapeutic innovation is a predominate theme within the profession. Not only are their patients' well-being and their own liability dependent on their knowledge of the latest developments in therapeutics, but the physician's self-image is also at stake.

Layered on top of the physician's demands for information is the desire of patients to learn about medications and new innovations in health care. Further, the passion of pharmaceutical manufacturers to increase sales of their products provides all the necessary ingredients for a well-greased channel for pharmaceutical information dissemination and receipt. However, pharmaceutical marketing also carries great responsibility. Although manufacturers are quite willing to make physicians and patients aware of net treatments and advocate their benefits, manufacturers must also be concerned about communicating the risks and limits of treatment. As a matter of United States law, advertising and labeling of prescription drugs requires that risk information be included as an integral part of pharmaceutical promotion. Promotional practices of the pharmaceutical industry are reviewed by the Food and Drug Administration (FDA) to assure the accuracy of the material and the dissemination of prescribing information. The purpose of this chapter is to briefly review the promotional practices and procedures of the pharmaceutical industry and describe how these practices are influenced by legal standards.

* The views expressed are solely those of the author and do not reflect the policy of the Food and Drug Administration

## Pharmaceutical Industry Communications

In recent years the pharmaceutical industry has broadened its communication base. While advertising in medical journals, direct mail promotion, and personal visits by representatives have remained the backbone of pharmaceutical promotion, new methods, media, and audiences have emerged as pharmaceutical companies expand their efforts to gain an edge on their competition. Advertisements may be delivered via computer, on videodisks, on television, or by facsimile transfer machine. Not only are other health professionals being targeted for pharmaceutical industry promotions, but patients and consumers are targeted as well. Furthermore, some areas that had not previously been considered to be under the influence of the pharmaceutical industry are becoming increasingly used to promote pharmaceuticals. Under certain circumstances, FDA considers communications to the press (i.e., press releases, press conferences, etc.) and educational seminars (i.e., presentations at or reports about scientific conferences) to be promotion. In response to these broadening efforts, FDA has expanded its view of what is considered pharmaceutical industry promotion.

Although the promotional efforts of the industry continue to encompass new areas of communications, the standards for prescription drug advertising remain stable. As required by the Food, Drug, and Cosmetic Act (FD&CA), there are two primary standards that control pharmaceutical industry promotions: 1. advertisements must not be false or misleading, and 2. there must be adequate stipulations made for the disclosure of prescribing (risk) information.

## The Package Insert as the Marketing License

One could spend many hours debating what is or is not "false or misleading" or what is meant by adequate disclosure. In pharmaceutical promotion, FDA utilizes the approved labeling as the primary standard for judging the content of pharmaceutical promotion. Advertising claims that are consistent with approved labeling are acceptable. Claims that are at variance with the approved labeling are considered false or misleading. Thus, the professional labeling or package insert establishes the basis of what FDA considers acceptable claims.

Of course, certain types of claims may not be covered by the package insert. FDA will not accept claims promoting new uses or new patient populations for the drug that are outside of labeling. However, claims that are not based upon the indications section of the label, but which are supported by adequate scientific data (e.g., bioavailability, quality of life, patient satisfaction) are permitted.

## False or Misleading Provisions

False or misleading statements about the advantages or uses of a product can have a profound impact on drug misutilization. Marketers frequently wish to introduce their products in the broadest possible terms to capitalize on the broadest possible patient base. FDA regulations prohibit such broadening of the patient base by requiring "fair balance" in product promotions.

Fair balance regulations require promotional claims to be placed in a proper context. If the product has advantages in certain populations, or if it is indicated for certain subgroups of patients, those limiting conditions or populations must be clearly stated in the promotional claims. Further, if there are significant limitations to the product's use, these too must be included in the advertisement to assure that the claims are not misinterpreted.

If manufacturers make false or misleading claims, FDA may require cancellation of the advertising. If such misleading claims persist or if the initial misrepresentation is egregious (threatening to the public health), FDA may require some corrective action. For example, FDA recently required a corrective advertisement for Cytotec, a drug used to treat ulcers induced by nonsteroidal anti-inflammatory drugs (NSAIDs). The purpose of the corrective advertisement was to "set the record straight" about the proper indications for the use of Cytotec. The original advertisement suggested that Cytotec can be used as a "co-therapy" with NSAIDs. The corrective advertisement reiterated the approved labeling that emphasized Cytotec is indicated for patients at "high risk" of gastric ulceration.

## Adequate Disclosure Requirements

The adequate disclosure requirements are based on the premise that a busy physician may not have an adequate opportunity to search for the prescribing information about a drug. Promotional materials are required to contain or make provisions for the dissemination of prescribing information.

This prescribing information takes several forms. In print advertisements, a "brief summary" of warning, precautions, and contraindications is required. In reality, the "brief summary" entails a thorough reprinting of the product's risks taken verbatim from the approved labeling. FDA regulations do not permit summarization of product risks; however, certain sections of the label may be omitted (e.g., dosage and administration, indications, clinical pharmacology).

Promotional materials that are sent directly to the physician or distributed by representatives are considered promotional labeling as opposed to advertisements. These labeling materials require that "full disclosure" (i.e., the package insert) be distributed with the promotional materials. Audiovisual materials require the dissemination of "full disclosure". In addition, audiovisual materials require that a "major statement" of product risks be included in both the audio and visual portions of the program. The scope of the "major statement" is usually quite brief, highlighting important prescribing risks and limitations.

## Preapproval Risk Disclosure Standards

Preapproval promotion is quite popular as marketers seek to lay the groundwork for a launch campaign once FDA approval is obtained. However, because there is no approved labeling, there is no basis for product claims. Preapproval promotion through product advertising is, therefore, quite limited. Manufacturers are permitted to inform prescribers that the company is working on a particular disease or doing research on a particular class of drugs (i.e., institutional advertising) or they are permitted to name the new drug entity, but make no claims or representations about the product (i.e., reminder advertising). Institutional and reminder advertising do not require "brief summary" disclosures.

Companies have also issued press releases about new products during research and development or at the time of FDA approval. FDA reviews these materials and applies promotional standards. Risk disclosure of two types is sought. First, it is required that significant known risks be described to fairly balance the promotional claims and assure disclosure of the meaningful material to the public. Second, information about the degee of testing is sought so that viewers of the press materials may make some judgment about the degree to which the drug's risks are known.

In conclusion, for the most part what we believe determines what we do. FDA standards for risk disclosure are intended to assure that people prescribing and using prescription drugs have an accurate and complete view of the benefits and the risks of the medications they use.

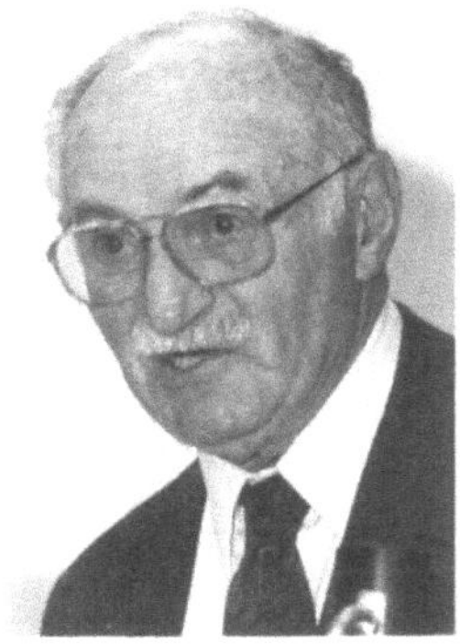

# 40. Health Behavior Change via Community Education

N. MACCOBY

Even with the devastation caused by AIDS, chronic disease has replaced infectious diseases as the principal source of morbidity and mortality in the Uinted States and most of the developed world. Much has been and is being done to prevent or control such devastating early cripplers and killers as cardiovascular disease, varieties of cancer, diabetes, and other chronic diseases through improvement in health care systems and pharmaceuticals. Much is also being done to help people alter their lifestyles in ways designed to reduce the risk of acquiring these diseases. Abstention from or cessation of smoking, a more healthful diet, and regular exercise habits can reduce risk of cardiovascular events and certain highly prevalent cancers such as lung and colon cancer. Some of these risk factors such as high vascular cholesterol and high blood pressure can also be lowered not only by adopting such behavior, but also via pharmaceutical therapy.

What all of these means of reducing risk of disease have in common is how people behave. Do people adopt styles of living which reduce risk? If not, what means may be employed to increase the likelihood of their adopting such behavior? I want to describe briefly the methods employed by us in the Stanford University Center for Research in Disease Prevention as well as those used by colleagues at other research centers in various parts of the world.

Some 20 years ago our group, led by John Farquhar [1, 2], and a Finnish group, led by Pekka Puska [3], independently began undertaking research on how best to educate communities to change their behavior in ways designed to reduce the risk of cardiovascular disease, then, and to a lesser extent still, the single biggest killer in those two countries and many other developed ones. Both employed mass media and community organization to help accomplish this task. Stanford's first main study in California [1] used mass media heavily and the North Karelia project in Finland [3] emphasized community organization. Later, when the researchers in the two countries came to learn of each other's work, Stanford and other United States projects, such as those in Minnesota [4] and Rhode Island [5], began using community organization methods more extensively, and North Karelia increased its use of mass media.

From the beginning, in order to effect behavior change the Stanford group relied upon behavior theory heavily, both that available and that which had to be devised. We borrowed from Cartwright's theory of mass persuasion in effecting behavior change [6]. Cartwright analyzed the failure and later success of a campaign designed to sell United States' bonds to help promote consumer savings in the United States in World War II. Cartwright posited that changes in what people knew and were motivated to do were not sufficient in themselves to achieve the objective. Means of tripping off the desired behavior when it was ready to occur were necessary. Thus mass media, if well designed and employed, could inform and motivate people *toward buying* such bonds, but frequently fell short of getting them to actually *buy* the bonds. However, when the foreman or the shop steward at the worksite asked workers individually to sign up on the sheet requesting payroll deductions for the bonds, no further communications were necessary. They signed up.

My Stanford colleague Albert Bandura has more recently formulated a social cognitive theory to describe and predict throughts and actions. His thinking and advice to us during the last 20 years have contributed much to our work [7]. He posits a triadic reciprocality in which the person, his environment, and his behavior interact and influence each other in a variety of ways.

Most efforts at health education have relied on the provision of information as the sole or principal means of achieving behavior change. Bandura's approach stresses the person's own role in developing self-management of behavior through training, manipulation of the immediate environment, and through self-observation or feedback. Self-efficacy is a cornerstone in this approach. Dr. Jean Mayer, a great nutritionist, once observed that American women practiced the rhythm method of *girth* control. Most New Year's resolutions have a very short life-span. Bandura states that by getting people to perform tasks successfully, their self-efficacy (confidence) improves for subsequent efforts at changing their behavior. Thus, a smoker who quits for a week and then resumes smoking can be shown how successful he/she has been – not a failure. His/her experience is that he/she can quit smoking. He/she needs now to learn how to avoid relapses.

Finally, McGuire [8] has formulated many principles of persuasion which we have found useful. Most significant is his work on social inoculation. Preceding a persuasive communication by first presenting a weak dose of counter-arguments serves not only to help make this communication effective, but more importantly tends to make subsequent real counterefforts less effective in destroying the initial effects of the persuasive communication. Well-informed people are generally more difficult to persuade to an idea contrary to one they hold. They argue against the persuasion attempt. We had shown this experimentally earlier [9, 10].

We applied this idea successfully in teaching many people not to start smoking. We found that many 12-year-olds starting middle school emulated their older peers and succumbed to pressures to begin smoking experimentally. This experimentation in smoking typically led to later addictive smoking. We employed an educative process that included getting the young students to invent and use counter-arguments in the presence of simulated pressures to smoke [11]. The rate of experimental smoking remained very low compared with that of uninstructed classes.

This method with variations has since been successfully employed by both us and others. For example, in a schools study [12] concerning reduction of risk of cardiovascular disease, a ten-session curriculum resulted in changed exercise, diet, and smoking behavior; reduced pulse rate, demonstrating exercise gains; reduced mass body indices, indicating diet changes; and carbon monoxide exhaled, confirming the smoking reports. We did not reduce addictive smoking, but did succeed in reducing the number of experimental smokers, of whom many were likely to become confirmed smokers. We are currently testing whether we can succeed in training regular classroom teachers to achieve similar results so that the course could be made generally available. These methods might prove useful in helping people to discriminate between false rumor and accurate information about the costs and benefits of pharmaceuticals.

As mentioned above, almost 20 years ago, a group of us at Stanford planned and, during the decade and a half since have carried out field experiments aimed at reducing the risk of cardiovascular disease in entire communities. We selected communities because these diseases and their precursers were very widespread in the United States as well as in many other developed countries – so widespread as to make individual education unfeasible. It is clear the risk factors for cardiovascular disease were exacerbated by human behavior. In addition to smoking, high blood cholesterol and high blood pressure were clearly influenced by diet, exercise, and adherence to an appropriate regimen of drug taking. The community contains a variety of sources of influence, such as schools, industries, health maintenance organizations, consumer organizations, clubs, churches, governmental agencies, and media. These all play a role in influencing citizens and families to behave in healthier fashion.

Drawing from the theoretical perspectives described above, we reasoned that in order for people to change their behavior a set of specifiable psychological processes had to occur.

1. Awareness. People need to become aware of the problem. Therefore, heart disease had to be moved from the periphery to the focus of attention.
2. There must be an increase in knowledge about the diseases and their associated risk behaviors.
3. Motivation to change must be present. One might surmise that these first three factors would be sufficient for changes in behavior to occur, but they are usually not enough. Knowing the need and being motivated to change often characterizes good intentions, but not necessarily good behavior.
4. Learning skills are often needed. Changing diet involves not only nutritional information, but how to shop for, prepare, present, and consume meals that are both heart healthy and also interesting and attractive to eat. Smoking cessation involves a high degree of skill in how to deal with pressure and tempting situations as well as how to cope with addiction to nicotine. Exercise, too, involves a great deal of skills acquisition.
5. Practicing the newly acquired thinking and response patterns is needed if these skills are really to be learned. Watching someone else hit a tennis or golf

ball can be helpful, but there is no substitute for guided practice and feedback for learning.
6. Finally, the new habits must persist in the face of all sorts of pressures and invitations to relapse. Mark Twain once observed that quitting smoking is easy; he had done it a great many times.
7. A great deal is understood now about the first six of these steps, but the last, the problem of *maintenance* of behavior change, is currently the topic of choice among researchers. Progress is being made in this area, but much remains to be found.

Our first study was the Three-Community Study [1, 2]. Since face-to-face communication would not be a feasible model for general use, we hoped to be able to change the two intervention towns by mass media. However, there was some evidence to suggest that mass media alone might not suffice. While the media might do well with our first three behavioral objectives – awareness, knowledge, and motivation – there was reason to be concerned about the potential success in the last four. However, we designed our media in such a way as to maximize their effectiveness on all our behavioral objectives. We then covered the possibility of their failure by employing in the second town a subsample of those at highest risk. These were given face-to-face intensive instruction in addition to the media exposure. A third town served as a reference.

We found that at the end of 2 years the community limited to mass media only did as well as the one supplemented by intensive instruction. By the end of the 3rd year, however, successful risk reduction was maintained much more in the supplemented town than in the one with mass media alone. Both communities evidenced more risk reduction than did the third town in which there was no intervention except to screen and test. One other important finding was that the behavior changes that brought about the increased risk reduction were greater in the maximum intervention town than in the controls, and they lasted longer. Clearly, if we were to be successful in maintaining risk reduction for long periods of time, we needed a feasible substitute for face-to-face instruction to supplement the mass media. We decided that community organization should be attempted. By mobilizing community leadership, we put even our mass media campaign efforts into the hands of the town facilities, with Stanford people serving as advisors.

The Five-City Study [13, 14], as this effort is known, consisted of two larger cities, in each of which the intervention was as similar as we could make it, and three comparison cities. One of these was eventually dropped from our sample surveys for budgetary reasons, although we are currently conducting morbidity and mortality surveillance in all five.

Education was carried out through four different channels of communication:
1. broadcast media (television and radio);
2. newspapers;
3. other mass-distributed print media (mass mailings of booklets and mass distribution through community organization);

4. direct education (combining both face-to-face and mediated education in classes, contests, and correspondence courses).

The broadcast media component included the repeated showing of 102 different public service announcements (PSAs), nine special television programs (one of which was an interactive viewer program and was 57 minutes long), five multipart news series, and 11 Spanish radio series (varying from 5 to 50 parts). Three television stations and two Spanish-language radio stations volunteered the broadcast time and expertise needed to carry out this effort. During the 5.5 years of education, two newspapers (one Spanish-language and one English-language) carried a weekly "doctor's column" which was written by project staff (total of 313 English-language columns and 224 Spanish-language columns). A third newspaper printed approximately 30 % of these columns. An additional 166 special features, food columns, news stories, and advertisements were presented in the four newspapers.

Direct education included over 800 professional education meetings, workshops, and seminars. These were attended by more than 15 000 health professionals, teachers, and worksite health promotion coordinators. An estimated 42 200 other individuals attended single or multiple-session risk reduction classes, and 890 enrolled in two correspondence courses on weight control and smoking cessation. In addition, 9 400 individuals participated in eight exercise, weight control, and quit-smoking contests. Risk reduction programs in worksites used contests, distribution of self-help materials, presentations and workshops, and consultation in establishing environmental and employee change programs in smoking, exercise, nutrition, and weight control. In the 3rd to 5th education years, 260 key personnel were contacted in 75 workplaces employing at least 100 employees. This led to educational programs for 7 500 employees in the 3rd year, followed by programs for 39 000 and 46 000 employees in the 4th and 5th years, respectively.

The education program also included components for children and their families. Cardiovascular risk reduction programs were designed for grades 3–7 and 10. These included special sessions on smoking and distribution of quit-smoking contest brochures, multifactor risk reduction classes for teachers and administrators, and complementary materials on exercise and nutrition provided for parents.

The total number of educational exposure episodes is the sum of those delivered by both mediated and direct channels; episodes vary in duration, intensity, and effectiveness. On average, each adult was exposed to 527 educational episodes. Of these 42 % were in the category of nutrition and weight. Blood pressure and smoking cessation each accounted for about 20 % of the messages, while about 8 % concerned either exercise or instructions pertaining to all risk factors. In all, 28 % of the total messages occurred in the first 2 years and 27 %, 21 %, and 25 % in the 3rd, 4th, and 5th years, respectively. When Spanish-language print, radio, and face-to-face messages are summed together and divided by the projected number of Spanish-speaking message recipients, these individuals were exposed to between 210 and 400 Spanish-language health messages in each year of the education program.

After 64 months of education, relative to mean changes from baseline measures in the control towns, the treatment cities show significantly increased knowledge about cardiovascular disease and significant decreases in plasma total cholesterol, risk of coronary heart disease, and total risk. Resting pulse, adiposity, and systolic and diastolic blood pressure also improved. Relative to the controls, knowledge was also significantly increased and total risk, resting pulse, percentage of smokers, and systolic and diastolic blood pressures were significantly decreased in the treatment cohort sample after 51 months of education. Thus, community-based education can be effective in achieving significant decreases in cardiovascular disease risk factors through changing behaviors.

It is evident from these studies that the health behavior of entire communities can be improved through appropriate methods of communication. The application of these and other relevant methods can perhaps be successfully applied to other problems of health education.

## References


1. Farquhar JW, Maccoby N, Wood PD, et al. (1977) Community education for cardiovascular health. Lancet i: 1192–1195
2. Maccoby N, Farquhar JW, Wood PD, et al. (1977) Reducing the risk of cardiovascular disease: effects of a community-based campaign on knowledge and behavior. J Community Health 23: 100–114
3. Puska P, Nissinen A, Tuomilehto J, et al. (1985) The community-based strategy to prevent coronary heart disease: conclusions from the ten years of the North Karelia Project. Ann Rev Public Health 6: 147–193
4. Lasater T, Abrams D, Artz L et al. (1984) Lay volunteer delivery of a community-based cardiovascular risk factor change program: the Pawtucket experiment. In: Matarazzo JD et al. (eds.) Behavioral health: a handbook of health enhancement and disease prevention. Wiley, New York, pp. 1166–1170
5. Backburn H, Luepker RV, Kline FG, et al. (1984) Lay volunteer delivery of a community-based cardiovascular risk factor change program: the Pawtucket experiment. In: Matarazzo JD et al. (eds) Behavioral health: a handbook of health enhancement and disease prevention. Wiley, New York, pp. 1171–1178
6. Cartwright D (1949) Some principles of mass persuasion. Hum Relations 2: 253–267
7. Bandura A (1986) Social foundations of thought and action. Prentice-Hall, Englewood Cliffs NJ
8. McGuire WJ (1964) Inducing resistance to persuasion: some contemporary approaches. In: Berkowitz L (ed) Advances in experimental social psychology, vol. 1. Academic, New York
9. Festinger L, Maccoby N (1964) On resistance to persuasive communications. J Abnormal and Social Psychology 68
10. Roberts DF (1974) Information processing and persuasion: counterarguing behavior. In: Kline F, Clark P (eds) Sage Communication Research Annuals, vol. 2. Sage, London
11. Telch MJ, Killen JD, McAlister A et al. (1982) Long-term follow-up of a pilot project of smoking prevention with adolescents. J Behav Med 5: 1–8
12. Killen JD, Telch MJ, Robinson T, Maccoby N (1988) Cardiovascular disease risk reduction for tenth graders: a multiple-factor school-based approach. JAMA 260 12: 1728–1733
13. Farquhar JW, Fortmann SP, Maccoby N, et al. (1986) The Stanford Five-City Project: design and methods. Am J Epidemiol 123: 656–669
14. Farquhar JW, Fortmann SP, Flora J, et al. (1990) The Stanford Five-City Project: effects of communitywide education on cardiovascular disease factors. JAMA 264 (3): 359–365

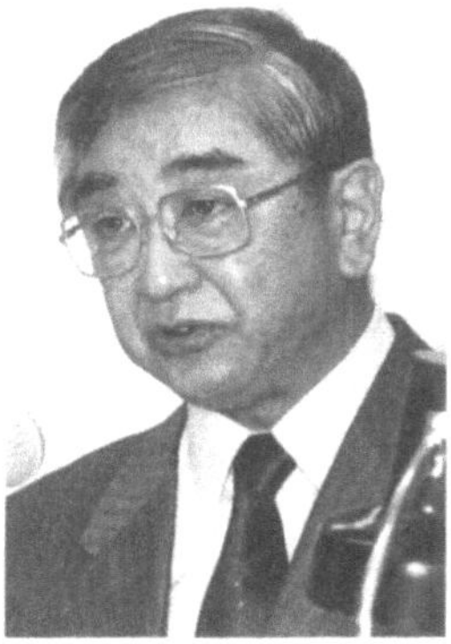

# 41. Risk Perception: Analyzing Images and Fears

Y. TANAKA

## Image, Reality, and Risk Communication

### *Image and Reality*

We cannot know what we call reality in the same direct fashion as a curious baby does, testing a bottle of milk by touch, by taste, by sniff, and by other manipulations. We know the evidence of our senses, but we also have the evidence that these senses are easily deceived. We make inferences about people from what they say and what they do, but these inferences often prove wrong, partly because the perceived image we have of people, their words, and their behavior, largely depend upon signs, or the indirect *pseudoenvironment,* which only fragmentally describes the object or person. The images we have of government, industry, or experts, therefore, might often contradict what they actually are. We also make inferences about things and events from what we hear other people say and what the mass media report about them. Again, these inferences often prove wrong, partly because the image we have of them, their nature and meaning, largely depend upon our pseudoenvironment. Thus we may perceive what is actually unsafe as safe and what is reasonably safe as unsafe.

Reality consists of numerous cognitive events, both physical and human. Of these cognitive events we have images, and these images in turn tend to be susceptible to distortion by a number of causes, such as preoccupation, misconception, prejudice, or inaccurate or inadequate information. Note, for example, how the nuclear reactor accident at Chernobyl on April 26, 1986 has eliminated the safety image of nuclear power worldwide. Because people had been told by government and industry that nuclear power was absolutely safe and because they believed what had been said, they now feel they have been maliciously deceived. They not only reject the safety image of nuclear power but distrust those who previously claimed its safety.

To the extent that almost all human behavior involves communication activities of some sort, and that humans make most crucial decisions for other humans as well as for themselves, there is good reason to believe that social and behavioral scientists share certain common research goals as well as research needs. During the past few decades, therefore, there have been a growing number of both theoretical and empirical investigations of the dynamics of human communication behavior in the conduct of interpersonal and social relations. Research that is relevant to such interpersonal and social communication problems has cut wide swaths through the social and behavioral sciences: attitude formations and change; the effect of context upon the interpretation of both perceptual and linguistic signs; interpersonal perception and group dynamics; and the interaction among beliefs, decisions, and social behavior [18, 19].

### *What Is Communication?*

From mentalists to behaviorists, over the last half century an intensive effort has been made to construct a general model of human behavior. Models which can explain human behavior have been developed by a number of behaviorists. Among these are a variety of cybernetic models that variably take into account the communication and control aspects of human behavior. In the simplest terms, these models presuppose a series of psychological processes in which one individual's or organizations's behavior, in the form of explicit *output* information produced by him or it, is dependent upon the *input* information that an individual or organization may receive from other people or organizations and from the environment. In order to examine their validity and discover their relevance to our problem, let us first look at some of these models.

As an initial point of reference, it is useful to keep Lasswell's [7] classic formula in mind. The scientific study of communication, he says, involves discovering:

Who says (the sender)
What (the message)
In which channel (the media)
To whom (the receiver), and
With what effect (the effect)

There is another type of model, the cybernetic one, first introduced by C. B. Shannon [17] for telephone communication and subsequently adjusted for human communication situations by C. E. Osgood [14].

On the basis of theory of these models, we now can make a more formal statement about the nature of human communication behavior. We can assume the existence of various processes of decoding and encoding between input and output events. *Decoding* here refers to the way in which the individual human (or organization) receives information from his environment – namely, the internal reaction caused by the input on the subject. *Encoding* designates these processes whereby the individual human (or organization) chooses some response, in the form of output, to the environment surrounding and affecting him or it. That which psychologists call *mediation process* is thus considered the bridge between decoding and encoding. In the simplest terms, it is the process which mediates between the sensory nervous process of decoding on the input side and the motor nervous process of encoding on the output side. Even in comparatively simple acts, such as making a speech, an individual's communicating behavior is complex, susceptible to many factors, as suggested above, and it is a continuously renewing process whereby the individual is always adapting to the environment.

### *Feedback Loop as the Building Block of the Social System*

At this point the term *feedback* is also relevant. It has been stated thus: "The action is initiated by an incongruity between the state of the organism and the state that is being tested for, and the action persists until the incongruity ... is removed" [11]. According to this view, the fundamental building block of the social system is the feedback loop [24].

Dealing with the complex organization and mechanisms of government, Karl Deutsch [1] defines feedback as "a communication network that produces action in response to an input of information, and includes the result of its own action in the new information by which it modifies its subsequent behavior". In other words, by this feedback mechanism, individual humans (or organizations) can correct errors and adjust their behavior to the continuously renewing environment.

Furthermore, in view of the present state of communication technology, interpersonal interaction is not necessarily limited to the face-to-face situation. The whole or part of an encoded message may be quoted in the newspaper, or broadcast by radio and television, or even relayed via communication satellite to the final destinations in foreign countries. It may also be possible for several individuals (and organizations as well) to exchange encoded messages continuously in a conversational mode, using the computer-communication (or "compunication") network. Today, thanks to the technological development of various electronic devices, a message can be encoded for literally universal mass consumption. Then, as the feedback loops become more complex and more diverse, the communication source will need some extended scanning devices or monitors to gather information. The communicator will continuously need to keep eye on local, national, and international communication channels and the messages transmitted through them, in order to meet with the communication need of the receivers.

### *Persuasion and the Effects of Communication*

Persuasion may be defined as the art of winning men's minds both by words and by deeds. The basic premise here is that persuasion is an act of communication. We must note, however, that it is a special kind of communication, often called purposive, and it is not involved in all communication situations in which behavior is influenced by a set of input stimuli. In order to be persuasive in nature, the communication situation must involve a conscious attempt by the communicator to influence the thought and behavior of the receiver through the transmission of some message.

Persuasive communication, therefore, implies a judgment of the situation and the receiver in terms of the intention of the communicator and the resultant thought or behavior change of the receiver. Persuasive communications can thus be judged with respect to their success in producing desired thought or behavior, or their failure to do so. Examples of success and failure of persuasive communication can be easily seen in advertising, public relations, election campaigns, or international diplomacy. In many cases successful persuasion involves two-way communication, the continuous process of feedback loops, between the source and the receiver.

Research on persuasive communication embraces the study of persuasiveness on the one hand, and persuadability on the other. It also involves the study of attitudes – how they are formed and how they can be changed. The focus of recent research on persuasion has been interrelationships among these variables, and the studies have been increasingly empirical or experimental, oriented toward the theory of attitude organization and change. Comprehensive reviews and summaries of the relevant literature can be found in publications by, e.g., McGuire [8,9,10], and Upmeyer [23].

## *The Nature of Risk Communication*

The science of human communication is a relatively young science. It is interdisciplinary, sharing its major methodologies and theories with adjacent disciplines such as psychology, sociology, political science, journalism, and media research [15]. It has constructed a number of general models of communication and developed its own vocabulary. The preceding sections of this chapter have shown some of the general models of communication and the key concepts frequently used in communication research. Within the science of human communication, risk communication constitutes a new, unique branch. The unique nature of risk communication may be summarized in its definition as "an interactive process of exchange of information and opinions, among individuals, groups, and institutions, involving messages about the nature of risk or expressing concerns, opinions, or reactions to risk messages or to legal and institutional arrangements for risk management" [13].

It must be noted here that the unique need for risk communication has arisen from the very fact that our modern life is increasingly surrounded by such hazards as pollutants in the air and in drinking water, pesticide residues in food and milk, threats from radiation and toxic chemicals, adverse drug reactions (ADR), or the new socioepidemiological hazard commonly known as AIDS. Government, industry, and people at large do not have sufficient experience and are incapable of knowing about and coping with the increasing lethal risks surrounding them. Hence, risk communication involves the elements of purposive communication, for its ultimate objective is to enhance the accurate knowledge of the risks and improve the ways in which government, industry, and

people can cope with those risks jointly and intelligently. The basic premise of risk communication should therefore:
1. Convey the messages containing information, concerns, and opinions about risk
2. Involve the continuing feedback loops between the source and the receiver
3. Be a process of purposive (or persuasive) social communication, involving a number of sociocultural and psychological factors.

During the last decade, there was a sharp increase in the number of both theoretical and empirical studies on risk perception and communication, notably in the United States. The emergence of research on risk perception and communication itself may be taken as an indication of the mounting public awareness and concern about various risks arising from environmental and man-made hazards. Comprehensive reviews and summaries of those studies on risk perception and communication can be found in various publications [2,3,4,12,13,16].

## Japanese studies on Risk Perception and Communication

Empirical research on risk perception and communication has a relatively short history in Japan. Early in the 1980s, some research began with investigating laypeople's perception of the nuclear risks and benefits compared with those of other natural and man-made hazards [20]. In the late 1980s and within the RAD-AR initiative, several empirical studies were carried out to examine the perceived risks of drugs and ADR. The results of earlier RAD-AR studies were summarized and reported by Fujino [5]. In the following sections, some of the major findings of relevant empirical research conducted in Japan of risk perception and communication will be briefly presented and discussed.

### *Risk/Benefit Perception Gaps Between Laypeople and Experts*

In a recent publication by the National Research Council [13], a group of American experts observed that a wide range of differences exist between laypeople and experts in their risk perception and communication, so that these differences obstruct effective communication between the two. Some examples may be quoted from their observation:
1. Laypeople and experts speak different languages
2. Laypeople and experts solve different problems
3. Laypeople and experts disagree about what is feasible
4. Laypeople and experts see the facts differently

The findings of Japanese RAD-AR surveys reported by Fujino [5] and Hirano [6] appear to support the foregoing observations made by the Americans:
1. Regarding physicians' explanation of both efficacy of drugs and ADRs, four out of five (83 %) physicians and seven out of ten (68 %) laypeople surveyed

were affirmative about physicians' explanations of efficacy, and seven out of ten (68 %) physicians and two out of five (44 %) laypeople were affirmative about physicians' explanation of ADR.
It is clear that, whether regarding efficacy or ADR, significantly more physicians believe physicians give an adequate explanation to patients than laypeople do.

2. With respect to the psychological need for information about drugs, as many as nine out of ten (88 %) laypeople, in contrast to only one out of three (37 %) physicians, regard information about efficacy as both necessary and desirable. Nearly all (92 %) laypeople and two-thirds (62 %) of the physicians regard information about ADR as both necessary and desirable. It is obvious that laypeople are more enthusiastic about obtaining information on drugs and ADR than physicians, who think they are already sufficiently giving such information to patients. Japanese physicians thus do not seem to be meeting with patients' information needs for various reasons.
3. Opinions about ADR are widely different between laypeople and physicians. For example, while nearly one out of two (46 %) laypeople and one out of five (20 %) physicians believe ADR should never occur, one out of ten (13 %) laypeople and two out of five (44 %) physicians recognize ADR as unavoidable. For a great majority of laypeople, ADR are something to be avoided at all costs, and should they occur even by chance, laypeople would prefer the drug not to be used for them. Generally, laypeople tend to reveal more stringent, negative attitudes against ADR than do physicians.
4. Laypeople and physicians tend to disagree about the causes of ADR. More than half (55 %) of the laypeople and nearly four out of five (74 %) physicians consider ADR occur only to certain people under certain disease conditions; two out of five (43 %) laypeople and one out of four (27 %) physicians think they occur only from taking an excessive dose. Thus, compared with laypeople, more physicians seem to believe ADR occur only by chance and are only attributable to the patients' particular conditions rather than to the physicians' responsibility.
5. In still another comparison, laypeople and physicians disagree as to who is responsible for ADR. For laypeople, the government (39 %) is more responsible for ADR than are individual physicians (32 %), and the pharmaceutical industry (31 %). For physicians, both the pharmaceutical industry (31 %) and the government (30 %) are more responsible than individual physicians (25 %).

Apart from the RAD-AR studies, Tanaka [20,21] found similar perceptual differences between laypeople and experts in his comparative studies on the perceived nuclear risks and benefits among the Japanese. Figures 1 and 2 display a two-dimensional representation of the perceived risks and benefits of various objects, Fig. 1 for nuclear experts ($n$=545) and Fig. 2 for nonexperts consisting of university students and their parents living in Tokyo ($n$=630). It is clearly seen from Figs. 1 and 2 that both groups significantly agree in their risk/benefit judgments on serious natural hazards and lethal illnesses. The two groups similarly perceive these hazardous objects as both risk and nonbenefit. On the

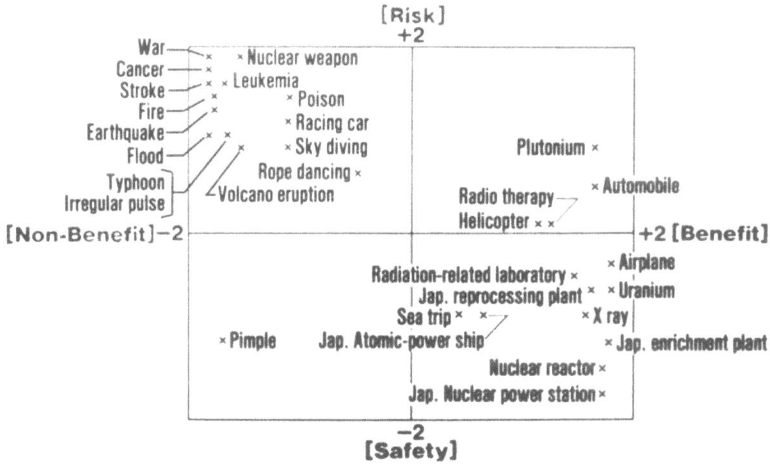


**Fig. 1.** Risk/benefit perception of nuclear experts [20]

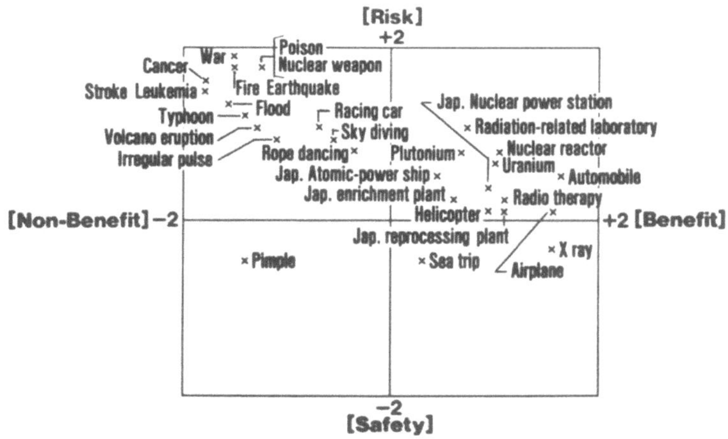


**Fig. 2.** Risk/benefit perception of nonexperts I [21]

other hand, while the nuclear experts perceive most nuclear objects as both safe and beneficial, with only the two exceptions of plutonium and radiotherapy which are both regarded as risky *but* beneficial, the nonexperts perceive the same nuclear objects as risky but beneficial with only one exception, X-ray, which is rated both safe and beneficial. We thus have an indication that laypeople tend to perceive the same nuclear objects as more risky than do nuclear experts. It may also be noteworthy that automobile is rated as risky but (far more) beneficial. The latter is true for groups.

In a recent RAD-AR study, [6,21] of which I was principal investigator, risk/benefit perceptions of various medical and pharmaceutical objects were examined with a total of 630 Japanese male and female university students

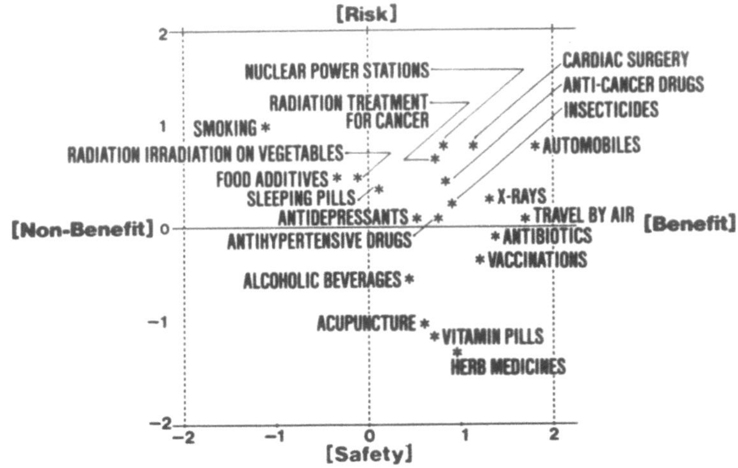


**Fig. 3.** Risk/benefit perception of nonexperts II [21]

serving as young, educated lay subjects. Figure 3 shows a two-dimensional representation of their risk/benefit perception. There are three objects – smoking, irradiation on vegetables, and food additives – which are perceived by the subjects as both risk and nonbenefit and, hence, to be rejected. Note, on the other hand, that the subjects regarded both nuclear power stations and radiation treatment for cancer as a risk but a benefit to almost the same degree and hence much more acceptable than smoking, for example. It is also interesting to find that acupuncture and herb medicine, both types of traditional Oriental medicine, are perceived by the Japanese youth as both safe and beneficial, similar to vitamin pills. Finally, automobile is again found to be risky but (far more) beneficial showing a steady cultural consistency operating in the risk/benefit perception among the Japanese.

### *Fears and the Personality Factors*

In the foregoing Japanese RAD-AR study [6], an attempt was also made to examine correspondence between fears and personality factors. To measure the varying intensity of fears toward different objects of judgment, subjects were asked to rate ADR, sickness, death, earthquake, and nuclear accident, on a five-point fearful-not fearful scale. They were simultaneously asked to check a battery of personality test items. The data were then submitted to multivariate analyses to examine the implicit structure and interrelationships among these variables.

First, by way of using factor analysis, a total of 14 meaningful factors were obtained. Those factors included, in order of their factor salience:

1. *Mysticism believing* (e.g., believe palm-reading; believe in fortune-telling; believe in astrology)

2. *Health attentiveness* (e.g., carefully read instructions on medicine; careful not to smoke too heavily; careful not to drink too much)
3. *Technology acceptance* (e.g., look forward to external fertilization of humans; advance genetic recombination and biotechnology; promote the ability to determine the sexes of fetus)
4. *Risk sensitivity* (e.g., fearful of diseases; fearful of ADR; fearful of death)
5. *Aggressiveness* (e.g., answer back whenever criticized; cannot stand being treated rudely; want to be conspicuous in everything)
6. *Inventiveness* (e.g., want to invent various things; like to play with new ideas)
7. *Food-safety consciousness* (e.g., do not eat food containing synthetic coloring agents, etc.; do not eat any foodstuff produced in areas radioactively contaminated; like to eat natural food); and
8. *Medication dependence* (e.g., currently taking prescribed medicine; currently taking medicine to maintain good health; like to see a physician to maintain good health)

Secondly, on the basis of the factor analytic result, factor scores were computed for each variable and for every subject along each factor dimension. Then, the data were submitted to multiple regression analysis, to examine the correspondence between the intensity of fear toward each object of judgment, as a dependent variable, and the factor scores of personality variables, as independent variables. In all cases examined, highly significant ($p < 0.001$) multiple correlations were obtained, even if the magnitudes of correlation were not very impressive. Those significant correlations appear to indicate that the intensity of fear toward a certain object may be predicted in part from personality traits. The result of this multiple regression analysis will be summarized in the following, with only the statistically significant ($p < 0.05$) independent personality variables mentioned.

1. *ADR*. The more health-attentive and aggressive people are the more they are inclined to fear ADR.
2. *Sickness*. The more medication dependent, inventive, and health-attentive people are, the more they are inclined to fear sickness.
3. *Death*. The more health-attentive and aggressive people are, the more they are inclined to fear death.
4. *Earthquake*. The more mysticism-believing, food-safety conscious, and health-attentive people are, and the less they are inventive and accept technology, the more they are inclined to fear earthquakes.
5. *Nuclear accident*. The more food-safety conscious and health-attentive people are, and the less they accept technology, the more they are inclined to fear nuclear accidents.
6. *All objects combined*. The more health-attentive, food-safety conscious, and aggressive people are, the more they are inclined to fear hazardous things.

Although further studies will be needed in this respect, particularly for cross-cultural comparisons, it is still interesting to note that the kind and magnitude of contribution of independent variables vary as the objects of judgment become different; the health-attentiveness factor seems to be a constant predictor across all the objects of judgment.

*Segmentation of the Risk-Communication Audience*

It is generally believed that women are more sensitive to risks than men. To test this and other hypotheses, a study was carried out by Tanaka [22] with a total of 500 housewives living in Tokyo serving as subjects.

*Risk/Benefit Perception Among Japanese Housewives.* Figure 4 summarizes the risk/benefit perception of nine common objects by 500 Japanese housewives. There seems to be a high degree of consensus about three high-risk/low-benefit objects; with over 80 % of subjects regarding food additives, spray using chlorofluorocarbon gas, and smoking as risks, while only less than 40 % of them seeing these as benefits. In a similar fashion, both herbal medicine and vitamins can be categorized as low-risk/high-benefit; and nuclear power plant, oil thermal power plant and travel by airplane, as medium-risk/high-benefit. Again, automobile proves to be high-risk/high-benefit, with nearly all the subjects perceiving it as both risky and beneficial.

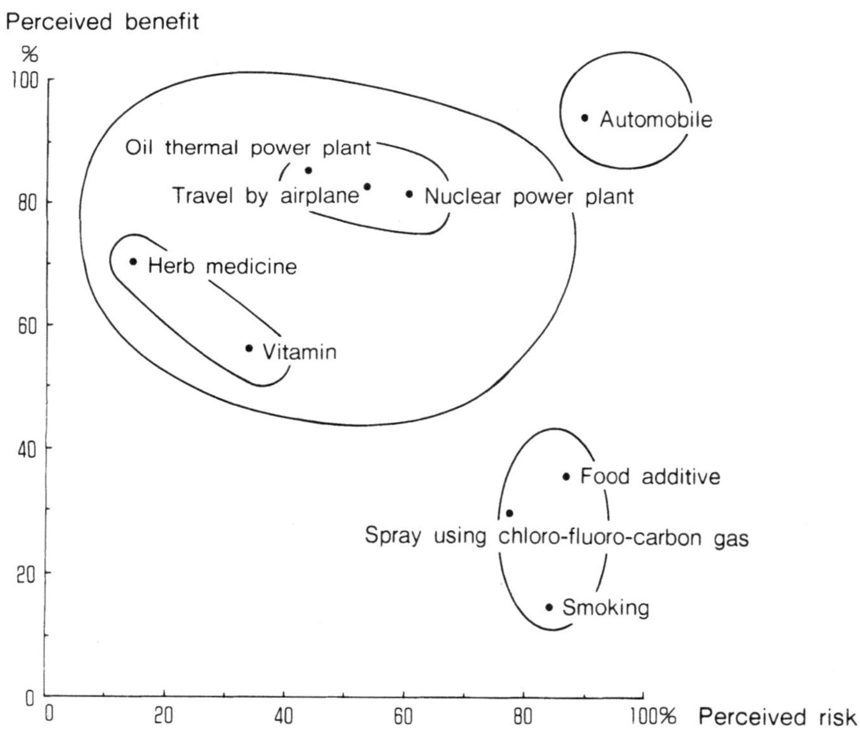


**Fig. 4.** Risk/benefit perception of Tokyo housewives [22]

Although no direct comparison between sexes was possible in this study, the result seems quite consistent with those of the earlier studies mentioned above which involved males only and both sexes. Such overall similarities may be partly attributed to the overwhelming influence of the mass media that serves to crystalize the public's attitudes and behavior into general cultural conformity.

*Segmentation of Japanese Housewives as the Communication Audience.* By using the same data obtained from the 500 Tokyo housewives, some correlational analysis was carried out in order to examine the interrelationship among the attitudinal variables. More than 200 attidudinal variables (question items) were thus submitted to factor analysis and a total of 29 factors were obtained as a result. Out of those factors, two salient factors – social participation and perceived risk and benefit – were then chosen for subsequent cluster analysis. The cluster analysis in this study was intended as a useful method for investigating how 500 housewives can be divided into independent groups on the basis of the subjects' personal attributes, such as age, education, and material status, and their various attitudes toward social participation and risk/benefit perception. Finally, five meaningful clusters were obtained. They are shown in Fig. 5 in a two-dimensional representation defined by the social participation and risk/benefit perception factors. Each cluster was then named, according to the unique attributive and attitudinal characteristics of component subjects. For reference to the specificity of each cluster, the name and some typical characteristics are shown below.

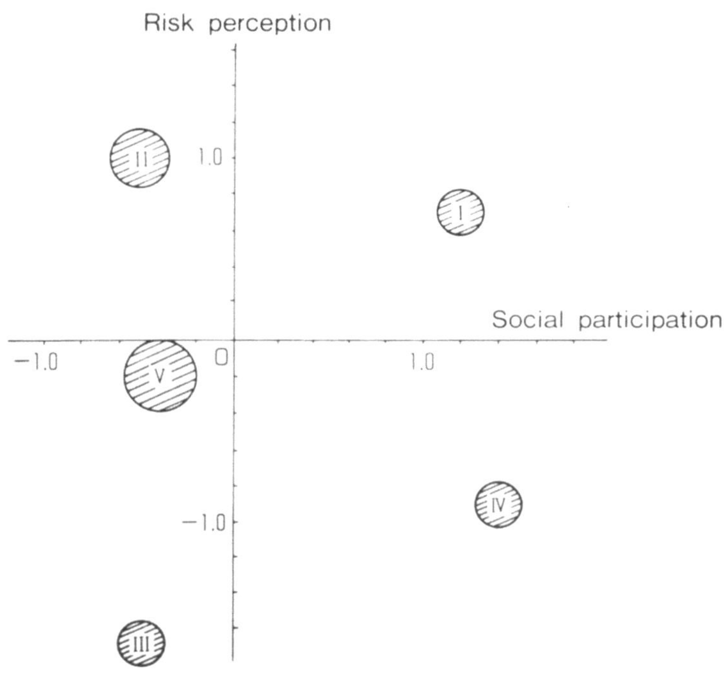


**Fig. 5.** Segmentation of receivers of risk communication (Tokyo housewives) [22]

- *Cluster-1* "Conservative activists"; ($n$=72); mostly in the 30–40 years age group; mostly highschool graduates; many working; interested in participating in anti-nuclear-weapon, anti-nuclear-power, antipollution protests; interested in political and economic affairs; perceive nuclear energy as dangerous but beneficial.
- *Cluster-2* "Optimistic silent majority"; ($n$=121); some in the 20–30 years and many in 30–40 years age groups; mostly highschool graduates; few working; not interested in environmental problems, political and economic affairs, and nuclear-energy issues; perceive nuclear energy as both safe and beneficial.
- *Cluster-3* "Socially indifferent"; ($n$=56); mostly in the 40–50 years age group; mostly highschool or trade-school graduates; not interested in environmental problems, political and economic affairs; not interested in participating in anti-nuclear-weapon, anti-nuclear-power, or anti-pollution protests; perceive nuclear energy as not needed.
- *Cluster-4* "Progressive activists"; ($n$=56); mostly in the 30–40 years age group; mostly university, college, and junior-college graduates; only a few working; interested in political, economic, and international affairs; interested in participating in volunteer activities, antinuclear-weapon and anti-nuclear-energy protests, and peace demonstrations; perceive nuclear energy as dangerous and not beneficial; criticize nuclear power plants as not being safe; believe science does not contribute to enrichment of life.
- *Cluster-5* "Average silent majority"; ($n$=195); mostly in the 30–40 years age group; many trade-school graduates; few working; interested in television sports programs and shopping magazines; not interested in anti-nuclear-weapon, anti-nuclear-energy and anti-pollution protests; perceive nuclear energy as beneficial.

The foregoing clustering of 500 Japanese women may illustrate the uniquenesses of the attributes and attitudinal system characteristic of each group. The findings may also present an important problem for the pursuit of effective risk communication. As has been pointed out, the audience of risk communication is never homogeneous, differing in personal attributes, values, beliefs, and attitudes to a wide variety of things and people. Effective risk communication, therefore, should take into account those differences in the target audience.

Finally, the result of the above-mentioned Japanese study suggests the need for further systematic studies in the social and behavioral science domains for examining

a) reasonable segmentations among the heterogeneous receivers;
b) the specific content of risk communication which might be appropriate and adequate to a particular segment of the receivers; and
c) the ultimate effectiveness and usefulness of risk communication in view of public acceptance of advanced science and technology and their products.

## References


1. Deutsch KW (1963) The nerves of government. Free Press, New York, p. 88
2. Fischhoff B (1990) Psychology and public policy. Am Psychol 45 (5): 641–646
3. Fischhoff B, Lichtenstein S, Slovic P, Derby SL, Keeney RL (1981) Acceptable risk. Cambridge University Press, London
4. Fischhoff B, Svenson O, Slovic P (1987) Active responses to environmental hazards: perception and decision making. In: Stokols D, Altman I (eds) Handbook of environmental psychology. Wiley, New York, pp. 1089–1133
5. Fujino S (1988) Risk perception of prescription drugs: report on surveys in Japan. In: Horisberger B, Dinkel R (eds) The perception and management of drug safety risks. Springer, Berlin Heidelberg New York Tokyo, pp. 112–116
6. Hirano H (1990) Public attidudes and perception. In: Shimizu N, Tanaka Y, Jones J, Taylor D (eds) Improving drug safety: the assessment, management, and communication of the therapeutic benefits and risks of pharmaceutical products. Pharma International, Tokyo pp 70–84
7. Lasswell HD (1948) The structure and function of communication in society. In: Bryson L (ed) The communication of ideas. Harper and Row, New York, p. 37
8. McGuire WJ (1964) Introducing resistance to persuasion. In: Berkowitz L (ed) Advances in experimental social psychology, vol 1. Academic, New York, p. 191
9. McGuire WJ (1969) The nature of attitudes and attitude change. In: Lindzey G, Aronson B (eds) The handbook of social psychology, vol 3. 2nd edn, Addison-Wesley, Reading, Mass, pp. 136–314
10. McGuire WJ (1985) Attitude and attitude change. In: Lindzey G and Aronson B (eds) Handbook of social psychology, vol 2. 3rd edn Random House, New York, pp. 233–346
11. Miller GA, Galanter E, Pribram KH (1960) Plans and the structure of behavior. Holt, New York, p. 26
12. Morris LA (1990) Communicating therapeutic risks. Springer. Berlin Heidelberg New York Tokyo
13. National Research Council (1989) improving risk communication. National Academy Press, Washington, DC
14. Osgood CB (1963) Psycholinguistics. In: Koch S (ed) Psychology: a study of a science, vol 6. McGraw-Hill, New York, p. 247
15. Schramm W (ed) (1963) The science of human communication. Basic, New York
16. Schwing RC, Albers WA (1980) Societal risk assessment: how safe is safe enough? Plenum, New York
17. Shannon CE (1949) The mathematical theory of communication. In: Shannon CE, Weaver W (eds) The mathematical theory of communication. University of Illinois Press, Urbana. Ill
18. Tanaka Y (1971) Psychological factors in international perception. Annals of the American Academy of Political and Social Sciences 398: 50–60
19. Tanaka Y (1976) What is communication? In: De McLaurin R, Rosenthal CF, Skillings SA (eds) The art and sciences of psychological operations: case studies of military application, vol 1, Headquarters, Department of the Army, Washington, DC, pp. 20–22
20. Tanaka Y (1985) Sociology of nuclear energy (in Japanese). Denryoku Shinpo Sha, Tokyo
21. Tanaka Y (1989) The Chernobyl syndrome (in Japanese). Denryoku Shinpo Sha, Tokyo
22. Tanaka Y (1990) An audience analysis of risk communication: segmentation of Tokyo housewives born in the Showa era. Proceedings of the XXXlst Annual Congress of the Japanese Social Psychology Association, Tokyo (in press)
23. Upmeyer A (ed) (1989) Attitudes and behavioral decisions, Springer, Berlin Heidelberg New York Tokyo
24. Wiener N (1960) The human use of human beings. Houghton Mifflin, Boston, p. 12

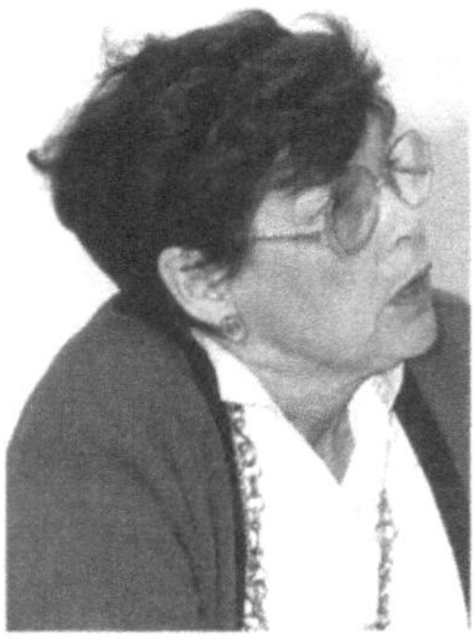

# 42. New Channels for the Patients

K. Whitehorn

Such innovations and improvements as I would like to suggest follow from the points I made in an earlier chapter (see "The Patients' View") about patient expectations, which are high, and their knowledge, which is low.

The pharmacist, now freed from having to spend time grinding up his pills and powders himself, is the most obvious link in the chain to strengthen. He is at the patient's level, speaks with a local accent, perhaps – or even the patient's language: there are over 100 languages in common use in London alone. If he has difficulty in checking back with the doctor when something has alerted his suspicion, we might consider an exdirectory line between surgery and dispensary; at any rate, we should aim for a closer understanding between doctor and dispenser, and in the words of one pharmacists: "It would help if the doctors knew our names."

I also wonder if there is a role for *a middle category of drugs* – not "on prescription" or "over-the-counter" but "prescribed by the pharmacist." If patients were encouraged to register with their pharmacists, as has been suggested, the ability to prescribe might be limited to those patients who were on that pharmacist's list. There is in Britain a class of drugs that are only to be sold if the pharmacist is on the premises, but the rule says nothing about how visibly present, helpful, or even awake the pharmacist has to be. A category to encourage the pharmacist to take a far more active part in the health care of his customers might have quite a few unexpected benefits.

More written information available to the patient would help. In Sweden there is the Patient-FASS (Pharmaceutical Specialties in Sweden); in France, there is a dictionary of drugs compiled by Professor Giroud; the nearest we have to it in Britain is a loose-leaf directory put out by the North East Thames Health Authority. It would be a good idea if these were available, not just in libraries, but in general practitioners' surgeries as well; then a patient could look up what the doctor had prescribed and find more detail than the doctor had probably had time to give him.

Patient groups, I am convinced, have a great future as channels of information. In Britain the single-disease groups for chronic sufferers are essential to people like diabetics, those with Parkinson's, multiple sclerosis sufferers, and so forth; they know more than anyone. Patient representatives can get together to put across a point of view, either to government, the pharmaceutical industry, or else. The Patients' Association, which I represent, has recently formed a Patients' Forum for other concerned national groups to meet – outfits like Age Concern, the National Association for the Welfare of Children in Hospital, MIND for the mentally ill, and so forth. I was much struck on a recent visit to Walton Hospital in Liverpool by the effectiveness of a group course run for pain sufferers (Walton has a renowned Pain Relief clinic). These were people for whom medicine could do no more, but simply by sharing their feelings and pooling their experiences, they were doing one another a power of good – and that was almost literally what it was: they had Tai Chi, they supported each other; the main change was that their feeling of control over their situation was increased.

Phone-ins are increasingly a source of information and shared experience among patients; phone lines, where a patient can ring a number and listen to a tape on a particular subject, are increasingly useful, and the Medical Advisory Service in Britain is beginning to market cassette tapes which will be sold over the counter at the pharmacist's.

When it comes to that invaluable source of information, the women's magazines, what is wanted, I think, is not a change of medium but a change of emphasis. Instead of going only to strictly medical journalists, the industry should try to involve the editors and the consumer writers, so that they may encourage patients to ask more questions and to be more vociferous. If we want to encourage a "culture of reporting" in which patients report the adverse or unexpected effects of drugs instead of just flushing them down the drain, it will have to emanate from the women's magazines as much as from anywhere.

As multiple dosing becomes more and more of a problem and since the elderly, the main drug takers, live longer and absorb more medicines, so patient-held records are becoming, to my mind, almost a necessity. Even if it is only a simplified form of record of what else the patient is taking which the patient presents to the pharmacist with the prescription, it might still help enormously. The medical profession looks askance at patient-held records. They are afraid the patients will lose them; however, the British experience is that wherever patient-held records have been tried out, the patients lose them a lot less often than the hospitals; computerization might enable backup data to be stored as well.

Finally, I would urge that questions about drugs, prescribing, and health habits be included in market research that is being conducted for other reasons. It is always hard to get straight answers out of people when they have a firm idea of what you want them to say, and nowhere more than in the field of health. More honest and unexpected answers might come from research done in a mixed context. And to this I would add that there is a serious need for far more test marketing of the information as well as the product.

But the industry should not expect the patients ever to take quite the same view of risk as they do: if I am feeling bad I may be only 0.06 % of the sample, but I am still 100 % of me. There will always be a different viewpoint – and more information than we can ever absorb; it is up to the industry to make sure it is accessible. It might follow the example of the United States Navy and try to devise "a system designed by geniuses to be run by idiots." I am not saying patients are idiots, only that they should not have to be geniuses to get information.

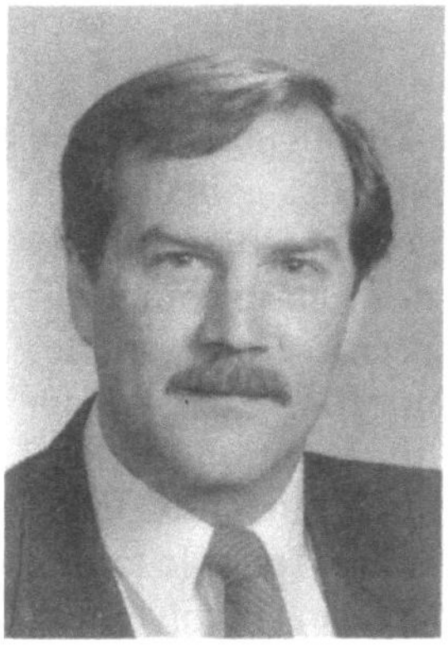

# 43. The Patients-in-the-Know Program

J. DOMEISCHEL

## Situation

Throughout the 1980s, consumer groups and the media led the demand to improve patients' understanding of medicines prescribed by their doctors. According to the National Council on Patient Information and Education (NCPIE), of the nearly two billion prescriptions filled annually in the United States, approximately half are taken improperly [2]. In addition, nearly 100 million prescription orders per year go unfilled or unrefilled. Two of every five patients skip doses or take "holidays" from their medication for 3 or more days. In a recent public opinion poll, approximately 75 % of the people reported that they stopped taking their medicine when they thought they "felt better"; 63 % said they "just forgot." More than 80 % said they were likely to take a little less medicine or take it less frequently than the physician prescribed [5]. Moreover, one-third of those patients who supplemented their prescription medication with over-the-counter medications did not seek their physician's advice before doing so [1].

## Noncompliance – The Other Drug Problem

All this adds up to what Dr. Robert Windom, the United States assistant secretary for health, calls "the other drug problem", one not as obvious as that of heroin and cocaine, but one that also threatens our health [2]. When people do not comply with their physician's instructions, they may not get well, they could suffer avoidable side effects, or could be hospitalized for drug misuse [4]. In short, quality health care is not attained.

In addition to the unnecessary human suffering, the cost of noncompliance is staggering – an estimated $ 22 billion a year in the United States alone for doctor and hospital visits, diagnostic tests, and additional drugs, according to research conducted by Dr. William Seidman, associate clinical professor of neurological surgery at the University of California, San Francisco [3].

## Health Care Professional/Patient Dialogue

To help eliminate the needless costs and illness that can result from improper use of prescription drugs, Paul Rogers, the Chairman of NCPIE, called for a dialogue between health care professionals and their patients in 1983 [6]. To prescription users, this dialogue with physicians and the information communicated about their medication is key to their therapeutic success. For example, nine out of ten prescription users believe it is very important to have an understanding from their health care professional about prescription medication, according to a recent national survey of 1000 people currently using prescription drugs. This finding is consistent with today's trend of people taking a more active role regarding their health. But despite the increasing involvement of patients with their own health care needs, patients must still rely on their physicians for prescription information.

## Assisting the Health Care Professional in Communicating with Patients

Patient's poor recall of information received from doctors about their drug regimen is a key factor in their poor compliance records. To help doctors overcome this problem with their patients and, thus, enhance patient compliance with treatment regimens, some consumer groups and the media have called for written prescription information which patients could take home from their physicians' offices. This information would be different in format and would serve as a supplement to the mandated package inserts already provided with pharmaceutical products. These consumer groups cite research which has shown that effective communication is a major component of patient satisfaction with the care received and their compliance with prescribed treatment regimens. The concept of information written in easily understood terms has been well received in a recent survey of 1000 prescription users – fully four out of five respondents thought this form of written information would be very useful.

## The Patients-in-the-Know Program

Despite past educational campaigns, the media have continued to call for more effective solutions to the prescription drug compliance problem. Thus, the Patients-in-the-Know program of Searle was developed to help meet this call. Searle wanted to take a leadership role in assisting the health care professional in effectively communicating to patients information about its prescription drugs on a global basis. Before launching such a program, Searle conducted research with its key audience on both the United States and international levels. This research was charged with determining the need for a patient information program, and its potential success with the program's target groups. On an international level, the research set out to determine the current requirements or climate in each country where Searle has a presence.

In the United States, the research included personal interviews with 248 office-based physicians, telephone surveys of 250 pharmacists, both chain and independent, and personal interviews with 800 consumers. All three audiences reacted favorably to the program concept, although physicians were less certain about using the program than were pharmacists. The overwhelming majority of consumers – 86 % – said they would read the information. Internationally, the research reported that an information program was already required in some countries for both prescription and over-the-counter medication, and not allowed in others.

This research provided the foundation for the Patients-in-the-Know program in the United States. The program was the third in Searle's series of United States social responsibility initiatives, or "Patients" programs. It follows the Patients-in-Need program in which Searle provides its products free to those who otherwise cannot afford them, and the Patients-Promise program in which Searle will refund the out-of-pocket cost for a product if it does not achieve the desired therapeutic benefit.

The Patients-in-the-Know program was among the first worldwide comprehensive efforts by a pharmaceutical company to make available through physicians and pharmacists easy-to-understand information about its prescription products. The initial United States version of this information, printed in English and Spanish, was on pads of tear-off Searle prescription information sheets for the medications Calan SR and Cytotec, with new products to be added as appropriate.

Unlike the technical package inserts which are required to inform doctors on all prescription drugs, the Searle prescription information sheets were designed for use by health care professionals in communicating information in lay terms and language that their patients can understand. They feature a photograph of the product, explain some of the reasons the doctor prescribed the medication, how the medicine should be taken, explain potential side effects and what to do if they are experienced, and give specific precautions about any potential drug interactions. The sheets also contain space for the doctor's additional personal instructions to the patient. The Searle prescription information sheets are designed to be distributed by physicians at their discretion – no specific drug information is given directly to patients. This recognizes the unique relationship between doctor and patient and is intended to build on that relationship.

Prior to the announcement of the Patients-in-the-Know program. Searle obtained program endorsements from the American Medical Association, the National Institute on Aging (NIA), the American Academy of Family Physicians, and the patient advocacy group, Medicine in the Public Interest. These endorsements helped lend stature to the program in the eyes of the medical community and the general public.

Two weeks before the launch of the Patients-in-the-Know program Searle notified physicians across the nation about the program. Even before the launch's public announcement, Searle received over 6000 requests from physicians for the Searle prescription information sheets. Physicians could request the information at no charge using a business reply card, a special toll-free number, or by asking their Searle sales representative.

Another element in the United States program addressed the needs of pharmacists. The Patients-in-the-Know program provided pharmacists with copies of a brochure to distribute to patients getting their prescriptions filled. The brochure contains important information applicable to all prescription pharmaceuticals. Like physicians, pharmacists were notified of the program 2 weeks in advance and demonstrated their enthusiasm by requesting over 12 000 pharmacy kits even before the program was publicly announced.

The elements in the Patients-in-the-Know program were designed to enhance communications and improve the relationship between patients and physicians and between patients and pharmacists, creating a partnership that maximizes patient compliance and the quality of health care. This improved communication has provided lasting benefits for both health care professionals and their patients. The Searle prescription information sheets reinforce patient confidence in the doctor even when patients are not in the office. The pharmacist benefits in that the brochure enhances his or her professional status. This take-home information benefits patients by encouraging them to comply with their drug regimen as prescribed and ultimately helps ensure their therapeutic success.

## Results

In the United States, the Searle Patients-in-the-Know program has been recognized for its leadership and value by congressional leaders and the medical community. The news media nationwide covered the announcement of the launch of the program and articles ran in major United States newspapers, including *The New York Times, The Chicago Tribune, The St. Louis Post-Dispatch,* and through syndicated columns such as *The People's Pharmacy*. The Associated Press carried the story nationwide. Total media coverage for the program exceeded 200 million impressions.

Even more important, the program has been used widely by health care professionals. More than 25 000 physicians have participated in the program and have distributed over 100 000 prescription information sheets. Participating pharmacists have distributed over 25 000 pharmacy kits. Searle has also launched the program on a worldwide basis, wherever appropriate. In addition to program participation, many health care professionals have added appreciative comments on their request cards for additional materials.

Given this enthusiastic participation on the part of health care professionals, Searle is confident that the Patients-in-the-Know program is meeting its overall objective of assisting in the improvement of the unique relationship between health care professionals and their patients, and helping our health care system operate safely and efficiently.

## Reference

1. Center for Economic Studies in Medicine (1989) Patients and their medications: the prescription information gap. Searle survey
2. Cohn V (1989) Confronting the other drug problem. The Washington Post, October 7

3. Heller LJ (1989) Taking care; playing dice with medicine. The New York Times, April 16, Sec. 6,8
4. Hinds M (1989) Consumer Saturday information on drugs for patient. The New York Times, February 26, Sec. 1,48
5. National Council on Patient Information and Education (1989) Fleishman Hillard press release, October 19
6. Wilke J (1983) Prescription drugs used improperly, FDA chief says. The Washington Post, July 30, A4

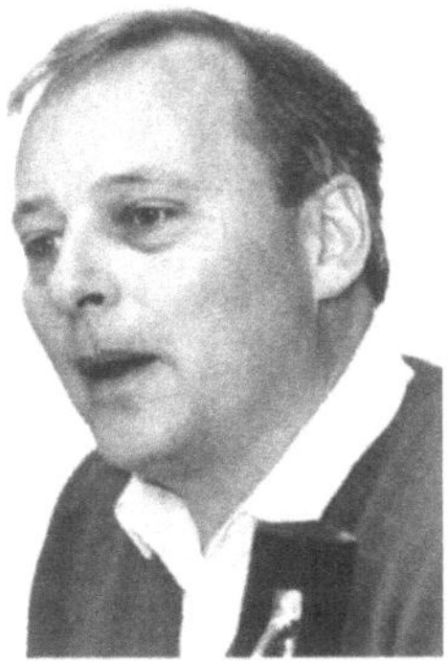

# 44. Information for the Public: A Swedish Example

B.-E. Wiholm and A.-G. Hedstrand

"The time is now past when health-encouraging precautions were a privilege for knowledgeable individuals who kept their professional secrets to themselves and gave doses of them to uninformed, passive patients who lined up for their health."

This 1983 statement by the former secretary general of the WHO, Dr. Mahler, indicated that people responsible for medical attendance had begun to realize that the patient has a legitimate need and right to be informed of his sickness and its treatment. The same attitude is reflected in the Swedish Health and Medical Care Act instituted in 1983, which states that patients have the right to be fully informed about their diseases, the consequences thereof, and the medical treatments available – including the risks involved. Here we will give an overview of some endeavors related to drug information through nontraditional channels, with special emphasis on three programs:

- *Patient-FASS* – a book sold to the public with comprehensive information on medicines available in Sweden.
- Drug information leaflets – limited practical information on the class effects and adverse reactions of the drug dispensed; handed out in pharmacies.
- The educational programs in schools and for the elderly run by the Swedish Medicines Information Council.

## Background

Health care in Sweden is mainly administered by the public sector. Only 2 000 out of 26 000 physicians work in the private sector. All 900 pharmacies are managed by The National Corporation of Pharmacies, which is a state-owned monopoly. About 2 850 pharmaceutical specialties have been approved for general marketing in Sweden by the Medical Products Agency (MPA). The total number of active substances in these pharmaceutical specialties is about 1 100, and there are relatively few pharmaceutical specialties with more than one active ingredient.

Comprehensive information on all marketed pharmaceutical specialties has been published since 1966 in a book called *FASS* (Pharmaceutical Specialties in Sweden). This book, which is the equivalent of the *Physicians' Desk Reference (PDR)* in the United States, the *Data Sheet Compendium* in the United Kingdom, *Die Rote Liste* in the Federal Republic of Germany, and the *Vidal* in France, is published by a company (LINFO) which is owned by the pharmaceutical manufacturers' associations. The texts in *FASS* are produced by the manufacturers, who have the legal responsibility for providing comprehensive and correct information, and they are approved by the MPA.

*FASS* has become a standard source of information within all Swedish health care. The book is delivered free of charge to all doctors, dentists, medical students, hospitals, health care centers, and pharmacies. *FASS* is also sold, for example, to students at nursing schools and the general public. The printrun is 155 000 copies, and in 1990 it comprised 1 300 pages.

## Patient-FASS

*FASS* has also been published in a version for patients, *Patient-FASS,* every second year since 1983, with the aim to:

1. Increase the level of general knowledge on pharmaceuticals so as to improve their use
2. Comply with the intent of the Health and Medical Care Act mentioned above.

The chapters of the *Patient-FASS* are depicted in Table 1.

**Table 1.** Main headings in *Patient-FASS* 1989/90

General Information

- Medicines, what are they?
- Prescribing and dispensing of medicines
- Different dosage forms of medicines
- Examples of different medication packages
- How to take your medicine
- Medicines and children
- Medicines and the elderly
- Your body and its functions
- What happens with the medicine in your body
- Side effects of medicines
- Additives in medicines
- Medicines and driving
- Medicines during pregnancy and breast feeding
- Interactions – how medicines influence each other
- Overdosing medicines – risk of intoxications
- Sports and medicines – risk of doping
- Vaccinations
- The medicine insurance and the patient insurance
- Before you see the doctor

List of Medical Terms

Product Descriptions

## *General Information Chapters*

*Patient-FASS* has 19 general chapters written by independent medical specialists. In these, information aiming at a rational use of the medicines is given in language tuned to laymen. There is also a list of medical terms to explain words which do not have an easily understandable Swedish synonym.

The main section of the book is the "Product Descriptions." All medicines approved, including those sold by prescription as well as those sold over the counter, are listed here in alphabetical order by brand name. The texts are based on those in *FASS,* but the information has been revised and simplified to avoid unnecessarily complicated medical language. The following headings are used:

*Dosage form,* in which the designation and strength of the medication, as declared on the pack are listed, and the color, shape, makings, and flavor, etc. are also described.

*Composition,* in which active ingredients and additives which could affect allergic patients are listed.

*Indications,* in which indications, together with information about the effects and mode of action of the product, are listed.

*Dosage,* in which a standard text for all pharmaceuticals available on prescription only is given, stating that the doctor should always determine the dosage. If possible, the normal dosages are stated. For medicines not requiring a prescription, the approved dosage is given.

*Side effects,* in which all adverse effects listed in *FASS* are mentioned. They are described in terms of symptoms whenever possible, e.g., respiratory difficulty instead of pulmonary fibrosis. The 1990 edition includes a new item: each product description contains a table presenting the side effects of that medicine according to the following frequency intervals: most frequent (has affected more than 1/100 patients treated), less frequent, and rare (less than 1/1000). An example of such information, information on the side effects of Ludiomil (maprotelin), is presented here:

Side effects

Many of the side effects experienced with Ludiomil medication occur only at the start of the therapy period and subsequently disappear. If the side effects cause real distress, the doctor should be contacted.

Most frequent: Tiredness, dizziness, dryness of the mouth which may increase the risk of damage to the teeth and mucous membranes during long-term treatment. Thorough oral hygiene is therefore important. Tremor, headache, dizziness (e.g., when you stand up). Difficulty in reading fine print, double vision, difficulty passing water (applies especially to elderly men), palpitations of the heart, usually transient. Weight gain, skin rash (a doctor should be contacted).

Less frequent: Constipation, liver changes, epileptic seizures.

Rare: Severe reduction of the number of white blood cells and platelets, severe allergic skin reactions, inflammation of the liver.

*Traffic warning,* in which a standard text is given for products which may negatively affect abilities to drive, etc., and that are included in a list of medical products set up by the national authority. On the packages of these products a red triangle is printed, and the same triangle appears in the text of *Patient-FASS*.

*Should not be taken,* which contains the contraindications.

*Caution* in which it is stated if the medicine is habituating and whether it can interact with other medicines. Any other appropriate precautions are also given here.

*Pregnancy and breast-feeding,* in which all medicines are classified in different categories according to what is known about their effects in these situations. The classification is made by a panel of experts and approved by the MPA.

Products mainly used in hospitals or issued to the patient by, for example, a nurse, are included in *Patient-FASS* to make it complete. However, not all headings are included and the indications are concluded by a standard text such as: "Bleomycine is given only by authorized medical personnel, who can provide further information."

## Distribution

*Patient-FASS* is sold to the general public in all pharmacies, in bookstores, and through a book club at a price of only 79 Swedish kronor, or US $ 12. It is also distributed free of charge to all general practitioners (6 500). The first edition sold 365 000 copies, corresponding to one in every thenth household. The following editions have sold about 250 000 copies altogether. The sales figures clearly indicate the interest and need for comprehensive information on medicines, both those requiring a prescription and those sold over the counter.

## Market Survey

In 1984 a survey was performed to evaluate acceptance and eventual influence on medication behavior of *Patient-FASS*. The survey was conducted as telephone interviews with 300 randomly selected members of the public, 200 doctors, 100 nurses, and 100 pharmacists. One of the questions put to the general public was: "Would you prefer information about your medicine to be given orally or in writing?"

For prescription drugs, 46 % wanted oral information. Almost 100 % of these persons wanted the information from their doctor; only a few percent preferred to be informed by pharmacy staff. A total of 30 % preferred written information, and 21 % spontaneously answered that they wanted both written and oral information. For medicine purchased without prescription, 30 % wanted to be informed orally. Almost 100 % wanted to be informed by pharmacists. In all 45 % preferred written information, and 18 % spontaneously answered that they wanted to be informed both orally and in writing. Thus, none of the information sources was predominant but there was a tendency to prefer oral information for drugs supplied on prescription and written information for drugs supplied without prescription.

The most common questions asked by the patients regarding their medicines, regardless of whether they were supplied with or without prescription, concern side effects. This was also confirmed by the health care staff (doctors, nurses, and pharmacists).

The questionnaire also gave an indication that *Patient-FASS* has affected relations between patients and health care staff. One-fourth of the doctors, nurses, and pharmacists thought that they had noticed a change in the patients' questions after *Patient-FASS* had been released. The patients put more questions to them, and many questions were more detailed than before the publication of the book. This was especially noticeable with regard to side effects.

The question to the general public on whether *Patient-FASS* had affected their attitude towards medicines was answered by 15% with yes. As an example, many mentioned that they were more careful when they used medicines and that they had cut down their use of painkillers. Among health care professionals 17% of the doctors, 41% of the nurses, and 66% of the pharmacists thought that *Patient-FASS* was of great help when they gave information to patients about drugs. Thus, *Patient-FASS* has contributed to the creation of an open dialogue between patients and health care staff. This is satisfactory as there is a need for an honest and open attitude concerning information to patients.

## Drug Information Leaflets

Another source of drug information for the patients are leaflets that have been produced by The National Corporation of Pharmacies since 1986. These leaflets were introduced as a less expensive alternative to patient package inserts. Patients who get their medicines in a pharmacy will receive both verbal and written information about these at the counter. The information leaflets cover groups of drugs – unlike *Patient-FASS,* where a product description covers just one single medicine. There are 72 different leaflets covering 90% of all prescriptions. The leaflets are produced by The National Corporation of Pharmacies together with medical experts and in cooperation with the pharmaceutical industry.

The leaflets contain general information about the medicines and are intended to repeat and supplement the verbal information given by the doctor. Each leaflet contains at least the following headings:

- How does your medicine work?
- How to take this medicine.
- For how long should your medicine be taken?
- If you have forgotten to take your medicine.
- The medicine may sometimes cause side effects.
  Only side effects that the patient can recognize himself and relate to the medicine, and those adverse reactions which call for an immediate contact with the doctor, are included.
- Pregnancy.
- How to store your medicine.

The pharmacist complements the written information verbally by stressing important information. The pharmacist also receives a reminder which leaflet should be given and what information should be stressed verbally by the computer, which also prints the label. All doctors have received a complete set of information leaflets, and these have also been discussed with them by the local pharmacists.

## Medicines Information Council

The Medicines Information Council (MIC) was initiated by the Ministry of Health and Social Welfare and consists of a panel of experts from the Ministry, The National Board of Health and Social Welfare, the MPA, The Consumers Agency, the County Councils (as responsible for health care), The National Corporation of Pharmacies, and the Pharmaceutical Manufacturers Organizations, but no representative from academia. The chairman is, however, a professor of medicine, and the secretary represents the Association of Swedish Pharmacists.

The MIC has during the years concentrated on delivering basic information on medicines and health-related behavior to youngsters and the elderly and on methodological questions. Already in 1980 a project was started to increase the knowledge of medicines among young people in cooperation with the Ministry of Education. In this project available literature on medicines for teachers was evaluated and a program for integrating information on medicines and their proper use at different school levels was designed. New study material was developed (books, slides, and videos) tuned to the four school levels and to special areas such as sports clubs. The teaching program was gradually implemented between 1982 and 1986. Material from the general chapters in *Patient-FASS* is integrated and used in the teaching program.

Another major project has been "Durgs and the Elderly." Here special teaching programs for health and social care personnel have been developed. Symposia for physicians and pharmacists on the subject have been held on several occasions throughout the country, and so-called study circles for elderly people have been designed and started through existing programs of continuing education organized by nonprofit, often labor-union-related organizations. These study circles have also been run in so-called service houses for elderly people.

The MIC has also been involved in the development of new techniques for giving information on medicines to laypeople, and in a project concerning the need for and feasibility of a special computer-based data bank on patient information on medicines. The project group concluded that it would be useful and feasible and suggested that such a data base be created under the auspices of The National Corporation of Pharmacies.

## Conclusion

In Sweden there is now a tradition of some years to give increased information on medicines and other health-related issues to the public, both as a means of increasing the level of knowledge in general and to promote an accurate and rational medication behavior. Overall, this has been appreciated by both the public and the health care providers, and there are no indications that an increased knowledge about side effects or other risks associated with pharmacotherapy has had significant negative effects on public health – instead, there are indications to the contrary.

# 45. Discussion

The centrality of the patient and the physician-patient relationship in the panelists' presentations initiated discussion about the importance of evaluation of communications to and from both the patient and the physician. For example, the labeling of pharmaceutical products should be evaluated more fully because it often is overly complex and poorly organized; greater professional feedback from primary care physicians would be especially useful. Package inserts also have become long and difficult to comprehend, with many readers unable to understand the information. Participants thought it was important to evaluate the extent to which drug information in such compendia as the *PDR* and the Swedish *FASS* is communicated effectively to physicians.

In many patient and physician studies, even poorly presented information gets communicated to a highly motivated audience. Nevertheless, more information could be received if the communication channels were improved through evaluation strategies and techniques proven to be useful in other areas of application (e.g., community studies). Unless as much attention is given to developing quality drug "software" (i.e., drug information and its communication) as to developing quality "hardware" (i.e., the pharmaceutical product itself), noncompliance and inadequate knowledge among physicians and patients will make it impossible to achieve the desired levels of drug safety.

Several questions arose from the observations that the primary mode of drug information communication is often the written word and that the intended receivers of this information are seldom attuned to hear messages that are widely broadcast. How can one open up, or improve, the listening function in physician-patient and pharmacist-patient communication? How can such one-to-one communication be reinforced over time and used more effectively? How important is it for an individual patient to receive personalized information when he or she talks about and receives a prescribed drug? The key to increasing people's attentiveness is often not to try to teach them something specific, but rather to get them to pay attention to materials and information they otherwise might ignore. For example, by observing what types of materials are selected for reading in a physician's waiting room, it may be possible to choose more effective drug information communication channels. The level of resources available for direct patient education (e.g., public service announcements) will never approach the level of resources used to market drugs, however, so the patient's relationship with his or her physician and pharmacist remains one of the most important channels through which communication of a personalized nature can be provided to a receptive individual.

The use of drug information as part of a therapeutic strategy is important. For most patients, it is not sufficient for them to have all the information about a drug they are taking. A patient needs to know how to assess the effectiveness of a prescribed therapy when he returns to his physician. For example, a patient with mild heart failure needs to know not only what drug he is taking (e.g., a diuretic) but also whether it will lead to short-term disabling or embarrassing consequences. Clear information about the potential interactions among all the drugs prescribed as part of the therapeutic strategy also is vital. Companies should consider tailoring the information they distribute about a drug to the likely therapeutic situations in which the drug is to be used.

Although the Patients-in-the-Know program's promotional materials were regarded by some participants as too focused on the sponsoring company, the program received high marks as a useful service for physicians and patients. The dilemma is how to encourage companies to act in ways which not only benefit themselves, but also meet the needs of physicians and patients. The hope is that factual information will be provided in ways that are not overly self-promotional. At the same time, participants acknowledged that when companies provide the resources to produce drug information materials, physicians and patients will likely need to accept references to these companies in the materials. In all communication initiatives, however, information and promotional materials must be produced and used in a manner sensitive to the cultural, social, and political context in which they are viewed.

Programs such as Patients-in-the-Know have been developed for use in the United States as a result of a 1981 federal government decision not to have a mandatory patient package insert program. Whereas in the continental European drug dispensing system, for example, with each drug prescription the patient receives standard information about the drug, the United States approach has been to encourage drug companies, consumer groups, health profession organizations, and others to develop their own programs to meet patients' needs for drug information. A large and effective program has been developed by the National Council on Patient Information and Education (NCPIE), supported by dozens of pharmaceutical companies and other organizations. But many other groups, including the American Association of Retired Persons and the Association of National Retail Druggists, also have developed their own systems – and each group is interested in promoting its own approach, including the Patients-in-the-Know progam.

What is important in the case of such programs as Patients-in-the-Know and its sponsoring company's other two well-publicized initiatives – providing drugs free to patients who cannot afford them and giving the patient his money back if he is not satisfied with the drug's results – is not that they are the only approaches or even the best approaches. Rather, what is important is that they are innovative approaches, new ways of trying to inform patients about the quality and use of pharmaceutical products. It is important that the pharmaceutical industry and other drug safety constituencies should not follow analysis with paralysis and become fearful of trying new, common sense ideas.

More broadly, participants emphasized the general need for innovation in drug information communication. For example, channels of communication between the pharmaceutical industry and editors, journalists, and reporters need to be reexamined. Women's magazines play a central role in providing pharmaceutical information to large numbers of people, yet their editors and writers have little background in the sciences and tend to focus on bad news. A decade ago, mass media coverage of environmental concerns was in a similar state, yet now the quality of reporting on environmental issues is generally excellent. What types of innovative communication strategies might the pharmaceutical industry develop to enhance the quality of mass media coverage of drug issues?

Innovative strategies could be used to expand drug education programs in the schools. By better informing young students about the basic elements of safe drug use and about drug risks and benefits, we will have a knowledge base to build upon when these children become independent adults making their own pharmaceutical decisions. Innovative approaches also are required to obtain better information about primary care physicians' information and communication needs. Whereas significant attention is being directed at generating additional information about patients' use and understanding of drugs, we lack adequate knowledge about what physicians need to know, what they would like to know, how they can speak most effectively with patients, how best to communicate information to them, and so on.

# *Part X*

# *RAD-AR Activities*

# 46. International Overview

The Wolfsberg meeting in 1988 reflected the existence of a strong sense of commitment to drug safety and to the RAD-AR initiative. In the period after that meeting, individual companies came together informally to decide on the best way of bringing the aims of the RAD-AR initiative to reality. An initial phase of research to gain a better understanding of the issues and a number of pilot projects were undertaken. It was decided that work would be carried out in national working groups and that international meetings would also be held to establish a framework for long-term collaboration.

A number of international meetings took place in order to define practical projects on issues discussed at the 1988 Wolfsberg meeting. The focus of discussions was on two areas: pharmacoepidemiology and patient-public communication. In the former, the first task undertaken was the assessment of all existing pharmacoepidemiological data bases in the United States, information which was then collated in a data resource handbook. The success of this project led to the compilation of further volumes for the United Kingdom, Continental Europe, and Japan. At the same time, efforts were made to expand rare disease registries and to develop record linkage data bases. Work also began in the area of pharmacoepidemiological training.

In the sphere of patient-public communication, work started more slowly as it was felt that a solid scientific foundation was necessary before discussion could start on what should be communicated and how. Substantial research needed to be undertaken not only in the area of understanding public attitudes, perceptions and expectations, but also in that of interaction between the patient-public and other health care providers. To complement this research, a number of national surveys were carried out to define the baseline from which work would start.

The exchange of information was further promoted by print, video, and electronic media in an effort to communicate some of the emotional as well as the scientific aspects of the issues.

Work began initially in the United States, the United Kingdom, the Federal Republic of Germany, and Japan. However, within a short time a number of other countries became involved. Each country organized its activities according to the needs and criteria recognized by its national working groups, but projects were all more or less in line with the priorities defined at the international working group level.

## United Kingdom

Companies based in the United Kingdom have actively supported RAD-AR. The pharmacoepidemiology group, made up of manufacturers, regulators and academics, meets six times a year and has a very crowded agenda. The group's greatest achievement to date is the expansion of MEMO, a record-linking scheme centered in Tayside, Scotland. The scheme links together hospital discharges and prescriptions through the patient's national health number. RAD-AR has provided 50 % of the funds for a research fellow for a 3-year period, and the group is keen to support the MEMO project further, possibly with housing and more staff.

The group also organized a weekend teach-in at Bath University so that general practitioners could get some insight into life from the pharmacoepidemiological point of view. This meeting was well attended, although industry was in the majority rather than prescribing physicians.

The group looking into risk perception and communication has also been active. It has established an annual meeting with patient groups to address matters such as the RAD-AR initiative, risk/benefit in general, the validity of patient information sheets, risk perception, and the European scene in terms of patient information.

There are also regular meetings with patient groups at which the topics discussed usually relate to specific diseases. Additionally, RAD-AR gives financial support and analyzes data from research projects on risk perception.

The RAD-AR group in the United Kingdom is currently looking at ways of putting RAD-AR on a better legal footing, perhaps in the form of a registered medical charity.

## Federal Republic of Germany

Although there is no formally recognized body to coordinate activities in the Federal Republic of Germany, there are two informal working groups dealing with pharmacoepidemiological and communication matters. It is very likely that these groups will be coordinated by the MPS – the society of the research-based German pharmaceutical industry, the "Big Seven."

The pharmacoepidemiological group is working on three projects. It is investigating the feasibility of creating registries for hematological disease, teratogenic questions and the epidemiology of liver disease. The communications group has concentrated on two projects. It did a second analysis of some already published surveys on risk perception and organized a workshop to look at the role of communication in drug safety problems. The results of the first project were discouraging as the study's criteria were not homogeneous and samples were not representative. However, further better-designed studies are planned. For the second project, experts on drug safety from institutions and industry got together with communication experts from the media and industry. Each group was asked to articulate its expectations of the other groups and make proposals to improve the existing situation. Among the proposals made were the establishment of a data bank for pharmacoepidemiology, the establishment of working groups, communications channels, and consistent standards within companies, the eventual publication of guidelines for good communication practice, and a substantial improvement in the standards and objectivity of journalistic reporting.

## The Netherlands

In 1987, the Dutch Federation of Physicians formed a working group with government representatives and a number of academics in order to discuss the possibility of implementing pharmacoepidemiology in the Netherlands. This group recommended the use of a catch-all record-linkage research program similar to those in operation in England. Further discussion resulted in a proposal for an institute of pharmacoepidemiology using information from Phase I and Phase III studies.

The Dutch RAD-AR council was recently established with members from the industry and academia. Representatives from the government will also be invited to join and the council will shortly begin fund-raising activities and a pilot study.

## The United States

The study of pharmacoepidemiology is well established in the United States and activities have been guided principally by the Clinical Safety Surveillance Committee of the Pharmaceutical Manufacturers Association. A part of this committee is the Evolving Epidemiological Monitoring Techniques (EEMT) Working Group which has worked in close collaboration with the RAD-AR project. This group is now preparing a white paper on automated, multipurpose data bases and strategies for their evaluation in use. This document will also include guidelines for the optimal utilization of these resources, including descriptions of common problems which affect their use or value as well as methods to overcome these problems. This committee also keeps track of existing and developing pharmacoepidemiological data bases.

At the same time, a subcommittee has been developing recommendations for a code of ethics for pharmacoepidemiologists. Areas covered so far include uses of multipurpose data bases, custodianship of the data, the peer review process, and conflict of interest issues.

In coordination with the clinical trials working group, the EEMT committee is developing and hosting a treatment R&D workshop. This program was designed to get experimental drugs more rapidly to people with critical illnesses. The committee wants to look at the type of contribution that epidemiology could make to the design and implementation of future treatment R&D programs.

The working group dealing with risk perception and communication in the United States has been trying to institutionalize that aspect of the RAD-AR program for a number of years, but with little success. The group's main objective is to establish a nucleus of companies which are prepared to contribute financially to the RAD-AR initiative and enable the funding of some significant projects in the risk perception and communication area.

The group plans to work with the National Council of Patient Information and Education to develop a project that deals with the risk aspect of communication between the patient and the prescriber. Work is also proceeding on a joint project between Columbia University and Georgetown University on prescription medicines, the results of which will be integrated into the risk communication center at Columbia University. The group is also considering collaboration with the Food and Drug Law Institute to sponsor a seminar on risk, and with the Media Institute and the Prescription Drug Advertising Coalition to find ways of providing the lay public with better information on prescription medicine.

# 47. RAD-AR Council Japan

The RAD-AR Council of Japan was founded in May 1989. Its membership has grown from 11 to 19 companies, only three of which are not based in Japan. The Council's objective is to increase the understanding and credibility of pharmaceutical drugs in society by promoting and supporting research, risk assessment, and communication activities in the area of drug safety. At the head of the Council is the governing board of company presidents, but the work is largely carried out by a steering committee and two committees devoted to pharmacoepidemiological and communications matters. These committees are supported by a number of expert committees made up of journalists, academics, and medical and pharmaceutical experts.

The RAD-AR Council took over responsibility for the planning of the Tokyo symposium which took place in October 1989. This event was very successful and attracted more than 400 participants from 13 countries. The two-fold objective of exchanging information through presentations and establishing the foundations of a Japanese RAD-AR program was very satisfactorily met.

After the Tokyo symposium, work began on developing a RAD-AR program that would be effective within the Japanese cultural context. Five expert committees looked at the drug safety issue from medical, pharmaceutical, economic, general risk management, and communications perspectives and were consequently able to identify new areas of concern and to define a number of practical approaches for action.

The Council's projects for 1990 include:
1. Development of pharmacoepidemiology data bases in Japan
2. Training in pharmacoepidemiology
3. Organization of media workshops and briefings
4. Preparation of publications and newsletters
5. Establishment of RAD-AR network in Japan
6. Development of communications programs to improve patient/physician interaction
7. Provision of grants for research and symposia
8. Support for the International RAD-AR Foundation

In 1989 the Pharmacoepidemiology Committee was involved in three areas: pharmacoepidemiological studies, studies to clarify the efficacy and benefit of drugs, and a pharmacoepidemiology workshop.

Studies were carried out by a research team at Tokyo University, whose primary goal was to coordinate existing data bases in Japan. The number of deaths caused by adverse drug reactions was extracted from demographic data, and those caused by pharmaceuticals were investigated. The team also examined the possibility of using the REZEPT data base – a type of invoice breakdown on medical care for health insurance reimbursement.

A research team from the Faculty of Economics at Chuo University undertook a study on society and the future role of drugs in Japan. The aim of this study was to clarify the efficacy and benefit of drugs by analyzing the impact of drug therapy on an illness and on population structures. Pharmacological causes and primary factors such as the rate of illness and mortality in tuberculosis and circulatory diseases, the mortality rate of infants, and the birth rate were also analyzed. The results of these studies showed that drugs had made a considerable and positive contribution to Japanese society.

At the pharmacoepidemiological workshop held during the Tokyo symposium and attended by some 350 people, presentations were made that provided some background on the history of pharmacoepidemiology, its basic methods and tools. The three areas on which the Pharmacoepidemiology Committee has concentrated in 1990 are the development of data bases for further studies, the completion of the Japanese edition of the *Data Resource Handbooks*, and the organization of training programs in pharmacoepidemiology.

The Communication Committee is involved in research projects and in the study of decision making models. The majority of its projects deal with drug safety and the production of drug information for the public. Public perceptions and sensitivity to drug risks are also being studied, and studies into the impact of risk/benefit information on patient decision making are being carried out. The group has been active in the production of RAD-AR publications in Japanese; articles on pharmacoepidemiology and the RAD-AR initiative have appeared in trade journals and daily newspapers. The communications priorities for 1990 included the development of a physician/patient program, the refinement of models for risk management decision making and the production of a RAD-AR Council newsletter.

# *Part XI*

# *Reports and Recommendations from the Working Groups*

# 48. Generating and Assessing Knowledge

To provide a basis for considering future actions, the last session of the conference began with summary reports and recommendations from the six discussion sessions involving the three working groups.

## Working Group A

*R. Bruppacher*

In addressing principles and needs in risk analysis, the group focused strongly on different aspects of spontaneous reporting of adverse drug reactions (ADRs). These reports are important, even though the systems used to collect, sort, quantify, and analyze them are imperfect. While such systems are necessary, they can only provide warning signals, which in turn need validation. It was agreed that physicians should be advised, trained, motivated, and encouraged to participate in spontaneous reporting programs. At the same time, physicians who provide ADR reports should be protected from legal consequences of their

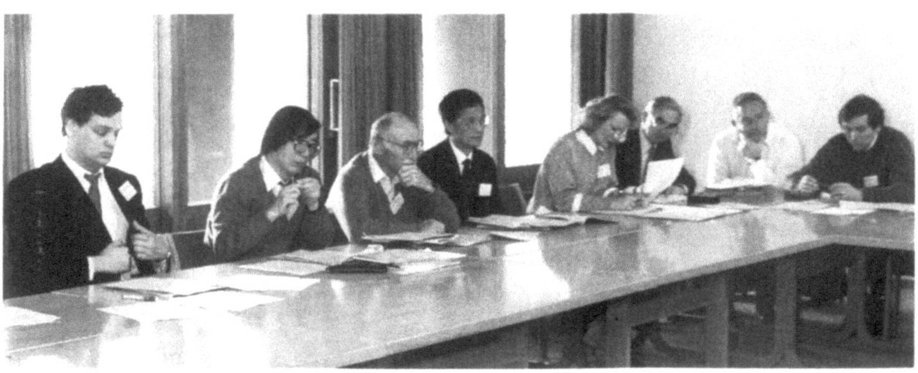

actions. The pharmaceutical industry also shares the responsibility for improving spontaneous ADR reporting.

The group emphasized the importance of accessing alternative data bases in addition to spontaneous ADR reports if one is to make rational decisions. There is an attendant need, however, for greater data base infrastructure and standardization and for greater expertise in the use of data bases.

An essential factor in risk assessment and prediction is background risk. Also important is international collaboration, and the group recommended broader international access to and funding support for the World Health Organization (WHO) data base currently maintained by the Swedish government. Risk/benefit assessments will continue to grow in importance, and international collaborative initiatives such as RAD-AR will be needed even more in the future. In particular, the group recommended the establishment of an international fund or foundation to support and encourage good problem-oriented studies.

## Working Group B

*B. Luce*

The primary issue addressed in the discussion of principles and needs in benefit analysis was quality of life (QOL). Although the group struggled to reach a consensus on the definition of QOL, it agreed that QOL is important in expanding the concept of efficacy, especially with respect to patient education and the patient-physician relationship. It also distinguished between abstract QOL measurements and the integration of QOL considerations into clinical assessments. Although QOL expands the concept of benefits, it does not necessarily follow that its inclusion exhausts all potential benefits. From the patient's point of view, the disease itself compromises QOL, and therefore a better understanding and measurement of QOL relative to specific diseases and geographic regions is essential.

On the issue of economic benefits, the group believed strongly that the analysis of such benefits should not be included in the drug approval process, but that it is appropriate for payment decisions. Another issue discussed was whether large numbers of patients should be exposed to risk for the benefit of a few patients. The group concluded that this issue could only be assessed on a case-by-case basis, but that the important principle is the concept of patient autonomy, with the patient being informed fully about the benefits and risks involved in the use of a drug.

The group agreed that the RAD-AR initiative should be involved in QOL studies. In particular, it should encourage the inclusion of QOL as a valid endpoint of pharmacological therapy. On the other hand, inclusion of economic analysis on the RAD-AR agenda at the present time could compromise the credibility of the RAD-AR initiative.

A member of the audience strongly endorsed the use of applied socioeconomics and decision theory to understand more fully the benefits of a drug, while at the same time recognizing the inappropriateness of its use in the drug approval process.

## Working Group C

*D. Henry*

In considering principles and needs in the risk/benefit assessment of drugs, the group expressed the view that the dictum "above all, do no harm" was no longer easily applicable. It is now more realistic to say "avoid situations in which, based on an understanding of the best available information, the likelihood of an adverse effect is disproportionate to the demonstrated benefits."

It was felt that remedies appearing to be free of ADRs are not necessarily harmless if there are no accompanying benefits to the patient. This, in effect, denies the patient possible alternative treatments that might carry certain risks, but also substantial benefits. Whatever the risk/benefit assessment on the part of the physician, the patient's right to choose is paramount. The physician's responsibility is to inform the patient of the risks and benefits, as far as they are known, in an understandable way.

An effort should be made to portray both risks and benefits in absolute as well as relative terms. Appropriate marketing plays an important role in assessing and maintaining the benefit/risk ratio. If marketing leads to patients using a drug from which they cannot get maximum benefit, then the benefit/risk ratio for that group of patients may change.

The group discussed appropriate marketing and the kinds of incentives necessary to achieve it. There is conflict between the medical view and the marketing view of what is appropriate, particularly if the latter approach appears to be succeeding in saturating a designated segment of the population. One of the penalties for poor marketing is adverse publicity.

Finally, there was agreement that if risk/benefit assessment is a process of comparative assessment with regard to different drugs and other interventions, then this cannot take place without access to full and reliable information on drug effects. Much useful information exists but is inaccessible due to questions of confidentiality. The group suggested that the RAD-AR initiative should look into the question of the level of confidentiality actually necessary, particularly with regard to the industry's data bases. A member of the audience added that accessibility of national health system and government regulatory authority data also needs to be improved.

# 49. Dialogue and Communication

## Working Group A

*K. Tolo*

The working group looked at the principles and needs for drug safety communication within traditional relationships between the industry, regulatory authorities, health professions, academia, and the patient community, as well as within emerging relationships between these parties and the media. One area of discussion was patient product information (PPI). Such information is desirable and even essential, but PPI objectives and the quality of current communication

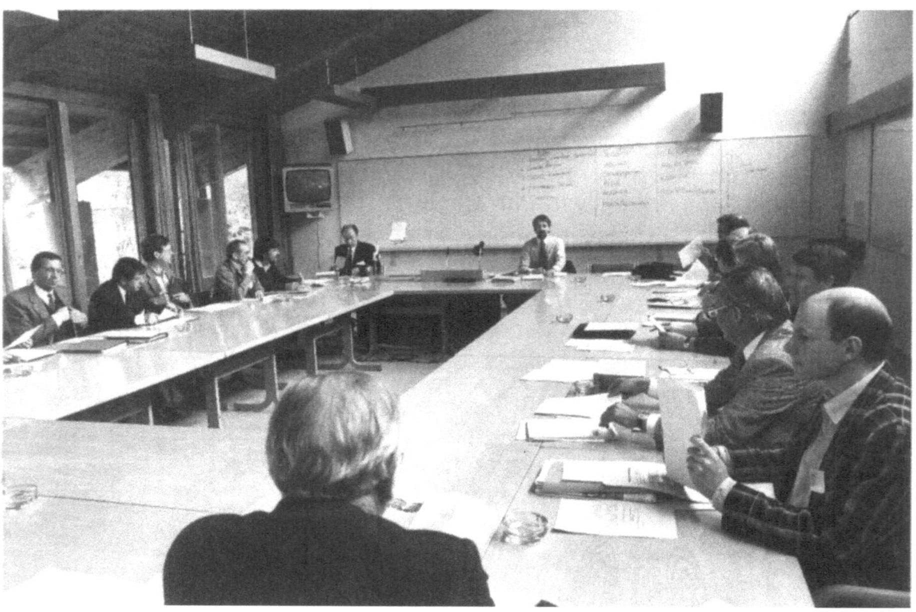

effectiveness measures (for example, readability measures) need to be assessed more systematically. The group questioned whether alternative or complementary means of communication exist to supplement the traditional forms of PPI. A form incorporating the five questions formulated by the National Council for Patient Information and Education (NCPIE) to improve physician-patient communication was suggested as a general instrument that could be used for all drugs in a particular setting, lessening the need for drug-specific information. NCPIE recommends that every patient *ask* the following *five questions* in order to obtain the minimum essential information needed to follow a drug regimen correctly and safely:

1. What is the name of the medicine and what is it supposed to do?
2. How and when do I take it – and for how long?
3. What foods, drinks, other medicines, or activities should I avoid while taking this medicine?
4. What are the side effects and what do I do if they occur?
5. Is there any written information available about the medicine to reference at home?

NCPIE also recommends that patients *volunteer* the *following information* to their doctor or pharmacist whenever a medicine is prescribed or dispensed:

1. The names of the medicines they are currently taking, including nonprescription medicines
2. Any problems they are having with their medicines
3. The medicines to which they are allergic
4. If they are, or think they might be, pregnant

Also recommended was a RAD-AR conference on drug safety and PPI use in the Third World.

Direct advertising was also discussed, and the group felt that advertising should undergo systematic comparison with other communication channels with reference to the quality of material produced. It was noted that there often is a very fine line between permissible mass media coverage of drug safety material and prohibited direct advertising of drugs. The expansion of satellite television and international networks crossing national boundaries could result in potential legal and institutional conflicts. Cited as examples were the Food and Drug Administration's (FDA's) intention to relax certain direct advertising guidelines in the United States at the same time as the European Community is considering banning drug advertising.

A suggestion to incorporate NCPIE's five questions into drug advertising was made. The industry should move from drug-specific and crisis-oriented communication to a more general ongoing communication strategy. There was a strong recommendation for workshops and exchanges, possibly organized by RAD-AR, to bring together journalists and industry scientists with the aim of understanding more clearly each other's needs and perspectives. RAD-AR also could play a lead role in developing good communication practices statements with respect to the industry and the media, and in coordinating a study group in communication strategy that would include legislators.

## Working Group B

*D. Taylor*

Before focusing on the new channels of drug safety communication, the group examined the traditional channels, especially physician-patient relationships. The physician is still the most important communicator of information to the patient, and any new channels should reinforce and support the physician's efforts.

The current medical situation was viewed as one of transition, with social relationships evolving, the authority of the physician being eroded, and the patient becoming a more active and often autonomous decision maker. The new channels of communication should be properly developed and exploited, and communication should be viewed comprehensively, with attention given to ethical issues as well as to proposed promotional principles. The mass media are increasingly important, and media representatives of all types have the responsibility to provide balanced information. In the case of public controversies, the media are in a position to provide alternative views that might allow those people wishing to do so to make their own pharmaceutical decisions. They also can be a direct channel of communication in times of drug crises, with the power to alert the public to potential problems and thus minimize damage and concern.

Another media role is that of motivation. Journalists are in a position to encourage the public to participate more actively in their own health care, teaching them which questions are important and how they can be asked. This is an important means of reinforcing the patient-physician relationship, with the patient taking a more responsible role.

The public education system is also a good channel of communication for health care matters, with a number of countries already having made a start in this direction. While PPIs are important, the written word is not sufficient; graphics and cartoons also need to be used.

Different types of risk/benefit information are needed by patients and the public at different times. The information needed prior to a prescription decision is different from that needed to use a drug intelligently. Although the task at hand is largely to educate consumers into becoming more autonomous, the group recognized the patient's right to defer to the physician if he or she so desired.

The group stressed that the efforts being made through the RAD-AR initiative to improve drug safety are important and should be continued through the structure of a formal body within which there is a broader sharing of responsibility and funding. A planning committee organized by an impartial body such as CIOMS should develop a business plan and map out future actions.

## Working Group C

*D. Burley*

The group's report focused on principles and needs to ensure competence, partnership, and dialogue in medical decision making. This was discussed with reference to autonomy, information, and channels of communication. There should be a middle road between total medical paternalism and total patient independence. The ideal situation would be one that would recognize patient autonomy, but nevertheless optimize the chance that the medication accepted by the patient would be used to its best advantage. At the same time, the group recognized potential problems with autonomy due to traditions in patient-physician behavior, differences in patient age and education, the nature of medicines prescribed, differences among country cultures, and financial and time constraints. The group also recommended that, each time a drug is prescribed, the patient ask the physician the five questions recommended by NCPIE as good guiding principles. Information must accompany medicine to ensure good dispensing practice.

To ensure as full an understanding of drug safety information as possible, the information must be repeated and passed on through multiple channels of communication, including the pharmacist. The value of this approach is to reinforce and repeat information, bearing in mind that the patient can only cope with a limited amount of information at a given moment. Further information should be available through education at school and access to simple drug compendia and other reference materials. Improved PPIs as well as workshops and seminars on historical case studies are effective, as are audiovisual channels of communication, in passing on good medical information.

# Part XII

# Ethical Perspectives Revisited

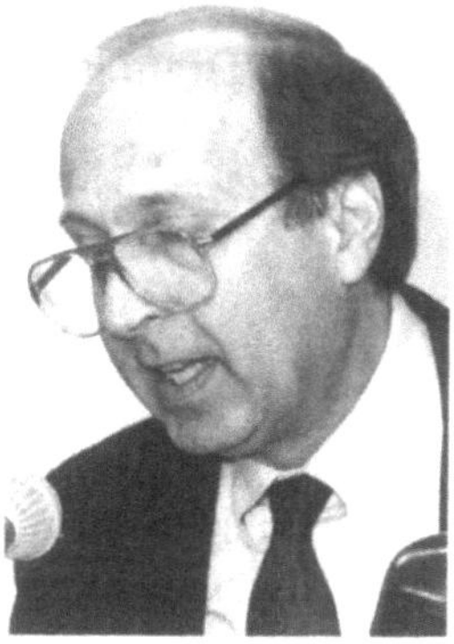

# 50. Applying Ethics

S. GOROVITZ

I will make ten brief points based on my reaction to the discussions I have heard.

1. Ethics, like the rest of philosophy, often involves – indeed even requires – a change in perspective, a willingness to stand back from the particularities of one's own immediate point of view, a willingness to transcend arrogance and complacency about how one sees and understands the world. Recall also that ethics is in large measure concerned with questions of character – of courage, candor, and willingness to contemplate the difference between self-interest and a larger truth. And this sometimes requires challenging one's own beliefs and assumptions.
2. Consider at this point a slight digression, which may nonetheless be usefully illustrative. Each year I greet 1300 new students, most of whom arrive believing that what a university education is primarily about is getting a good job after graduation and having a good career. I begin by inviting them to contemplate their own obituaries. The message I want them to understand is that it is not our goal to prepare them for employment, and it is not our concern what becomes of them immediately after they finish school. It is our goal instead that as they approach the ends of their lives, they can look back on those lives with a sense of pride at having been the kinds of people they most admire and can feel gratified at the choices they have made in their various roles as spouses, parents, friends, neighbors, and citizens, and also in their careers. This is not an idle exercise. When the students take that longer view, they achieve a new understanding of the choices immediately before them. It changes what they do. The same may be said for ethical reflection.
3. Professor Lowrance emphasized that benefit/risk evaluation is really applied ethics. I hope you thought carefully about that important remark, about what it means and why he said it. I want to emphasize and extend that point. Risk assessment and all that relates to it is a fundamentally value-laden activity with ethical assumptions and consequences. Even to speak of a risk is to refer to a possible outcome as having a negative value. If we are rigorous, we will not only be concerned with the probability of and the conditions that lead to

such an outcome, we will also be concerned with how negative the outcome is, for whom, and for what reasons. And that is a consideration of values.

4. Dr. Faich reminded us that regulations focus on the law. But ethics is not merely a matter of law. It is much broader, much deeper. It is in part reflected in law, but no one would suggest that the difference between what is ethical and what is unethical is entirely captured by the law. Much that is unethical is not covered by the law and should not be covered by the law. Gratuitous rudeness, for example, is unethical, but not the sort of behavior we want to see prohibited as a matter of law. The moral order succeeds largely by virtue of substantial consensus, not by the imposition of laws, regulations, or guidelines, but rather with their assistance and the willing acceptance of them when they reflect widely shared values. Now I turn to several points that pertain more specifically to pharmacology.
5. It is important to ask what basic values package inserts are designed to serve. Do they exist just to meet some regulatory requirement, or do they meet some real human need? As effective communication to patients, they are for the most part a ludicrous mockery of successful information transfer. There is an analogue in what those who do not know any better call the ivory tower. Professors reading final examinations are often astonished and bewildered. How is it possible, they wonder, for the students to know so little when I said it so well? The point is, of course, that communicating effectively involves much more than saying it in what, from one's own point of view, is a complete, accurate, and perhaps even elegant way. So it is very instructive and sometimes humbling to read those final exams. It is not clear to me that the pharmaceutical industry has that corrective of having to read final exams.
6. There is a substantial overlap between the pharmaceutical industry's interests and the public interest. In the long run, it is very much in the interest of any company to act with integrity. A conflict of interest can exist, especially in the short run. This is not evidence of evil, but it is wrong to pretend that there can be no conflict between corporate interests and the public interest. Of course there can. Such conflicts require careful scrutiny and honest reflection.
7. The issue of coercion of the media by the threat to withdraw advertising money was raised here yesterday. Any problem can be viewed as an opportunity; this problem provides an opportunity to respond with candor and courage. One possible response to that corporate advertiser is acquiescence, withdrawal of the offending material, and maintenance of the advertising revenue stream. Another possible response is to confront the advertiser with the prospect of a major exposé about how a corporation which ostensibly cares about its reputation in fact tries to bully the press into suppressing the truth. I suggest that any responsible media manager who is acting with integrity would seriously contemplate the latter, and not think very seriously about the former.
8. The desire was expressed yesterday to hear what the "ethics guys" think about the refund policy for pharmaceuticals that fail to meet expectations. My immediate interest on hearing about that program was to wonder how

often the claim for a refund is made. Often, for promotional purposes, companies provide guarantees in the full confidence that their exposure is extremely small because the likelihood that claims will be lodged against that guarantee is minuscule. I would be interested to know how much has been paid out in response to that guarantee, which may be just an attractive and inexpensive promotional gimmick.

But I have a much deeper concern. A policy of providing refunds for pharmaceuticals that fail to live up to the aspirations with which one uses them sustains the illusion that in health care it is reasonable to expect the same kind of warranty and the same kind of certainty that one can seek in the world of consumer goods. This is a socially destructive illusion.

9. There does exist a considerable amount of drug-specific information. As you know better than I, there could exist much more. We have paid much attention at this meeting to postapproval, long-term pharmacoepidemiology, and that certainly is important. But it is also important not to forget the power of simple, general information. Dr. Burley's workshop summary precisely addresses that power. I want to suggest three additional points – simple, obvious points, which, I believe, require and deserve sustained attention.

   First, all prescription drugs have both intended benefits and some risks. Second, it is possible to reduce, but not to eliminate, those risks by the proper use and monitoring of the drugs. Third, it is prudent for patients to obtain information about the specific benefits, risks, and indications of adverse reactions of the drugs that they are using. If those three simple points could be effectively conveyed, a tremendous amount of progress would have been made. I urge investing more in the effective transmission of that single message along with that of Dr. Burley. The point that risk cannot be entirely eliminated is precisely the point that is undermined by the likening of pharmaceuticals to "guaranteed-or-your-money-back" products.

10. Finally, despite the skepticism of those who have a dismissive attitude toward ethics – or toward poetry, for that matter – I submit that ethics is the most practical of disciplines. It deals with what we ought to do, with how one ought to lead one's life. What could be more practical than that? Let me cite two examples of its immediate practicality, however. First, in reviewing the history of liability litigation in the United States, pay attention to the effect on the size of judgments of a jury's perception of wrongdoing on the part of the defendants. I submit that the ethical integrity of the actors in any drama that is scrutinized in litigation has a profound effect on the outcome. Second, consider the entire social enterprise of institutional review boards which protect the interests of human subjects of pharmacological research. This is fundamentally an exercise in applied ethics. It arises out of basic value commitments and is structured to protect those values. It is that social construct that allows research in pharmacology to continue at all. Only by paying careful attention first to the ethics is it possible to proceed to the science. I add, as a footnote, that sloppy science is itself unethical.

In conclusion, I hope to have made at least plausible the position that the ethical dimensions of the world in which you work are too important to ignore and should be an essential ingredient in your continuing dialogues.

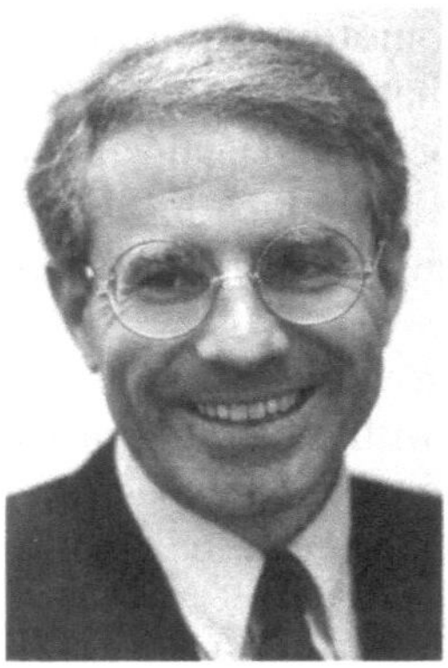

# 51. Moral Common Sense

K. M. Leisinger

During this conference I have had the impression that we all are convinced we are subject not only to biological, pharmacological, and financial laws but also to moral ones, which cannot be violated with impunity. All our discussions revealed a profound concern to humanize the interactions between the pharmaceutical industry and the patient, and this in itself is of moral value.

We have discussed how a business enterprise can respond to the challenge of corporate ethics. We have reflected on four elements of a pragmatic approach to this end, namely:

1. Moral common sense
2. Personnel policy (selecting people according to holistic criteria and enlarging performance appraisal and reward systems)
3. Corporate policies and codes of conduct (reflecting state-of-the-art knowledge and broad public consensus)
4. Management development (including ethics as a discipline and involving middle and lower management)

While the elaboration of criteria for personnel policies, corporate policies and codes of conduct, and management development systems would have gone beyond the scope of this seminar, we were able to find concrete examples for Goodpaster's moral common sense rules, which are presented in the following.

*Avoid Harming Others.* Be it in our personal lives or in our business lives, the avoidance of harming others is an ideal which we can only strive for but never reach. Yet the goal to at least minimize the risk of harming others is realistic and attainable, and this is the very aim and objective of RAD-AR. Our participation in this initiative is a step on the way to accomplishing this task.

*Respect the Rights of Others.* We have identified at least one pronounced right of others that the pharmaceutical industry has to respect. This is the *right to know* for patients, regulatory authorities, academia, and the media. But this right to know has a corresponding duty, which is the *duty to inform*. This implies the task of constantly monitoring drug use, objectively assessing new findings, and acting accordingly.

*Do Not Lie or Cheat.* The commandment requiring that we should not lie or cheat must be applied first and foremost in our information policy, in which we should follow some basic principles:

- Provide sober, comprehensive, and accurate information to all parties
- Admit if you do not know something
- Clearly state when you are only assuming something

Those principles are worth heeding, not only in our business lives but also privately.

*Keep Promises and Contracts.* Promises and contracts, we have to add, must also be kept if they are not put down in writing. There are lots of unwritten rules which are naturally obeyed. Anyway, I still think it would make sense if all those involved in health care, and not just doctors, took the Hippocratic oath.

*Obey the Law.* As said before, there are many unwritten rules; we cannot find laws forbidding certain actions. Consequently, we have reached agreement on a common policy: To act legally is only the ethical minimum.

*Prevent Harm to Others.* The commandment requiring us to prevent harm to others again touches our information policy. It obliges us to help others make an informed choice and avoid mistakes by having accurate and honest information.

*Help Those in Need.* In connection with helping those in need, the Third World was mentioned several times. Somebody suggested devoting another RAD-AR conference specifically to Third World issues. In view of the fact that there are 3 billion people living in poverty and sickness, I can only support this idea. It is important that the pharmaceutical industry commits itself not to take advantage of this situation, but to take it as a challenge and try its little bit to improve it. Professor Gorovitz mentioned Rawls' theory in this context: "One should treat things and people equally, but if one deviates from this equality aspect, it must be to the advantage of the least privileged."

*Be Fair.* Concrete examples of fairness in the pharmaceutical business were related to safety and quality standards with regard to both products and information. What is unsafe and inappropriate for an industrialized country should not be good enough for a developing country. Particularly in areas like industrial and environmental safety, standards that embody state-of-the-art knowledge and the highest morality must be brought to bear consistently, wherever in the world they apply and regardless of whether this is required by the law.

*Reinforce These Imperatives in Others.* As I said in the beginning, it is intellectually fun and edifying to talk about ethics abstractly, which is essentially what we have done over the past few days. Now comes the tough part: actually doing what we have been talking about. Unless concrete actions follow, we have all wasted our breath. Now we have to take ourselves at our words, carry the messages home, and set examples by our own actions.

In conclusion, I wish to quote from the Encyclical Letter *Sollicitudo Rei Socialis* of Pope John Paul II: "One would hope that also men and women without an implicit faith would be convinced that there are more profound attitudes and higher values than economic goals." And a second quote from this Encyclical Letter: "Though it be with sorrow it must be said that just as one may sin through selfishness and the desire for excessive profit and power, one may also be found wanting through fear, indecision, and basically through cowardice." In other words, if we all wait for the right direction to come from above (whatever "above" may be), the waiting will be as fruitless as the waiting for Godot.

I am convinced that, if we all start to do whatever little we can do, many little things will change. But it takes time, and we need to be patient. As the African proverb states, "The grass doesn't grow faster if you pull on it." And citing another African proverb: "If many little people in many little places do many little things, this will change the face of the world."

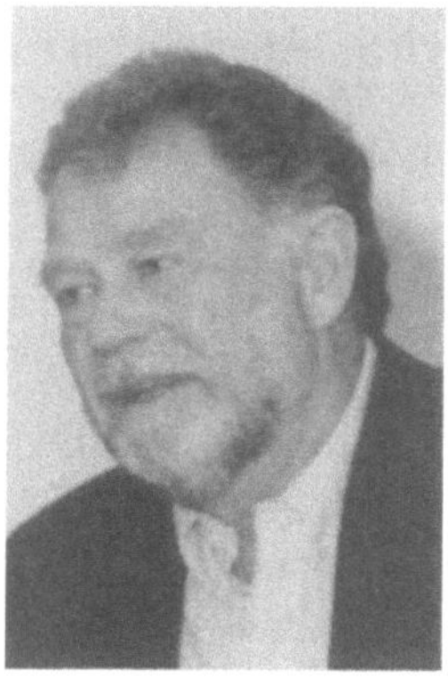

# 52. Guiding Principles

E.W.D. Young

I commend all of the contributors for the openness, honesty, and care with which they have addressed the various tasks and issues of the conference. It has been a complex and difficult process, but the spirit in which it has been undertaken epitomizes what it means to do ethical work; it means proceeding with care, with openness, with honesty, and with rigor.

On the first day of the conference I conducted three experiments (see "A Biomedical Ethical Perspective"). Of course, the speed with which the questionnaires I handed out had to be completed, to say nothing of the fact that the language used was English rather than the five or more other languages represented here, immediately detracts from any scientific validity they might have had. Nevertheless, the results are interesting, and I will present them here.

The first experiment asked each participant to rank the four ethical principles of *nonmaleficence, beneficence, autonomy,* and *justice* in order of priority at the various stages of the process of improving drug safety. I was surprised that autonomy figured so highly in the early stage of knowledge generation; I would have expected concerns about whether a drug works (whether it is going to be beneficial) and what are its likely problems to have loomed larger. Likewise, at the point of knowledge utilization, autonomy was ranked highly, but justice surprisingly low; if justice presents us with questions about access and fairness in distribution, as well as cost-effectiveness, one would have expected it to be higher on the scale at the time products are being used.

With respect to the players, the principals involved, several findings from the second experiment are of note. Media representatives seemed to be more concerned about bad things that happen than good things. This appears to indicate that harm is more important to media representatives than benefits (although a good product can be killed either with too much praise or by exaggerated statements about its potential for harming). This finding says something important to the pharmaceutical industry, which it would do well to heed. Under the category of patients, the results were as I predicted they would be: when one has what might be described as a mild problem, concerns about beneficence rank lower than when one has a more major problem; likewise, with a major problem, the question of harm ranks lower than when the problem is minor. On other words, someone with a slight malady does not expect to be severely harmed! As far as manufacturers are concerned, I was surprised that justice was ranked as low as it was.

In the third experiment, there were some interesting mixed responses. Far and away the group placed most often at the center of the pentagon of ethical principles was that of patients. The physician ranked second to the patient. However, there was an enormous spread and range of opinion, indicative of the way in which national, ethnic, and cultural differences influence our ranking of important moral principles.

These moral principles should be viewed more as guiding lights than as destination points. They do not present the harbor that you are necessarily trying to reach as much as they do the lighthouse that is there to keep you off the rocks. This puts the whole discussion about whether nonmaleficience is either attainable or relevant into some perspective; it may not be attainable, but it certainly is relevant. Even though it is more of a lighthouse than a harbor light, it still serves an indispensable function.

With reference to who should be at the center of the pentagon, I need to make the point that the relationship between physician and patient will assume different forms in different places. The traditional form of the relationship was that of the wise and beneficent parent-like physician dealing with a childlike, frightened, and often ignorant patient, as a good parent might deal with a child. In some countries, there was a consumer revolt against this paternalism, which led to a reversal of roles. Now the consumer assumed the dominant position, attempting to reduce the physician to childlike compliance. This was as demeaning to physicians as paternalism on the part of the doctor had been to patients. Ideally, what we are striving for is an adult-adult form of the relationship, in which both the physician and the patient collaborate from their different perspectives and with different sources of expertise in order to achieve an appropriate result. As was beautifully said during one of the panels, the patient knows more about his or her body than anyone else. Patients have this primary, subjective expertise, whereas the physician's or pharmacist expertise is more objective and scientific. There is nothing wrong with both physician and patient wanting a parent-child form of the relationship. But transactions become tangled when the physician wants to treat the patient as an adult, and the patient insists on assuming a childlike role. The important point is not that the form of the relationship should always and everywhere be the same, but that the partners to the transaction should agree on the form the relationship will take.

One point that emerged during a discussion session is that facts are a resource in short supply. It is inevitable that values should enter into the selection of what we choose to regard as facts, as well as how we interpret, communicate, and act upon them. One of the major lessons of this Wolfsberg conference, for me at least, has been the reminder of how patient and thorough we have to be in the quest for factual knowledge, as well as how important it is that we be honest about what are merely assumptions and about what we simply do not know. Because values are implicit in this enterprise, in selecting, interpreting, and communicating information, it necessarily becomes a moral endeavor. As

Professor Leisinger put it, morality undergirds everything we have been doing this week and will be doing when we depart.

Much was said about feedback during the conference, particularly from the patient to the physician in reporting adverse drug reactions. I want to suggest that feedback is equally important as part of the process of obtaining an informed consent. After the attempt has been made to explain risks, benefits, and alternatives, and to put these into perspective, and once the physician has made a recommendation (which is not inappropriate, providing reasons for the recommendation are given), then it is terribly important to ask the patient, "Will you please tell me what you have heard me say?" Frequently, in the hospital setting, I have been astounded at the gap between what has been said by the physician and what has been heard by the patient. Unless we build into the informed consent process a feedback mechanism, this gap could exist without our ever knowing about it.

Let me comment on our discussion of quality of life. Here, too, values impinge because, ultimately, we all have to decide for ourselves what quality of life is acceptable in light of the capacities and opportunities we value. Anthony Shaw, an American pediatrician, proposed what he calls a "formula without numbers." Shaw writes with the pediatric situation in view, but his proposal has other applications as well. His formula is that $QOL = NE \times (H + S)$, with $QOL$ representing quality of life, $NE$ natural endowment, $H$ and $S$ what the home and the society, respectively, are able to provide. In other words, if a baby is born with disabilities, and neither the home nor the society into which she has been born is able or willing to devote substantial resources of money, love, and affection to the child, the net result in terms of quality of life will be poor. Shaw's point reminds us that, inevitably, there is a social dimension to life and that, therefore, everything we do, whether as manufacturers or media representatives, whether as pharmacists or physicians, has social consequences, either diminishing or enhancing the quality of life of those who use our products.

Now I come to a final point, and then a proposal. Professor Leisinger aptly expressed the point I want to make: Integrity has its own inevitable and inescapable moral force. He concluded his remarks by quoting African proverbs. I shall end mine by reminding you of one of my African heroes, Nelson Mandela. He spent twenty-seven-and-a-half years in prison, many of these in solitary confinement. When he came out, he was saying exactly the same things he had said at his trial, twenty-nine years earlier! And he said these things gently and compassionately, with enormous dignity and equally impressive strength. It was then that we saw the moral force of a human being with integrity. By what he is, Mandela challenges us to go forth to act with equal integrity, not allowing ourselves to be sidetracked by what is expedient or popular.

There is an analogy between what has been happening in this conference and, I imagine, in the pharmaceutical industry as a whole, and what is going on in the environmental movement. My final remarks in this regard come from *The Wall Street Journal*, in which there is a wonderful editorial entitled, "Oh, Holy Day." The holy day refers to Earth Day (April 22, 1990) observed by environmentalists around the world. Let me read excerpts from this editorial:

> "Those of us attuned primarily to concerns of the secular world have trouble fitting the environmental movement into our usual categories. Thus, we are coming to see environmentalism as a religion. As much as anyone else, we are in favor of clean air, blue water, wholesome food, verdant parks, neat streets, pristine mountains, and unspoiled deserts. Having set these ends, we turn to the usual means, cost/benefit analysis, emission taxes, economic growth, technology (clean nuclear power, for example). Yet consensus with environmentalism seems to take no roots. Indeed, our very efforts seem to make it more and more remote. So perhaps we could comprehend more by taking environmentalism not as a movement to protect the materials of the planet, but as an effort to cleanse the souls of its inhabitants. In Europe we live on a prosperous continent, in a prosperous epoch, but as we hurry to the airport or to the tennis club or to the supermarket, even the sternest of materialists is nagged by an anxiety. Amidst all the luxuries and the machinery, perhaps something is lost, as well as gained, some simple goodness. Environmentalism emerges as a faith that appeals to a community that is uncomfortable with its prosperity and fears that wealth has created a chasm between it and natural goodness."

Now, my proposal. I would like to see the process that has begun here this week continue on an ongoing basis, with the types of people represented in this conference continuing to talk to one another. Therefore, perhaps the time has come for the RAD-AR initiative to become the RAD-AR Institute.

# *Part XIII*

# *An Agenda for Action*

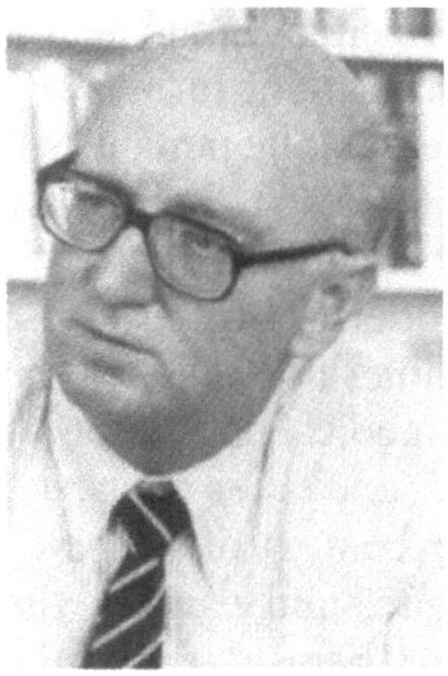

# 53. Future Directions

W. P. von WARTBURG

In closing, I would like to return briefly to the objectives as they were defined by the planning committee of this Wolfsberg conference, and to see to what extent we managed to meet them.

The first objective was to bring the parties involved in drug safety together for a mutual dialogue. This objective has been met, as evidenced by the discussions that took place during both the plenary and working group sessions. Not only were these exchanges frank and open, but they were also highly productive.

We also had the objective to look at the various elements involved in drug safety. It is important to recognize that drug safety has many aspects, as there is a tendency to see this issue in absolute terms. If you ask someone their opinion of a drug, they may say they think it is safe or unsafe. But if we delve deeper, we begin to see the difficulties of data generation, data evaluation, and communication that make us aware of the existence of the many shades of gray implicit in this complex subject and, equally, make us realize that snap decisions in this area should be avoided. We hoped that, by breaking the drug safety concept down into elements such as ethical considerations, risk analysis, benefit qualifications, the evaluation of the weighing-up process, and the communications aspect, we would learn more about this complex field. And in this context, I think we have achieved a good deal.

Another objective was to test the RAD-AR spirit in a viable context. It was by no means certain that the spirit released from the bottle 2 years ago at the first Wolfsberg meeting would spread beyond the industry and infect the other constituencies so vital to the cause of drug safety. But the feedback that I have had leads me to believe that this spirit has not only survived, but will flourish.

We hoped also to identify some issues of common concern. Many came to light during the conference. It is clear that we will have to deal with each issue individually in order to achieve tangible results. Finally, we aimed at gathering proposals for further action culled from a broader audience; I have a whole bag of them as a result of this conference.

Our main concern has always been the patient. This was underlined in the test which conference participants completed for Professor Young when most of them placed the patient in the middle of the pentagon of principles in the health care environment. I feel this is only common sense. If the patient turns away from drugs, saying he no longer likes this technology, he fears it, he perceives it as negative, it is to the manufacturer's detriment. This applies also to regulatory authorities because the removal of approved drugs indicates that, in the patient's opinion, the authorities have not been doing their job properly. Likewise, if a patient does not benefit from a prescribed medicine blame also falls on the physician, who is deemed to be a bad representative of the medical profession. It is in our interest that medicines are understood, prescribed, and taken properly, and that health care be understood better in the broader context of society.

Many concerns have come to light during this dialogue, and each of the constituencies present has played a part in expressing them. I think the conference provided an opportunity for the exchange of information, on the one hand, and the transfer of convictions, on the other. From what people have been telling me, it started with listening and ended with learning, and that process when we are involved in this kind of undertaking, is as important as concrete results. Professor Young pointed out to us that it is the lighthouse guiding our actions which is important, not the harbor to which we are sailing. When we talk about improving drug safety, we will never be able to sit back and say "Well, we've done that. What's next?", because improvement is an open-ended continuing exercise for which we need lighthouses to keep us on the right course.

Let us move on the future. The first step, proposed and reiterated by many of the participants, should be the formalization of the RAD-AR structure. This should take place on a national scale with the formation of national and even regional RAD-AR councils, as well as on an international scale. I have been a little hesitant about taking this step up to now, as I felt we should learn to walk before we started running. And, to my mind, it is not the institution that really counts, but the flow of information between the various members within it. This flow of information must increase to a flood in the coming decade as I am convinced that only by intensive networking between individuals and bodies can we influence a change for the better. I hope that we can fulfill the need for an open structure and the need for networking in such a way that no individual or body will feel isolated or locked out. We should aim at combining forces wherever it makes sense.

In addition, we should work on what has been called a "business plan." This should be a plan of action that will indicate not only what should be done in both pharmacoepidemiology and communication, but also which resources are available and who would be responsible for what. To achieve this, we will need considerable time and effort. We will have to allocate priorities to our actions, so that we do not spread ourselves too thin and disperse our energies on too many areas. I think we are now in a position to structure the existing RAD-AR Consortium more formally, and I hope that it will include members of all the constituencies represented in this room.

When we planned this conference so that ethical considerations would underpin the proceedings, we had no idea how it would all fit together. But the results, I feel, have been gratifying. We should now continue what has been started here, and work at breaking down the barriers that exist between the various constituencies, so that those who *know* interact with those who need to communicate. All of this is to the ultimate benefit of the patient.

It remains only for me to thank you for your wholehearted participation, and to look forward to our next Wolfsberg conference in 1992. The intervening 2 years will allow us to take stock of what we have discussed, and to begin incorporating it into our daily lives, concentrating not so much on the harbor towards which we are moving, but on the beam of the lighthouse that is guiding us.

# 54. Wolfsberg Think Pieces

The 1990 Wolfsberg dialogue conference raised many issues and points that were energetically debated during the working group meetings. The diversity of opinions voiced reflected the range of professions and interests represented. The think pieces are the concentrated essence of these meetings, and summarize the areas in which the participants agreed that change must be effected. The think pieces also propose principles and guidelines for the way in which responsibility for action can be shared.

**Think Piece 1**

*Above All, Do No Harm?*

Constituencies expressed their belief that *"above all, do no harm"* is no longer unreservedly applicable to risk/benefit assessment. The dictum is misleading because it implies that safety, as an absolute value, is attainable. It was proposed, instead, that the probability of benefit must outweigh the likelihood of harm, while taking into account the severity of harm and degree of benefit, as well as the context and relevant perspective from which the assessment is made. The illusion that drugs do no harm should be replaced by a climate in which risk and benefit are balanced against each other.

**Think Piece 2**

*Spontaneous Reports of Risk.*

Spontaneous reports continue to be central to the generation of signals of warnings of potential risk, but other types of data are needed to quantify and understand the risk mechanism. Spontaneous reports and their generation can be improved, among other things, by:

- Educating physicians to observe and provide useful reports
- Protecting physicians who provide these reports from the legal consequence of their action

- Analyzing reports received, standardizing methods of coding, and summarizing multiple reports
- Using the information contained in the reports properly
- Preventing the misuse of such information
- Making decisions about which reports merit studies and are the most important for public health concerns

Various constituencies affirmed the importance of monitoring patterns of use and effects. To this end, manufacturers should not aim to penetrate a market with drugs at a rate faster than their effects can be measured and assessed. Continued shared responsibility on the part of manufacturers and regulators in solving these problems is necessary. To further research in this area, a center for studies and the coordination of spontaneous reports should be set up. Such a center would be able to address not only the points listed above, but also be instrumental in helping to avoid the duplication of effort in many countries.

## Think Piece 3

*Data Resources.*

Greater access to a wider variety of data sources which carry data on the experiences of populations exposed to pharmaceuticals is necessary. Industry should provide access to full information on drug effects. Dialogue on the issue of confidentiality should continue in view of the industry's argument that confidentiality must be maintained in order to avoid misuse of information, which could lead to good drugs being damaged and ultimately to patients being harmed. Although health insurance data banks have demonstrated their usefulness, there is limited access to the data contained in them. Access to such data could lead to significant improvements to public health, not only in detecting and quantifying health risks and putting them into perspective, but also in identifying the magnitude of certain public problems which could serve as a catalyst to stimulate new therapies. A number of specific actions are called for, including:
- Standardization of certain data to allow comparative studies
- Formation or identification of a committee or body to develop, communicate, and update standards which are of particular relevance to data gathering in pharmacoepidemiology
- Development of models demonstrating the usefulness of health insurance data which incorporate optimal protection of privacy
- An infrastructure to coordinate these efforts and the development of data sources, such as registries of known drug-induced diseases

## Think Piece 4

*Quality of Life Assessment.*

The assessment of quality of life (QOL) was considered to be a valid concept which should be employed in order to broaden the understanding of the overall efficacy of pharmaceuticals. The perception and measurement of QOL is affected by the type of disease and is also a function of prevailing cultural factors. The assessment of QOL should ideally be included in the patient-physician interaction, and in that setting it would become part of the assessment of the patient's physical, mental, and cognitive functioning. Further studies are necessary with regard to:

- The role of QOL assessment incorporated in medical practice
- The importance and way in which the type of disease and certain cultural settings affect assessment of QOL, using standard measurements
- Understanding and measuring how QOL can be practicably translated into information which is broadly and consistently useful in understanding the benefits of pharmaceuticals

## Think Piece 5

*Health Care Economics.*

The economics of health care and pharmaceuticals have taken on greater importance with the advent of rising costs and constraints. The analysis of economic endpoints as a measure of a pharmaceutical's effectiveness and the analysis of relative costs of comparable but dissimilar pharmaceuticals are considered to be indicative of this trend. Constituencies questioned whether it was reasonable to assess economic endpoints for each indication and for each drug. Economic analysis, it was agreed, should not be part of the drug approval process, but its role in payment decisions was acknowledged.

There is considerable potential for economic studies of pharmaceuticals, particularly as automated insurance claims provide enormous amounts of data on billed and paid costs in different settings. However, judgment should be exercised as to the appropriateness of such studies, as it is not clear whether overall costs are helpful to understanding the meaning of health outcomes. Investigation is needed into which types of studies are appropriate and in which context they are necessary.

## Think Piece 6

*Risk/Benefit Assessment: Considering Risks and Benefits in Preventive Therapies.*

Constituencies agreed that one of the most problematic areas for the appraisal of benefit and risk relates to drugs which yield their primary benefits only after long-term use. The proportional likelihood of the benefits of such drugs is often unknown, while taking them entails risks which may lead to the appearance of side effects long before any benefits can be appreciated.

The dilemmas posed by this problem are how to balance the benefit/risk appraisal, particularly when only a proportion of those using the drug will benefit directly, and how to explain this to the patient. The inherent problems of marketing such drugs need to be addressed in a collaborative effort in order to find the most appropriate approach.

## Think Piece 7

*Risk/Benefit Assessment: The Physician-Patient Perspective.*

When prescribing drugs, the physician's decision should be based on the best available information, and he should avoid, where possible, situations which would predispose the patient to an adverse effect (while taking into account its severity and outcome relative to the clinical need and context). It is the responsibility of both the physician and the drug manufacturer to ensure that the patient is in a position to make a benefit/risk appraisal on the basis of sound and clear information. To this end, manufacturers must hold themselves responsible for supplying the physician with adequate information about the balanced risks and benefits of drugs (in the context of therapeutic alternatives), thus enabling the physician to communicate this information to the patient. Likewise, physicians should be more aware of their role in this process and improve their communication skills, possibly through medical training programs.

## Think Piece 8

*International Issues.*

Understanding the risk of a particular pharmaceutical requires an awareness of the qualitative list of its effects, both dose dependent and independent. The frequency and public health impact of adverse effects where they are serious and not exceedingly rare must be analyzed. It is important to reach agreement about which risks merit close study, as many of them, although they generate public concern, are relatively rare. This should be arrived at through international collaboration and data sharing. The WHO and the Collaborating Center in Sweden have already made advances in pooling data from the various regulatory centers of member countries. However, if this information is to have a significant public health impact, mechanisms by which other interested parties could have access to such data should be explored.

There should also be active investigation of means by which worldwide data on morbidity, including drug effects, and mortality in populations can be made accessible on an international scale and in a standardized format to those involved in understanding the benefits and risks of pharmaceuticals. This data should serve as a means of improving the understanding of baseline morbidities and assist both regulators and manufacturers in defining the priorities for dealing with the wide array of problems with which they are faced.

## Think Piece 9

*Direct Advertising.*

Direct industry advertising of pharmaceutical products is an issue too important for government regulatory bodies to ignore. A systematic assessment of direct advertising in comparison with and contrast to other forms of industry communication is necessary. Particular attention should be paid to legal, economic, technical, and effectiveness criteria, and to the quality of the assessment measures used. National and regional authorities should foster dialogue and collaborative studies on the impact of satellite-based telecommunication networks on national direct-advertising regulations, as current trends are likely to lead to an unmanageable and contradictory mix of national policies. Companies should be encouraged by authorities to conduct well-designed experiments using non-massmedia channels. Authorities should employ external expertise to evaluate their direct advertising policies in order to gain fresh perspectives on how they could be used to promote drug safety.

## Think Piece 10

*Industry-Patient Communication.*

Communication between the industry and patients through patient product information (PPI) and other means is highly desirable and should be systematically assessed as to its objectives and effectiveness. Dispensing medicines without written PPI is considered to be bad medicine. The assessment of PPI should encompass, but not be limited to, the analysis of samples of current PPI, the development of "How to .." manuals, and the evaluation of the quality of the various communication measures (e.g., readability) used to produce PPI. This assessment should also consider:

- Alternatives to traditional PPI formats
- PPI strategies consistent with the legal and liability implications of interpreting PPI as a "license"
- Improvements and innovations in the ways physicians and other health professionals facilitate industry-to-patient communication of drug-safety information

Conferences and other ways of stimulating dialogue on PPI issues with the Third World should also be considered as a means of improving drug safety worldwide.

## Think Piece 11

*Industry-Media Communication.*

Improved communication between industry and the media requires that each group reach a better understanding of the other's communication strategies and professional standpoints, as well as drug safety concerns in general. Companies should move beyond target-oriented communication with the media and establish regularly used communication channels. They recognize that a single media strategy cannot satisfy the differing needs of the varying media branches, nor those of journalists with a specific brief (e.g., news, science, business). Journalists and industry scientists, either directly or using the services of a third party (e.g., a university), should consider planning and conducting workshops on neutral ground to lay the foundations for good communication. Other joint initiatives should include the establishment of short-term, two-way sensitivity programs (e.g., internships or exchanges) between industry and the media, and the promulgation of jointly developed guidelines for good communication practices.

## Think Piece 12

*Multiple Communication Channels.*

Multiple and repeated channels of communication are essential to provide the amount of drug safety information necessary to ensure patient autonomy and reasoned compliance in medical decision making. Apart from the physician, other important channels of communication are pharmacists, women's magazines, simple drug compendia, materials produced by pharmaceutical companies, school programs, and related educational materials. Each approach should be systematically assessed as to its potential effectiveness in providing the various categories of patients with information, as well as to its effectiveness relative to alternative channels of communication. Possible initiatives should include:

- The compilation of unbiased and validated reference sources of patient materials
- The organization of broad-based workshops and seminars to conduct historical case studies on significant drug issues
- The production of multimedia materials containing sound medical information
- The creation of a task force to develop improved patient product inserts
- The formation of an international network between industry and health care organizations to foster improved drug safety information

## Think Piece 13

*Patient Participation.*

Effective patient participation in medical decision making requires a balance between the extremes of medical paternalism (where the patient is told what to do) and complete patient autonomy (where the patient is given information and left to make up his or her mind). The patient's right to choose must be protected, even if the choice does not fit in with the expert's assessment of the best decision. Responsibility must be shared in order to ensure that decisions are based on reliable and valid information that has been clearly and understandably communicated, ultimately leading to the optimal use of drugs by patients. Studies should be carried out on the role of factors such as traditional physician-patient behavior patterns, age and educational differences among patients, the relative importance of prescribed medicines to patient well-being, national and ethnic cultures, and how financial and time constraints influence perceived and actual patient autonomy. Initiatives for improving collaboration and dialogue in medical decision making might include programs to broaden physicians' and other health professionals' understanding of why, how, and when patients seek greater or lesser autonomy, as well as case studies to ascertain what type of information communicated in which way best enables different types of patients to reach their respective and desired dependency-autonomy balance.

## Think Piece 14

*New Communication Channels.*

Through new channels and technologies of communication, the media are shaping physicians' messages and patients' receptivity by informing the public about drug safety issues and medical developments. This is done by alerting the public to drug crises and by motivating the public to participate more actively in their own health care and in their relationships with physicians. While the physician remains the most important communicator of drug safety information to the patient, it was, however, acknowledged that the exploding information environment has changed the context dramatically and permanently within which physician-patient dialogue occurs. Ethical as well as technical and contextual issues of drug safety information should be assessed, differentiating between advertising, promotional communication and nonpromotional education. Both physicians and patients should note not only the information communicated, but also the credibility of the source and the degree of public trust in the information communicated.

**Think Piece 15**

*Empowerment for Decision Making.*

An informed medical decision making partnership requires not only that patients receive basic drug safety information, but also that they are able to interpret it in such a way so as to result in competent and autonomous behavior. Each patient should know or seek to find out the following information (supplied by the National Council for Patient Information and Education) about each drug that he or she is proposed:

- The drug's name and its intended purpose
- How and when to use it and for how long
- Which foods, liquids, and other medicines and activities to avoid while taking the drug
- Possible side effects and what to do should any occur

Pharmaceutical companies, government regulatory authorities, health professionals, the media, citizen groups, and patients, both separately and collectively, should encourage the more regular provision of such information to patients through whatever means are determined to be the most effective, as well as encouraging the active involvement of patients in seeking out such information if it is not routinely provided.

# *Appendix*

# 55. Bibliography

## Ethics


Arnold RM et al. (1987) Ethical issues in a drug information center. Drug Intell Clin Pharm 21(12):1008–1011

Baier H (1987) Benötigen wir eine Ethik der Medizin? Der Freiraum des Arztes zwischen Markt, Politik und Recht. In: Bress L (ed) Medizin und Gesellschaft. Springer, Berlin Heidelberg New York Tokyo, pp. 132–147

Bankowski Z (1988) Genetics, medicine and ethics. World Health, WHO, Geneva

Beauchamp TL, Childress JF (1989) Principles of biomedical ethics. Oxford University Press, New York

Brett AS (1984) Ethical issues in risk factor intervention. Am J Med 76(4):557–561

Brett AS (1986) The modification of cardiovascular risk factors: ethical issues. Cardiol Clin 4(1):163–168

Bryant JH, Bankowski Z (1985) Health policy, ethics and human values – an international dialogue. Highlights of the Athens conference. Council of International Organizations of Medical Sciences, Geneva

Beauchamp TL, Bowie NE (eds) (1988) Ethical theory and business. Prentice-Hall, Englewood Cliffs

Beauchamp TL, Childress JF (1989) Principles of biomedical ethics. 3rd edn. Oxford University Press, New York

Darr K et al. (1986) The ethical imperative in health services governance and management. Hosp Health Serv Adm 31(2):53–66

Davidson DL, Goodpaster KE (1984) Managing product safety: the Ford Pinto. In: Goodpaster KE (ed) Ethics in management. Harvard Business School Publishing Division, Boston MA, pp. 111–119

De George RT, Pichler J (eds) (1987) Ethics, free enterprise and public policy. Prentice-Hall, Englewood Cliffs

Deutsch E (1989) The functions of ethical committees. Drug Res/Arzneim Forsch 39(II) (8a):1049–1053

Dollinger MJ (1988) Confucian ethics and Japanese management practices. J Bus Ethics 7(8):575–584

Engelhardt HT (1989) Bioethics in the People's Republic of China. In: Veatch RM (ed) Cross cultural perspectives in medical ethics: readings. Jones Bartlett, Boston

Fletcher JC (1984) Ethical and social aspects of risk predictions. Clin Genet 25(1):25–32

Follesdal D (1986) Risk: philosophical and ethical aspects. Prog Clin Res 208:41–52

Forrow D et al. (1988) Science, ethics and the making of clinical decisions: implications for risk factor intervention. JAMA 259(21):3161–3167

Gellerman SW (1986) Why "good" managers make bad ethical choices. Harv Bus Rev Jul/Aug:85–90

Gerber P, Eadie M (1988) Ethics in drug trials. Med J Aust 149(5):229–230

Gorovitz S (1984) Why you don't owe it to yourself to seek health. J Med Ethics 10:143–146

Gorovitz S, MacIntyre A (1976) Toward a theory of medical fallibility. J Med Philos 1(1):51–71

Graber GC (1988) Ethical issues in medicine. Survey of Business 24(1):15–20

Guerrette RHH (1988) Corporate ethical consulting: developing management strategies for corporate ethics. J Bus Ethics 7(5):373–380

Haney CA, Colson AC (1980) Ethical responsibility in physician-patient communication. Ethics Sci Med 7(1):27–36

Harris RL (1986) 1985 Henry F. Smyth Jr. Award lecture: Information, risk and professional ethics. Am Ind Hyg Assoc J 47(2):67–71

Harrison PJ (1989) Ethics and drug safety. Pharm Med 4(2):155–157

Howard-Jones N (1982) Human experimentation in historical and ethical perspectives. Soc Sci Med 16:1429–1448

Jonas H (1984) Das Prinzip Verantwortung. Versuch einer Ethik für die technologische Zivilisation. Suhrkamp, Frankfurt

Jones TM, Gautschi FH (1988) Will the ethics of business change? a survey of future executives. J Bus Ethics 7:231

Jonsen AR (1988) Ethics of drug giving and drug taking. J Drug Issues 18(2):195–200

Kee F (1989) Risk management, public policy and informed consent: a case study. Public Health 103(4):281–287

Kersting F, Seybert HW (1986) Eine internationale Ethik-Kommission. Neun Jahre Erfahrungen in der Beurteilung von Protokollen zur Arzneimittelprüfung. Med Klin 81(11):405–408

Leisinger KM (1989) Business ethics and transnational corporations. In: Proceedings of the conference on "A developing world economy – the ethics of international corporations", Sep 28–Oct 1, San Rafael, CA

Leisinger KM (1989) Proverty, sickness and medicine: an unholy alliance? Developmental policy, health and the role of the pharmaceutical industry in the third world. IFPMA, Geneva

Leisinger KM (1990) Unternehmensethik als Führungsaufgabe. Unternehmen und Strafrecht. In: Umwelt-Aussagen zum strafrechtlichen Risiko der Unternehmen und ihrer Mitarbeiter. HRV Hannover Rechtsschutz AG, Hannover, FRG
Levine RJ (1988) Post-marketing surveillance – some ethical considerations. J Rheumatol 15 [suppl 15]:34–39
Lewis PV (1985) Defining "business ethics": like nailing jello to a wall. J Bus Ethics 4:377–383
Logsdon JM, Palmer DR (1988) Issues management and ethics. J Bus Ethics 7(3):191–198
Lowrance WW (1986) The ethics of access to health care. The Bridge 16(10):14–18
Main R (1988) Performing drug studies in the elderly – a personal view on the ethical issues. J Clin Pharm Ther 13:307–312
Matley J, Greene R (1987) Ethics of health, safety and environment: what's "right"? Chem Engineer 94(3):40–46
Miller AB (1988) The ethics, the risks and the benefits of screening. Biomed Pharmacother 42(7):439–442
Parker LM (1989) Doctor-patient communication and ethical issues (editorial). J Clin Oncol 7(9):1182–1183
Pochin E (1982) Risk and medical ethics. J Med Ethics 8:180–184
Poumadere M (1989) Scandalous need for an honest policy in risk communications. Intern Manage 44(7):49
Rich A (1985) Wirtschaftsethik. Mohn, Gütersloh
Rothman DJ (1987) Ethical and social issues in the development of new drugs and vaccines. Bull N Y Acad Med 63(6):557–568
Sass HM (1985) Medizinethik in den USA. Münch Med Wochenschr 127(34):779–801
Sass HM (1986) Schwerpunkt Bioethik. Von der wachsenden Bedeutung ethischer und kultureller Wertfragen in biologischer und medizinischer Wissenschaft und Praxis. Mensch Medizin Gesellschaft 11:229–230
Sass HM (1989) Ethics of drug research and drug development. Drug Res/Arzneim Forsch 39(II)(8a):1041–1047
Shapiro S (1985) The decision to publish ethical dilemmas. J Chron Dis 38(4):365–372
Smith D (1984) Politics, ethics and safety. Safety Pract 2(6):19
Thompson WG (1988) The ethics of physician-pharmaceutical company relationships. Can Med Assoc J 139(9):835–836
Tomlinson T, Brody H (1988) Ethics and communication in do-not-resuscitate orders. N Engl J Med 318(1):43–46
Tunkel V (1989) Drug trials: who takes the risk? Lancet 2(8663):609–611
Vere DW (1988) The ethics of adverse drug reactions. Adverse Drug Reaction Bull 128:480–483
Vitell SJ, Festervand TA (1987) Business ethics: conflicts, practices and beliefs of industrial executives. J Bus Ethics 6:111–122
von Wartburg WP (1989) Political issue management with common sense. Industrial Crises Quarterly 3(4):303–318

Wall DW (1987) Ethics and the pharmaceutical industry: some ideas for general practitioners. J R Coll Gen Pract 37(299):267–269
Watterson A (1986) Ethics and the safety practitioner. Safety Pract 4(7):30–31
Weller S (1988) The effectiveness of corporate codes of ethics. J Bus Ethics 7:389–395
Wertheimer MD et al. (1985) Ethics and communication in the surgeon-patient relationship. J Med Educ 60(10):804–806
World Health Organization (1988) Ethical criteria for medicinal drug promotion. WHO, Geneva
Young EWD (1986) Current ethical issues in emergency care. J Emerg Nurs 12(5):301–304
Young EWD (1987) An ethical approach to risk-benefit assessment. RAD-AR conference, Jan 26–28, Basel
Young EWD (1989) Alpha and Omega: ethics at the frontiers of life and death. Addison-Wesley, Reading, MA

## General Risk/Benefit Topics

Anonymous (1987) Acceptable degrees of therapeutic risks. Scrip 24 Jun:22
Aronow WS et al. (1987) Risk factors for atherothrombotic brain infarction in persons over 62 years of age in a long-term health care facility. J Am Geriatr Soc 35:1–3
Bajgier SM (1982) An interactive model of attitude and risk-benefit formation regarding social issues. Policy Sci 14:257–278
Berando FM (1986) Survivor education: the role of habits, attitudes and risk taking. Death Stud 10:391–409
Blomquist G (1986) A utility maximization model of driver traffic safety behavior. Accid Anal Prev 18:371–375
Bolton NE (1988) Risk management today. Am Ind Hyg Assoc J 49(Nov):A698–A700
Brauers WK (1986) Essay review article: risk, uncertainty and risk analysis. Long Range Plann 19:139–143
Breyer F, Fuchs VR (1982) Risk attitudes in health: an exploratory study. National Bureau of Economic Research, Working Paper 857
British Medical Association Guide (1987) Living with risk. Wiley, Chichester
Bühlmann H, Loeffel H, Nievergelt E (1969) Einführung in die Theorie und Praxis der Entscheidung bei Unsicherheit. 2nd edn Springer, Berlin Heidelberg New York
Carpenter PF (1982) Risk assessment. Meeting on risk assessment, National Academy of Science, Feb 10
Chelemer MJ (1987) The hazardous substances initiative: working to create safer tomorrow. MIT Report May:4–7
Clarke L (1988) Politics and bias in risk assessment. Soc Science J 25(2):155–165

Covello VT (1987) Decision analysis and risk management decision making: issues and methods. Risk Anal 7:131–139

Covello VT, Mumpower J (1985) Risk analysis and risk management: a historical perspective. Risk Anal 5:103–120

Covello VT et al. (1982) Risk analysis, philosophy and the social and behavioral sciences. Risk Anal 2:53–58

Covello VT et al. (1986) Risk evaluation and management. Plenum, New York

Crone HD (1988) Dose, content, risk: can we instruct the public. Regul Toxicol Pharmacol 8:1–3

Deisler PF (1988) The risk management-risk assessment interface. Environ Sci Technol 22(1):15–19

Ehrlich PR, Ehrlich AH (1989) Intelligent planning for safety. Society 27(1):15–16

European Community (1980) Nuclear and non-nuclear risk – an exercise in comparability. Final Report, EUR 6417 EN. Pollution Prevention (Consultants), Crawley, UK

Finkel AM (1990) Confronting uncertainty in risk management. Resources for the Future, Washington DC

Fischhoff B, Lichtenstein S, Slovic P et al. (1981) Acceptable risk. Cambridge University Press, Cambridge

Fritzsche AF (1986) Wie sicher leben wir? Risikobeurteilung und Bewältigung in unserer Gesellschaft. TÜV Rheinland, Cologne

Goodman J (1986) On criteria of insignificant difference between two risks. Risk Anal 6:235–244

Haight FA (1986) Risk, especially risk of traffic accident. Accid Anal Prev 18:359–366

Hanley JW (1981) Monsanto's early warning system. Harv Bus Rev Nov/Dec:107–122

Heimer CA (1988) Social structure, psychology and the estimation of risk. Ann Rev Sociol 14:491–519

Helal B (1984) Physical risks in modern sport. Med Sci Law 24:247–248

Hollaender A (1986) Acceptance of the distinguished contribution award of the society for risk analysis. Risk Anal 6:113–115

Imhof AE (1981) Die gewonnenen Jahre. Von der Zunahme unserer Lebensspanne seit dreihundert Jahren oder von der Notwendigkeit einer neuen Einstellung zu Leben und Sterben. Beck, Munich

Jasanoff S (1987) Cultural aspects of risk assessment in Britain and the United States. In: Johnson BB, Covello VT (eds) The social and cultural construction of risk. Reidel, Boston, pp. 359–397

Johnson BB, Covello VT (eds) (1987) The social and cultural construction of risk: essays on risk selection and perception. Reidel, Boston

Keller, LR, Sarin EK (1988) Equity in social risk: some empirical observations. Risk Anal 8(1):135–146

Kimbrough RD, Grandhean PA (1988) Risk assessment: extrapolation to individual risk. Basic Life Sci 43:245–253

Knoepfel P (ed) (1988) Risiko und Risikomanagement. Helbing Lichtenhahn, Basel
Krauer A (1988) Acceptable risk in society. In: Horisberger B, Dinkel R (eds) The perception and management of drug safety risks. Springer, Berlin Heidelberg New York Tokyo, pp. 5–8
Krauer A (1988) Chemie und Umwelt. Paper, Jan 6
Kuhlmann A (1981) Einführung in die Sicherheitswissenschaft. Vieweg/TÜV Rheinland, Cologne
Kunreuther H et al. (1984) A decision-process perspective on risk and policy analysis. Manage Sci 30:475–485
Lane JC (1987) Social epidemiology: directions for the future in academic and "shoeleather" risk analysis. J Community Health 12(2, 3):130–136
Lave LB (1987) Health and safety risk analysis. Science 236:291–295
Lowrance WW (1976) Of acceptable risk. Kaufmann, California
Lowrance WW (1986) The ethics of access to health care. Bridge 16:14–18
Luce BR, Elixhauser A (1990) Standards for socioeconomic evaluation of health care products and services. Springer, Berlin Heidelberg New York Tokyo
Lund AK et al. (1986) Perceived risks and driving behavior. Accid Anal Prev 18:367–370
Lynn FM (1986) The interplay of science and values in assessing and regulating environmental risks. Science Technol Human Values 11(2):40–50
Mackinnon B (1986) Pricing human life. Science Technol Human Values 11(2):29–39
Meadows D (1972) Die Grenzen des Wachstums. Bericht des "Club of Rome" zur Lage der Menschheit. Deutsche Verlags-Anstalt, Stuttgart
Medawar C (1986) No news, good news? Scrip 1162:18–19
Medawar C (1987) Failings of the pharmaceutical industry. Pharmaceut Med 2:259–263
Miller SA (1984) Introductory remarks to session on risk assessment and risk management. Fundam Appl Toxicol 4:380–382
Mills W (1988) The process of risk management .. and the pitfalls! AARN News Lett 44(4):14–15
National Research Council (1982) Risk and decision making: perspectives and research. National Academy Press, Washington DC
National Research Council (1983) Risk assessment in the federal government: managing the process. National Academy Press, Washington DC
Nelkin D (1987) The culture of science journalism. Society Sept – Oct: 18–25
Orleans M, Haverkamp AD (1987) Are there health risks in using risking systems? The case of perinatal risk assessment. Health Policy 7:297–307
Paehlke R (1989) The criteria of net benefit. Society 27(1):13–14
Pedroni G, Zweifel P (1988) Chance und Risiko: Messung, Bewertung, Akzeptanz. Pharma Information, Basel
Peets JI et al. (1987) The assessment of major hazards: the density and other characteristics of the exposed population around a hazard source. J Hazard Mater 14:337–363

Quarantelli EL (1988) Disaster crisis management: a summary of research findings. J Manage Studies 25(4):373–385
Rosen S (1981) Valuing health risk. AEA Papers Proc:241–245
Rothschild L (1987) Risk. Listener, Nov 30
Royal Society Study Group (1983) Risk assessment. Royal Society, London
Ruckelhaus WD (1983) Science, risk and public policy. Science 221:1026–1028
Ruckelhaus WD (1984) Risk in a free society. Vital Speeches Day 1:354–358
Samson DA (1987) Corporate risk philosophy for improved risk management. J Bus Research 15(2):107–122
Schneider T (1981) Grundgedanken und Methodik moderner Sicherheitsplanung. Sicherheitsingenieur 8:26–30/9:18–29
Starr C et al. (1980) Risk of risk decisions. Science 208:1114–1119
Swedish Drug Information Council (1987) The elderly and medicines. Swedish Drug Information Council, Stockholm
Teeling-Smith G (1983) Measuring the social benefits of medicine. Office of Health Economics, London
Tenner E (1987) Warning: nature may be hazardous to your health. Harvard Magazine Sept–Oct:34–38
von Winterfeldt D, Edwards W (1984) Patterns of conflict about risky technologies. Risk Anal 4:555–568
White GF (1988) Path to risk analysis. Risk Anal 8(2):171–175
Wildavsky A (1988) Searching for safety. Social Philosophy and Policy Center/Transaction Books, New Brunswick NJ, USA
Wildavsky A (1989) The secret of safety lines in danger. Society 27(1):4–5
Wilde GJS (1987) Theorie der Risikokompensation der Unfallverursachung und praktische Folgerungen für die Unfallverhütung. Unfallheilkunde 130:134–156
Wilson R, Crouch EAC (1987) Risk assessment and comparisons: an introduction. Science 236:267–270
Wittmann W (1982) Risikobewältigung: Gratwanderung zwischen Sicherheit und Freiheit. Informationstagung der SVA. In: Neue Zürcher Zeitung, Zeitfragen 289, Dec 11/12
Wynne B (1983) Technologie, Risiko und Partizipation: Zum gesellschaftlichen Umgang mit Unsicherheit. In: Conrad J (ed) Gesellschaft, Technik und Risikopolitik. Springer, Berlin Heidelberg New York Tokyo
Yadigaroglu G, Chakraborty S (eds) (1985) Risikountersuchungen als Entscheidungsinstrument. TÜV Rheinland, Cologne
Young EWD (1987) An ethical approach to risk-benefit assessment. RAD-AR conference, Basel, Switzerland, Jan 26–28
Young FE (1987) Risk assessment: the convergence of science and the law. Regul Toxicol Pharmacol 7:179–184

## Drug Risks

Amrein R et al. (1988) Antidepressant drug therapy: associated risks. J Neural Transm 26 Suppl:73–86

Anonymous (1984) Measuring drug risk: Ciba-Geigy's monitoring. Scrip 951:14–15

Anonymous (1987) ABPI issues post-marketing surveillance guidelines. Market Lett 7 Nov:13

Anonymous (1987) Intrauterine devices maker gambles on the informed consumer. Washington Post, March 13

Anonymous (1987) RAD-AR program analyzes risk for Ciba-Geigy. Market Lett Sept 21:25

Anonymous (1987) Risk management meeting: conference report, Brighton. Br Med J 294:1678–1679

Azarnoff DL, Herting RL (1984) Drug development: risks and problems. Ann N Y Acad Sci 432:279–285

Baichwal RS (1988) Benefits of biotechnology to pharmaceutical industry. Hindustan Antibiot Bull 30(3–4):51–53

Biscos-Garreau M, Girard M (1988) Comparison of benefits and risks of drug treatments: methodological problems. L'Encephale XIV:365–369

Borda IT, Bernecker GC (1985) The pharmaceutical industry – drug monitoring by Ciba-Geigy. In: Inman WHW (ed) Monitoring for drug safety. MTP, Boston, pp. 173–200

BPI (ed) (1985) Drugs – potential and risks. BPI, Frankfurt/Main

Brest AN (1987) Malpractice liability and drug therapy. Clin Ther 9(2):138–140

Brown P (1987) Ciba-Geigy's risk assessment. Scrip 1227:15

Burley D, Inman WHW (eds) (1988) Therapeutic risk: perception, measurement, management. Wiley, New York

Burley D, Silverstone T (eds) (1988) Medicines and road traffic safety. CNS, London

Burley DM (1986) Risks: in broad perspective. Adverse Drug Reactions, proceedings of a symposium, London, Mar 6, pp. 145–175

Cadieux RJ (1989) Drug interactions in the elderly. Postgrad Med 86(8):179–186

Campbell RWF (1988) Assessment of the risk-benefit ratio for antiarrhythmic drug use. Drugs 36:616–632

Carpenter PF (1982) Risk assessment. Meeting of National Academy of Sciences, paper, Feb 10

Carroll NV et al. (1986) Perceived risks and pharmacists' generic substitution behavior. J Consumer Aff 20:36–47

Carson FL, Strom BL (1986) Techniques of post-marketing surveillance. Med Toxicol 1:237–246

Champion GD (1988) A perspective on the cost-effectiveness and risks of nonsteroidal anti-inflammatory drug therapy. Med J Aust 147(7):346–349

Chetley A, Gilbert A (1986) Problem drugs – introduction. HAI, The Hague:1–4

Council for International Organizations of Medical Sciences (1986) Monitoring and assessment of adverse drug effects (working group report). CIOMS, Geneva

Destevens G (1987) The risk and benefits of drug therapy. Med Res Rev 7:173–181
Diamond LD, Laurence DR (1985) Product liability in respect of drugs. Br Med J 290:365–368
Eadie MJ (1987) The risk-benefit ratio of anticonvulsant drugs. Med Toxicol Adverse Drug Exp 295:324–337
Faich GA (1986) Adverse drug reaction monitoring. N Engl J Med 314:1589–1592
Faich GA (1986) Analgetic risks and pharmacoepidemiology. JAMA 256(13):1788
Fitzgerald JD (1986) Innovative drug discovery: what is an acceptable risk for a pharmaceutical company? 3rd World Conference on Clin Pharmacology, Stockholm, Jul 15
Gingell JC (1986) Non-steroidal anti-inflammatory drugs and serious gastrointestinal adverse reactions–2. Br Med J 292:1190–1191
Girard M (1988) Risk-benefit ratio of drugs: antidepressive agents. L'Encephale 14(3):97–99
Haire D (1984) How the FDA determines the "safety" of drugs. National Women's Health Network, Washington DC
Hallett C, Dean BC (1984) Bromazepam: acute benefit-risk assessment in general practice. Curr Med Res Opin 8:683–688
Harper CM et al. (1989) Drug-induced illness in the elderly. Postgrad Med 86(2):245–256
Hawkey C (1989) Non-steroidal anti-inflammatory drugs in patients with peptic ulcer disease: rarely justified in terms of cost or patient benefit. Br Med J 298:177–178
Heilmann K (1986) Impact of professional and lay media on patients and physicians. Am J Med 80 (Suppl 6a):5–7
Henry JA, Martin AJ (1987) The risk-benefit assessment of antidepressant drugs. Med Toxicol Adverse Drug Exp 2(6):445–462
Horisberger B, Dinkel R (eds) (1988) The perception and management of drug safety risks. Springer, Berlin Heidelberg New York Tokyo
Hull CJ (1989) The safety of new drugs. Br J Anaesth 62(6):587–589
Inman WHW (1984) Risks in medical intervention – balancing therapeutic risks and benefits. Pem News 2:15–36
Inman WHW (1985) Let's get our act together. In: Dukes G (ed) Side effects of drugs annual 9. Elsevier, Amsterdam, pp. XV–XX
Inman WHW (1987) Requirements for risk-benefit assessment of drugs before withdrawal. Pem News [Suppl] (March) 4
Inman WHW (1987) Prescription-event monitoring. Its strategic role in postmarketing surveillance for drug safety. Pem News 4:16–29
Jones JK, Kennedy D, Piper J, Rosa F (1984) Judging risks vs benefits of oral contraceptives. Clin Pharm 3:521–522
Karch FE, Lasagna L (1977) Toward the operational identification of adverse drug reactions. Clin Pharmacol Ther 21:247–254
Keown CF (1985) Contextual effects on people's ratings of seriousness for side effects of prescription drugs. Percept Mot Skills 61:435–441

Keown CF, Slovic P, Lichtenstein S (1984) Influence of information about side effects on perceived risk of prescription drugs. In: Winston WJ (ed) Marketing for mental health services. Haworth, New York, pp. 111–123

Keown CF et al. (1984) Attitudes of physicians, pharmacists and laypersons toward seriousness and need for disclosure of prescription drug side effects. Health Psychol 3:1–11

Lane DA, Hutchinson TA (1987) The notion of acceptable risk: the role of utility in drug management. J Chronic Dis 40:621–625

Lasagna L (1987) Post-marketing surveillance of multisource drugs – report of a conference, 9–10 July 1986. Center for the Study of Drug Development, Tufts Univ (ps 8711), pp. 1–58

Laurence DR, Black JW (1978) The medicine you take. Croom Helm, London

Lewandowski G (1988) What can be learned from drug safety issues? In: Horisberger B, Dinkel R (eds) The perception and management of drug safety risks. Springer, Berlin Heidelberg New York Tokyo, pp. 158–160

Mann RD (1988) From mithridatium to modern medicine: the management of drug safety. J R Soc Med 81(12):725–728

Mann RD (ed) (1989) Risk and consent to risk in medicine: the proceedings of a conference organized by the Management Forum Ltd, London. Parthenon, Park Ridge, NJ, USA

Markenson J (1987) A panel discussion on the safety of non-steroidal anti-inflammatory drugs. Semin Arthritis Reum 17(3, suppl 2):1–6

Mattison N (1984) Regulatory scene. Pharmaceut Med 1:13–16

Mazanec DJ (1988) Nonsteroidal anti-inflammatory drug therapy. Cleve Clin J Med 55(5):419–425

McMahon FG (1983) How safe should drugs be? JAMA 249(4):481–482

Medawar C (1987) Failings of the pharmaceutical industry. Pharmaceut Med 2:259–263

Michocki RJ, Lamy PP (1988) A “risk” approach to adverse drug reactions. J Am Geriatr Soc 36:79–81

Montagne M, Bleidt BA (1987) Social forces in the premature removal of drug products from the marketplace. Clin Res Practice Drug Affairs 5(2, 3):83–127

Montamat SC et al. (1989) Management of drug therapy in the elderly. N Engl J Med 321(5):303–309

Napke E (1986) Adverse reactions: some pitfalls and postulates. Center for Study of Drug Development, Boston

Naranjo C, Jones JK (1990) Drug induced disease: a symposium. Elsevier, Amsterdam

Palminteri R (1988) Benefit-risk ratio of new drugs: for whom? J R Soc Med 81:155–157

Pedroni G (1982) Drugs and adverse reactions. Pharma Information, Basel

Petri H, Leufkens H, Naus J, Silkens R, van Hessem P, Urquhart J (1990) Rapid method for estimating the risk of acutely controversial side effects of prescription drugs. J Clin Epidemiol 43(5):433–439

Pinder RM (1988) The benefits and risks of antidepressant drugs. Hum Psychopharmacol 3(2):73–86

Richard BW (1987) Drug regulation in the United States and the United Kingdom: the depo-prover story. Ann Intern Med 106:886–891

Sachs RM, Dieck GS (1988) The Feldene experience: a case study. In: Horisberger B, Dinkel R (eds) The perception and management of drug safety risks. Springer, Berlin Heidelberg New York Tokyo, pp. 81–89

Shapiro S (1986) Risks of agranulocytosis and aplastic anemia – their relation to drug use with special reference to analgetics. JAMA 256:1749–1757

Smith CG (1985) Past, current and future safety and efficacy trends in the drug industry. Regul Tox Pharmacol 5:241–254

Snell E (1987) How adverse are reactions to medicines? Scrip 1190:22–23

Spitzer WO, Hutchinson T, Lane D (1987) Post-marketing management of drug use: toward rational public policy. Can Med Assoc J 136:1022–1024

Spivey RN, Lasagna L, Trimble AG (1987) New indication for already-approved drugs: time trends for the new drug application review phase. Clin Pharmacol Ther 41:368–370

Stonier PD (1988) Road traffic safety and the pharmaceutical industry. Int Clin Psychopharmacol 3(suppl 1):133–140

Swedish Drug Information Council (1987) The elderly and medicines. Swedish Drug Information Council

Tallarida RJ et al. (1984) Non-physicians and physicians assess severity of disease states and adverse drug reactions: application to drug benefit-risk measurement. Pharmaceut Med 1:41–46

Teeling-Smith G (1983) Measuring the social benefits of medicine. Office of Health Economics, London

Tilson HH (1986) Social policy and drug safety. Clin Geriatr Med 2(1):165–179

Tootelian DH et al. (1988) Branded vs generic prescription drugs: perceptions of risk, efficacy, safety and value. J Health Care Mark 8(3):26–29

Turner P (1984) Food and drugs: why different approaches to their safety? Lancet i:1116

Ueberla K (1984) Sicherheit und Risiko im Arzneimittelbereich – Fiktion und Realität. In: Lange S (ed) Ermittlung und Bewertung industrieller Risiken. Springer, Berlin Heidelberg New York Tokyo

Urquhart J (1987) Assessing adverse reaction reports on old drugs in new dosage forms. Proceedings: The latest developments in drug delivery systems:32–34

Urquhart J, Heilmann K (1985) Drugs: Risk vs benefit. Agrippa, Cologne

Vale JA, Meredith TJ (1986) Acute poisoning due to nonsteroidal anti-inflammatory drugs. Med Toxicol 1:12–31

Vance MA, Millington WR (1986) Principles of irrational drug therapy. Int J Health Serv 16:355–362

Venning GR (1983) Identification of adverse reactions to new drugs I–IV. Br Med J 286:199–202, 289–292, 365–368, 458–460, 544–547

Venning GR (1984) Priorities in the benefit-risk assessment of new drugs. Adverse Drug React Acute Poisoning Rev 3:113–121

Venning GR (1987) Rare and serious adverse reactions. Med Toxicol Adverse Drug Exp 2(4):235–241
Venulet J (1984) Functioning of the side effect surveillance system at Ciba-Geigy Basel. Industrie Santé Jan:49
Venulet J (1987) Informativity of adverse drug reactions data in medical publictions. Center for Study of Drug Development (rs 8709), Tufts Univ, Boston (reprinted from Drug Inform J 19:357–365)
Volans GN (1987) Monitoring the safety of over the counter drugs. Br Med J 295:797–798
von Wartburg WP (1985) Ten aspects of risk as applied to pharmaceuticals. Ciba-Geigy J 2
Walker SR, Gelzer J et al. (1986) A comparative retrospective analysis of data for short- and long-term animal toxicity studies on 40 pharmaceutical compounds. Center for Study of Drug Development, Boston
Wardell WM (1978) History and application of drug safety and efficacy requirements in the United States. Agents Actions 8(4):420–421
Wehrauch TR, Philipp E (1989) Reduction of risk to patients through optimized planning of clinical drug development. Drug Res/Arzneim Forsch 39(II)(8a):1054–1055

## Drug Epidemiology

Bem JL et al. (1988) Review of yellow cards (1986): report to the Committee on the Safety of Medicines. Br J Clin Pharmacol 26(6):679–689
Borda IT, Bernecker GC (1985) The pharmaceutical industry – drug monitoring by Ciba-Geigy. In: Inman WHW (ed) Monitoring for drug safety. MTP, Boston, pp. 173–200
Carson JL, Strom BL (1986) Techniques of post-marketing surveillance. Med Toxicol 1:237–246
CIOMS Working Group Report (1986) Monitoring and assessment of adverse drug effects. CIOMS, Geneva
Clinch D (1988) Why not have definitive trials of gastrointestinal safety for nonsteroidal anti-inflammatory drugs? J R Soc Med 81(3):158–160
Crooks J (1983) Drug epidemiology and clinical pharmacology: their contribution to patient care. Br J Clin Pharm 16:351–357
Edlavitch SA (1988) Post-marketing surveillance methodologies. Drug Intell Clin Pharm 22:68–78
Faich GA (1986) Adverse drug reaction monitoring. N Engl J Med 314:1589–1592
Faich GA (1986) Analgetic risks and pharmacoepidemiology. JAMA 256(13):1788
Faich GA, Lawson DH, Tilson HH, Walker A (1987) Clinical trials are not enough: drug development and pharmacoepidemiology. J Clin Res Drug Dev 1(1):75–78
Faich GA et al. (1988) National adverse drug reaction surveillance 1986. Arch Intern Med 148:785–787

Faich GA, Stadel BV (1989) The future of automated record linkage for postmarketing surveillance: a response to Shapiro. Clin Pharmacol Ther 314:387–389

Fisher S (1987) Patient-initiated postmarketing surveillance: a validation study. J Clin Pharmacol 27:843–854

Fries JF (1988) Postmarketing drug surveillance. J Rheumatol 15(3):389–390

Fries JF (1989) Toward an epidemiology of gastropathy associated with non-steroidal anti-inflammatory drug use. Gastroenterology 98:647–655

Gaffey WR (1985) Use of epidemiology in risk assessment. In: New approaches in toxicity testing and their application in human risk assessment. Raven, New York, pp. 247–251

Gingell JC (1986) Non-steroidal anti-inflammatory drugs and serious gastrointestinal adverse reactions – 2. Brit Med J 292 May 3:1190–1191

Goldberg A (1985) Drug safety – the role of doctors, pharmaceutical companies and the medical press. Br J Clin Pract 39(1):5–6

Gordis L (ed) (1988) Epidemiology and health risk assessment. Oxford Univ Press, New York

Guess HA (1988) Limitations of available sources of data on prescription drug safety. In: Horisberger B, Dinkel R (eds) The perception and management of drug safety risks. Springer, Berlin Heidelberg New York Tokyo, pp. 51–56

Guess HA et al. (1988) Beyond pharmacoepidemiology: the larger role of epidemiology in drug development. J Clin Epidem 41(10):995–996

Hall GC, Luscombe DK, Walker SK (1988) Post-marketing surveillance using a computerized general practice data base. Pharmaceut Med 2:345–351

Hanft R (1989) Intensivierte Risikoüberwachung bei ausgewählten Arzneimitteln. Munch Med Wochenschr 131(7):109–112

Hartzema AG, Porta MS, Tilson HH (1987) Introduction to pharmacoepidemiology. Drug Intell Clin Pharm 21:739–747

Hartzema AG, Porta MS, Tilson HH (1988) Pharmacoepidemiology – an introduction. Harvey Whitney, Cincinnati OH

Hinderling PH (1988) Detection of populations at risk and problem drugs during drug development and in pharmacotherapy. Ther Drug Monit 10(3):245–249

Inman WHW (1985) Let's get our act together. In: Dukes G (ed) Side effects of drugs. Annual 9, Elsevier, Amsterdam, pp. XV–XX

Inman WHW (1987) Non-steroidal anti-inflammatory drugs assessment of risks. Eur J Rheumatol Inflamm 8(1):71–85

Inman WHW (1987) Requirements for risk-benefit assessment of drugs before withdrawal. PEM News 4 [Suppl] (Mar)

Inman WHW (1987) Prescription-event monitoring. Its strategic role in postmarketing surveillance for drug safety. PEM News 4 (Mar), pp. 16–29

Jick H (1985) The Boston collaborative drug surveillance program and the Puget Sound Health Maintenance Organization. Drug Inf J 19:237–242

Jonsson B (1983) The social costs of adverse drug reactions. Skandia Intern Symposia 3:31–48

Juengst G, Mohr R (1987) Side effects of ofloxacin in clinical trials and in postmarketing surveillance. Drugs 34 [Suppl 1]:144–149

Karch FE, Lasagna L (1977) Toward the operational identification of adverse drug reactions. Clin Pharmacol Ther 21(3):247–254

Kraynak MA, Kier KL (1988) Selected references on adverse drug reaction reporting. Drug Inf J 22:573–580

Langman MJS (1989) Epidemiologic evidence on the association between peptic ulceration and anti-inflammatory drug use. Gastroenterology 96:640–646

Lasagna L (1987) Postmarketing surveillance of multisource drugs – report of a conference held 9/10 July 1986. Center for the Study of Drug Development, Tufts Univ (ps 8711):1–58

Lawson DH (1984) Pharmacoepidemiology: a new discipline. Br Med J 289 Oct:940–941

Letzel H (1988) Statistics in drug risk research: the background of pharmacoepidemiology. In: Horisberger B, Dinkel R (eds) The perception and management of drug safety risks. Springer, Berlin Heidelberg New York Tokyo, pp. 70–76

Levine RJ (1988) Postmarketing surveillance – some ethical considerations. J Rheumatol 15 [Suppl 15]:34–39

Lunde PKM, Baksaas I (1988) Epidemiology of drug utilization – basic concepts. Acta Med Scand [Suppl] 721:7–11

Mann RD (ed) (1989) Risk and consent to risk in medicine: the proceedings of a conference organized by the Management Forum Ltd., London Apr 1988. Parthenon, Park Ridge NJ

Medical Department Ciba-Geigy (1985) The drug surveillants. Ciba-Geigy J (1):16–19

Nelson RC (1988) Drug safety, pharmacoepidemiology, and regulatory decision making. Drug Intell Clin Pharm 22:336–344

Pharma Corporation, The Degge Group (1988) International drug benefit/risk assessment data resource handbook, vol 1: North America. Pharma Corporation, Washington DC; The Degge Group, Arlington VA

Pharma Corporation, The Degge Group (1989) International drug benefit/risk assessment data resource handbook, vol 2: United Kingdom. Pharma Corporation, Washington DC; The Degge Group, Arlington VA

Porta MS, Hartzema AG (1987) The contribution of epidemiology to the study of drugs. Drug Intell Clin Pharm 21:741–747

Porta MS, Ruiz XM, Hartzema AG (1988) Pharmacoepidemiology: the name is new – what else is new? Drug News and Perspectives 1(4):243–245

Ray WA, Griffin MR (1989) The use of medicaid data for pharmacoepidemiology. Am J Epidemiol 129:837–849

Rogers AS (1987) Adverse Drug events: identification and attribution. Drug Intell Clin Pharm 21:915–920

Shapiro S (1984) The epidemiological evaluation of drugs. Acta Med Scand [Suppl] 683:23–27

Shapiro S (1989) The role of automated record linkage in the postmarketing surveillance of drug safety. Clin Pharmacol Ther 46(4):371–386

Shapiro S et al. (1986) Risks of agranulocytosis and aplastic anemia – their relation to drug use with special reference to analgesics. JAMA 256(13):1749–1757

Sibergeld E (1988) Epidemiology versus risk assessment: resolving some old controversies. Risk Anal 8(4):555–557

Spitzer WO (1988) Strategies, designs, criteria, tactics to be considered when evaluating scientific evidence. In: Horisberger B, Dinkel R (eds) The perception and management of drug safety risks. Springer, Berlin Heidelberg New York Tokyo, pp. 57–69

Spitzer WO, Hutchinson T, Lane D (1987) Postmarketing management of drug use: toward rational public policy. Can Med Assoc J 136 May:1022–1024

Stergachis AS (1988) Record linkage studies for postmarketing drug surveillance: data quality and validity considerations. Drug Intell Clin Pharm 22:157–161

Stolley PD, Strom BL (1986) Evaluating and monitoring the safety and efficacy of drug therapy and surgery. J Chron Dis 39(12):1145–1155

Strom BL (1987) The promise of pharmacoepidemiology. Am Rev Pharmacol Toxicol 27:71–86

Strom BL (1988) Overview of different logistical approaches to postmarketing surveillance. J Rheumatol 15 [suppl 17]:9–13

Strom BL (1989) Pharmacoepidemiology. Churchill Livingstone, New York

Swaen GMH (1988) The use of epidemiological data in risk assessment. Regul Toxicol Pharmacol 8:422–430

Tilson HH (1986) Post-marketing surveillance – the way forward. CMR annual lecture, Centre for Medicines Research

Tilson HH (1988) Pharmacoepidemiology: the future. Drug Intell Clin Pharm 22:416–421

Tilson HH (1988) Pharmacoepidemiology: the industry's perspective. J Rheumatol 15 [Suppl 17]:28–33

Tilson HH, Whisnant J (1985) Pharmacoepidemiology – drugs, arthritis and neoplasms: industry contribution to the data. Am J Med 78 [Suppl 1a]:69–76

Urquhart J (1987) How can we involve patients in drug epidemiology? 47th Int congress of pharmaceutical sciences of the Int Pharmac Federation, Netherlands, 1 Sep 1987, pp. 1–13

Venulet J (1984) Functioning of the side effect surveillance system at Ciba-Geigy Basel. Industrie Santé Jan, p. 49

Venulet J (1987) Informativity of adverse drug reactions data in medical publications. Center for the Study of Drug Development (rs 8709), Tufts Univ, Boston (reprinted from Drug Inf J 19:357–365)

Venulet J (1988) Possible strategies for early recognition of potential drug safety problems. Adverse Drug React Acute Poisoning Rev 7(1):39–47

Volans GN (1987) Monitoring the safety of over the counter drugs. Br Med J 295:797–798

Walker SR, Gelzer J et al. (1986) A comparative retrospective analysis of data for short- and long-term animal toxicity studies on 40 pharmaceutical compounds. Center for the Study of Drug Development, Boston

Wayne AR, Griffin MR (1989) Use of Medicaid data for pharmacoepidemiology. Am J Epidemiol 129(4):837–849

Wells F et al. (1988) Guidelines on postmarketing surveillance – joint committee of ABPI, BMA, CSM, and RCGP. Br Med J 296 Feb:399–340

World Health Organization (1988) The role of epidemiology in attaining health for all. WHO, Executive Board

## Risk/Benefit Perception

Bastide S et al. (1989) Risk perception and social acceptability of technologies: the French case. Risk Anal 9(2):215–223

Battelle-Institut (1981) Untersuchungen über die technischen, organisatorischen und gesellschaftlichen Voraussetzungen für Risikostrategien im Bereich technologischer Entwicklung (Endbericht) RS I/2-510321, SR 70. Battelle, Frankfurt

Borman SA (1983) Origin of risk assessment. Anal Chem 55(14): 1438a – 1440a

Brown J (1987) Risk perception: expert opinion versus public understanding. ESRC Newslett 59:17–19

Brown MS et al. (1990) Patient perceptions of drug risks and benefits. Center for the Study of Drug Development, Tufts Univ, Boston MA

Burger EJ (1988) How citizens think about risks to health. Risk Anal 8(3):309–313

Burley DM (1988) Understanding how the public understand risk. Management Forum meeting, Apr 27, paper

Carpenter PF (1983) Understanding risk. Med Device Diagn Industry 5(6):24–26

Carroll NV et al. (1986) Perceived risks and pharmacists' generic substitution behavior. J Consumer Aff 20(1):36–47

Ciba-Geigy (Japan) (1987) Report on public awareness survey on medical care and drugs (summarized edition). Ciba-Geigy, Japan

Covello VT (1987) Decision analysis and risk management decision making: issues and methods. Risk Anal 7(2):131–139

Covello VT et al. (1982) Risk analysis, philosophy, and the social and behavioral sciences. Risk Anal 2(2):53–58

Drabek TE (1986) Human system response to disaster: an inventory of sociological findings. Springer, Berlin Heidelberg New York Tokyo

Fishburn PC (1984) Foundations of risk measurement. Manage Sci 30:396–406

Freudenburg WR (1988) Perceived risk, real risk: social science and the art of probabilistic risk assessment. Science 242:44–49

Fritzsche AF (1986) Wie sicher leben wir? Risikobeurteilung und -bewältigung in unserer Gesellschaft. TÜV Rheinland, Cologne

Fujino S (1988) Risk perception of perscription drugs: report on surveys in Japan. In: Horisberger B, Dinkel R (eds) The perception and management of drug safety risks. Springer, Berlin Heidelberg New York Tokyo, pp. 112–116

Gafni A et al. (1984) Risk attitude and time preference in health. Manage Sci 30:440–451
Gardner GT, Gould LC (1989) Public perception of the risks and benefits of technology. Risk Anal 9(2)
Hammond K, Victor D (1988) Annotated bibliography for risk perception and risk communication. Center for research on judgment and policy, Univ of Colorado, Boulder
Harris L and Associates (1987) Risk perception research. Harris L and Associates, Inc
Heilmann K (1987) On the perception of drug-related risk. Drugs made in Germany 30(3):122–125
Heilmann K, Urquhart J (1983) Keine Angst vor der Angst. Risiko – Element unseres Lebens und Motor des Fortschritts. Kindler, Munich
Horisberger B, Dinkel R (eds) The perception and management of drug safety risks. Springer, Berlin Heidelberg New York Tokyo
Jung CG (1975) Über die Psychologie des Unbewußten. Fischer, Frankfurt/Main
Kasperson RE, Slovic P et al. (1988) The social amplification of risk: a conceptual framework. Risk Anal 8(2):177–187
Kishchuk NA (1987) Causes and correlates of risk perception. Risk Abstraction 4:1–4
Kletz TA (1983) The mathematics of risk. Interdisciplinary Sci Rev 8:114–119
Kuhlmann A (1978) Sicherheit als Wert in Technik und Gesellschaft. In: Ropohl G et al. Maßstäbe der Technikbewertung. Vorträge und Diskussionen, VDI Tagung, 18/19 Nov 1977. VDI Prints, Düsseldorf
Lave LB, Menkes J (1985) Managing risk: a joint US-German perspective. Risk Anal 5:11–23
Lee TR (1981) The public perception of risk and the question of irrationality. Proc R Soc Lond 376a:5–16
Lerch I (1980) Risk and fear. New Sci Jan:8–11
Lowrance WW (1983) The agenda for risk decision making. Environment 25(10):4–8
Lowrance WW (1985) Modern science and human values. Oxford University Press, New York
Macgregor D, Slovic P (1986) Perceived acceptability of risk analysis as a decision-making approach. Risk Anal 6(2):245–256
O'Donnell M (1986) The media and their influence on public attitudes to drug development and use. Br J Clin Pharmacol 22:101s–102s
Otway H, Thomas K (1982) Reflections on risk perception and policy. Risk Anal 2:69–82
Pochin EE (1975) The acceptance of risk. Br Med Bull 31:184–189
Sangeorge R (1987) Public perceptions of risk. National Audubon Society, paper
Schneider SL, Lopes LL (1986) Reflection in preferences under risk: who and when may suggest why. J Exp Psychol 12:535–548

Schuh H (1988) Risikoangst und Risikolust (with a German version of Slovic's graphs). Die Zeit, Apr 8

Slovic P (1987) Perception of risk. Science 236:286–290

Slovic P (1987) Ripples in a pond: forecasting industrial crises. Ind Crisis winter:34–43

Slovic P (1989) The perception and management of therapeutic risk. CMR annual lecture. Center for Medicines Research, Carshalton, Surrey, UK

Slovic P et al. (1984) Modelling the societal impact of fatal accidents. Manage Sci 30:464–474

Slovic P et al. (1987) Risk perception and risk regulation. Administrative Conference of the U.S., Washington DC, Mar 5

Slovic P, Fischhoff B, Lichtenstein S (1980) Facts and fears: understanding perceived risk. In: Schwing RC, Albers WA (eds) Societal risk assessment: how safe is safe enough? Plenum, New York, pp. 181–214

Slovic P, Fischhoff B, Lichtenstein S (1981) Perceived risk: psychological factors and social implications. Proc R Soc Lond 376:17–34

Slovic P, Kraus N, Lappe H, Major M (1989) Risk perception of perscription drugs: report on a survey in Canada. Decision Research, Eugene, Oregon (unpublished manuscript)

Slovic P, Kraus NN, Lappe H, Letzel H, Malmfors T (1989) Risk perception of prescription drugs: report of a survey in Sweden. Pharmaceut Med 4:43–65

Stallen PJ, Tomas A (1988) Public concern about industrial hazards. Risk Anal 8(2):237–245

Starr C (1985) Risk management, assessment, and acceptability. Risk Anal 5:97–102

Starr C et al. (1984) A perspective on health and safety risk analysis. Manage Sci 30:452–463

Teigen KH, Brun W (1988) Societal risks as seen by the Norwegian public. J Behav Decision Making 1:111–130

Toepfer K (1987) Risikoakzeptanz – Aufgabe der Politik oder der Wissenschaft? AGF-Meinungen. Special Issue (Dec)

von Wartburg WP (1984) Drugs and the perception of risk. Swiss Pharma 6(11a):21–23

Wheelock W, Conning D, Grosse D (1988) Public perception of food safety. J Royal Soc Health 108:130–141

Wildavsky A (1984) Die Suche nach einer fehlerlosen Risikominderungsstrategie. In: Lange S (ed) Ermittlung und Bewertung industrieller Risiken. Springer, Berlin Heidelberg New York Tokyo

## Risk/Benefit Communication

Alvan G, Ohmann B, Sjöqvist F (1983) Problem-oriented drug information: a clinical pharmacological service. Lancet II:1410–1412

Anonymous (1987) NRC launches study on risk communication. Risk Newslett June:13–14

Arnold RM et al. (1987) Ethical issues in a drug information center. Drug Intell Clin Pharm 21(12):1008–1011
Arntson PH (1989) Improving citizens' health competencies. Health Communication 1:29–34
Arntson PH (1990) Doctor-patient communication and decision making about prescription drugs. In: Shimizu N, Tanaka Y, Jones J, Taylor D (eds) Improving drug safety: the assessment, management and communication of therapeutic benefits and risks of pharmaceutical products. Pharma International, Tokyo:180–185
Arntson P, Makoul G et al. (1989) Patients' perceptions of medical encounters in Great Britain: variations with health loci of control and sociodemographic factors. Health Communication 1(2):75–95
Baldwin HJ, Cosler LE, Schulz RM (1987) Opinion leadership in medication information. Communication Quarterly 35:84–102
Birkhead D (1989) An ethics of vision for journalism. Critic Stud in Mass Communication 6(3):283–294
Bogaert M, Vander Stichele R, Kaufman JM, Lefebvre R (eds) (1989) Patient package insert as a source of drug information. Excerpta Medica, Amsterdam
Borchert G (1989) Drug information in TV-advertising. J Consumer Policy 12(3):371–380
Brown PJ (1988) Reporting adverse drug reactions: the media approach. In: Horisberger B, Dinkel R (eds) The perception and management of drug safety risks. Springer, Berlin Heidelberg New York Tokyo, pp. 149–157
Brushwood DB, Simonsmeier LM (1986) Drug information for patients – duties of the manufacturer, pharmacist, physician and hospital. J Leg Med 7(3):279–340
Bullman RW, Rowland F (1985) Directory of prescription drug information and education programs and resources. Washington DC
Carpenter PF (1988) Going patient, going public. In: Horisberger B, Dinkel R (eds) The perception and management of drug safety risks. Springer, Berlin Heidelberg New York Tokyo, pp. 141–148
Ciba-Geigy (Japan) (1988) Report on physician's survey on drugs and ADR. Ciba-Geigy Japan
Covell DG, Uman GC, Manning PR (1985) Information needs in office practice: are they being met? Ann Intern Med 103:596–599
Covello VT et al. (1988) Effective risk communication – the role and responsibility of government organizations. Plenum, New York
Cox GV, Strickland GD (1988) Risk is normal to life itself. Am Ind Hyg Assoc J 49:A223–A227
Crawshaw R (1989) Medicine and the media. J Clin Epidemiol 42(8):815–816
Davies JC, Covelllo VT, Allen FW (eds) (1987) Risk communication. Conservation Foundation, Washington DC
Desvousges WH, Smith VK (1988) Focus groups and risk communication: the "science" of listening to data. Risk Anal 8(4):479–484

Farquhar JW, Fortmann SP, Flora J et al. (1990) The Stanford Five-City Project: effects of communitywide education on cardiovascular disease risk factors. Jul 18

Food and Drug Administration (1987) Studies of reported adverse effects of marketed drugs; availability of grant; request for applications. Federal Register, Jul 10: 52:26086-8

Glaeske G (1989) Stiftung Warentest and the pharmaceutical market. J Consumer Policy 12(3):357–370

Gotsch AR, Kashdan RG (1988) Risk communication. N J J Med 85(11):954–958

Greenberg MR et al. (1989) Network evening news coverage of environmental risk. Risk Anal 9(1):119–126

Grieshop JI, Stiles MC (1989) Risk and home-pesticide users. Environ Behav 21(6):699

Hammond K, Victor D (1988) Annotated bibliography for risk perception and risk communication. Center for research on judgment and policy, Univ of Colorado, Boulder

Hance BJ (1989) Setting a context for explaining risk. Risk Anal 9(1)

Haney CA, Colson AC (1980) Ethical responsibility in physician-patient communication. Ethics Sci Med 7(1):27–36

Hannsson SO (1989) Dimensions of risk. Risk Anal 9(1):107–112

Heilmann K (1986) Impact of professional and lay media on patients and physicians. Am J Med 80 [Suppl 6a]:5–7

Herxheimer A, Davies C (1982) Drug information for patients: bringing together the messages from prescriber, pharmacist and manufacturer. J R Coll Gen Pract 32:93–97

Heussner RC, Salmon ME (1989) Where medicine and media clash. Minn Med 72(3):141, 143–145

Ibrekk H, Morgan MG (1987) Graphical communication of uncertain qualities to nontechnical people. Risk Anal 7(4):519–529

Johnson FR (1988) Economic costs of misinforming about risk: the EDB scare and the media. Risk Anal 8(2):261–269

Johnson FR, Fisher A (1989) Conventional wisdom on risk communication and evidence from a field experiment. Risk Anal 9(2):209–213

Jungermann H et al. (1988) Mental models in risk assessment: informing people about drugs. Risk Anal 8(1):147–155

Kasperson RE (1986) Six propositions on public participation and their relevance for risk communication. Risk Anal 6:275–281

Keeney RL, von Winterfeldt D (1986) Improving risk communication. Risk Anal 6:417–424

Keown CF (1985) Contextual effects on people's ratings of seriousness for side effects of prescription drugs. Percept Mot Skills 61:435–441

Keown CF, Slovic P, Lichtenstein S (1984) Influence of information about side effects on perceived risk of prescription drugs. Marketing for Mental Health Services:111–123

Keown CF et al. (1984) Attitudes of physicians, pharmacists and laypersons toward seriousness and need for disclosure of prescription drug side effects. Health Psychol 3(1):1–11
King M et al. (1989) Medicine and the media: social and legislative issues. Symposium of the Society of University Surgeons. Surgery 105(4):549–552
Konheim CS (1988) Risk communication in the real world. Risk Anal 8(3):367–373
Lexcin J (1989) Doctors and detailers: therapeutic education or pharmaceutical promotion? Intern J Health Serv 19(4):663–679
Maccoby N, Farquhar JW, Wood PD et al. (1977) Reducing the risk of cardiovascular disease: effects of a campaign on knowledge and behavior. J Community Health 23:100–114
Macpherson G (1988) Where is medicine heading? Medical media. N Z Med J 101(846):350–351
Makoul G (1990) Health locus of control and concern as predictors of health information attention and acquisition. Communication in Health Care Conference, Oxford University
McCallum DB, Yenney SL (1989) Communicating the benefits and risks of prescription drugs. Inst for Health Policy Analysis, Georgetown University, Washington DC
Medawar C (1988) Professional drug information: a consumer perspective. In: Horisberger B, Dinkel R (eds) The perception and management of drug safety risks. Springer, Berlin Heidelberg New York Tokyo, pp. 135–140
Mehta K et al. (1989) Prescription drug advertising trends: a study of oral hypoglycemics. Soc Sci Med 29(7):853–857
Morris LA (1982) A survey of patients' receipt of prescription drug information. Med Care 20:596–605
Morris LA (1990) Communicating therapeutic risks. Springer, Berlin Heidelberg New York Tokyo
Morris LA, Grossman R, Barkdoll GL, Gordon E, Soviero C (1984) A survey of prescription drug information. Am J Public Health 74:1161–1162
Morris LA, Grossman R, Barkdoll G, Gordon E (1987) A segmentational analysis of prescription drug information seeking. Med Care 25(10):953–964
Mumpower JL (1988) Lottery games and risky technologies: communications about low-probability/high-consequence events. Risk Anal 8(2):231–235
National Research Council (1989) Improving risk communication. National Academy Press, Washington DC
Nelkin D (1987) The culture of science journalism. Society Sep/Oct:18–25
Nelkin D (1988) Communicating the risks and benefits of technology: the case of pharmaceuticals. In: Horisberger B, Dinkel R (eds) The perception and management of drug safety risks. Springer, Berlin Heidelberg New York Tokyo, pp. 19–36
Nelkin D (1988) Risk reporting and the management of industrial crises. J Manage Studies 25(4):341–351
Nelkin D (1989) Communicating technological risk: the social construction of risk perception. Ann Rev Public Health 10:95–113

O'Brien BJ (1989) Words or numbers? The evaluation of probability expressions in general practice. J R Coll Gen Pract 39 Mar:98–100
O'Donnell M (1986) The media and their influence on public attitudes to drug development and use. Br J Clin Pharmacol 22:101s–102s
O'Riordan T et al. (1989) Themes and tasks of risk communication: conference report, KFA Juelich, 1989. Risk Anal 9(4):513–518
Otway H, Wynne B (1989) Risk communication: paradigm and paradox. Risk Anal 9(2):141–145
Parker LM (1989) Doctor-patient communication and ethical issues (editorial). J Clin Oncol 7(9):1182–1183
Patterson RM (1989) Drugs in litigation. Mitchie, Charlottesville VA
Peters JD (1989) Satan and savior: mass communication in progressive thought. Critic Stud in Mass Communication 6(3):247–263
Renn O (1989) Risk communication at the community level: European lessons from the Seveso Directive. J Air Waste Manage Assoc 39(10):1301–1308
Röglin HC (1984) Kommunikationsrisiken der Großtechnologien. In: Lange S (ed) Ermittlung und Bewertung industrieller Risiken. Springer, Berlin Heidelberg New York Tokyo
Rogers AS, Israel E, Smith C, Levine D, McBean AM, Walente C, Faich GA (1988) Physician knowledge, attitudes and behavior related to reporting adverse drug events. Arch Intern Med 148:1596–1600
Scherwitz L, Hennrikus D, Yysim S, Lester J, Vallbona C (1985) Physician communication. Pat Educ Couns 7:121–136
Scott HD, Faich GA et al. (1990) Physician reporting of ADR's – Rhode Island. JAMA 263:1785–1788
Shapiro S (1985) The decision to publish dilemmas. J Chron Dis 38:365–372
Sharlin HI (1986) EDB: a case study in communicating risk. Risk Anal 6(1):61–68
Shimizu N, Tanaka Y, Jones J, Taylor D (eds) (1990) Improving drug safety: the assessment, management and communication of therapeutic benefits and risks of pharmaceutical products. Pharma International, Tokyo
Sills JM, Faich GA, Milstien JB, Turner WM (1986) Postmarketing reporting of ADR's to FDA: an overview of the 1985 FDA guideline. Drug Inf J 20(2):150–156
Slovic P (1985) Risk perception and risk communication. Stanford HSR Seminar, April 29
Slovic P (1986) Informing and educating the public about risk. Risk Anal 6(4):403–415
Speeding EJ, Rose DN (1985) Building an effective doctor-patient relationship: from patient satisfaction to patient participation. Soc Sci Med 21(2)
Thompson WG (1988) The ethics of physician-pharmaceutical company relationships. Can Med Assoc J 139(9):835–836
Tomlinson T, Brody H (1988) Ethics and communication in do-not-resuscitate orders. N Engl J Med 318(1):43–46
Valente CM et al. (1988) The importance of physician-patient communication in reducing medical liability. Md Med J 37(1):75–78

Vander Stichele R, Bogaert MG (1989) Patient package inserts: the Belgian experience with a mandatory program. Drug Inf J 23:673–677
Wall DW (1987) Ethics and the pharmaceutical industry: some ideas for general practitioners. J R Coll Gen Pract 37(299):267–269
Wertheimer MD et al. (1985) Ethics and communication in the surgeon-patient relationship. J Med Educ 60(10):804–806
Weterings RA, van Eijndhoven JC (1989) Informing the public about uncertain risks. Risk Anal 9(4)
World Health Organization (1988) Ethical criteria for medicinal drug promotion. WHO, Geneva

**Regulation**

Albert RE (1985) Risk assessment in regulatory decision making in the EPA. In: Homburger (ed) Safety evaluation and regulation of chemicals 2. Karger, Basel, pp. 146–149
Beauchamp TL (1978) The regulation of hazards and hazardous behaviors. Health Educ Monogr 6:242–257
Bier VM (1988) The U.S. Nuclear Regulatory Commission safety goal policy: a critical review. Risk Anal 8(4):563–568
Bogen KT (1983) Quantitative risk-benefit analysis in regulatory decision making. J Health Polit Policy Law 8:120–140
Broekhuijsen-Molenaar A, Stocker CJ (1988) Liability for drugs in the Netherlands. Med Law 7(3):219–231
Clouse EH (1987) Social awareness and its effect on removal of drugs from the marketplace. Clin Res Practices Drug Reg Aff 5(2, 3):165–175
Dardis R (1988) Risk regulation and consumer welfare. J Consumer Aff 22(2):303–318
Deutsch E (1986) Compensation for subjects of clinical trials and strict products liability in German pharmaceutical law. Med Law 5(6):445–448
Deutsch E (1989) The functions of ethical committees. Drug Res/Arzneim Forsch 39(II) (8a):1049–1053
Fuelgraff G (1988) Scientific and political components of regulatory decision making: general considerations. In: Horisberger B, Dinkel R (eds) The perception and management of drug safety risks. Springer, Berlin Heidelberg New York Tokyo, pp. 117–120
Green W (1987) Odyssey of Depo-Provera: contraceptives, carcinogenic drugs and risk management analyses – a review of the drug approval process. Food Drug Cosmet J 42:567–587
Hall RC (1988) Drug trials and the role of ethics committees: a regulator's point of view. Med J Aust 149(5):262–264
Hart D (1989) Drug safety as a means of consumer protection: the approximation of laws in the EC medicinal products market and its limitations. J Consumer Policy 12:343–355
Hayakawa T (1987) Some aspects of the preclinical safety of drugs produced by recombination DNA technology: Japanese government regulatory position. Prog Clin Biol Res 235:15–29

Hayes AHJr (1981) Food and drug regulation after 75 years. JAMA 246(11):1223–1226
Huber P (1985) Safety and the second best: the hazards of public risk management in the courts. Columbia Law Rev 85:277–337
Hyman PM (1987) Regulatory risks of marketing drugs and cosmetics. Drug Inf J 21:393–401
Knauer TE (1987) The regulation of drugs on the basis of relative effectiveness. Food Drug Cosmet Law J 42:323–345
Lasagna L (1988) Scientific and political components of regulatory decision making: the United States experience. In: Horisberger B, Dinkel R (eds) The perception and management of drug safety risks. Springer, Berlin Heidelberg New York Tokyo, pp. 121–127
Laughren TP (1989) The review of clinical safety data in a new drug application. Psychopharmacol Bull 25(1):5–8
Lave LB, Males EH (1989) At risk: the framework for regulating toxic substances. Environ Sci Technol 23(4)
Lowe MF (1989) Risk assessment and the credibility of federal regulatory policy: an FDA perspective. Regulat Toxicol Pharmacol 9:131–140
Mattison N (1984) Regulatory scene. Pharmaceut Med 1:13–16
Meyer HM (1987) Risk and the FDA. PMA Med Section meeting, Florida, Mar 17
Mitchell JP (1988) Strict liability for products utilized in medicine and biology. J R Soc Med 81(4):200–202
Montesano R, Tomatis L (1977) Legislation concerning chemical carcinogens in several industrialized countries. Cancer Res 37:310–316
Myers A, Moore SR (1987) The drug approval process and the information it provides. Drug Intell Clin Pharm 21:821–825
Nelson RC (1988) Drug safety, pharmacoepidemiology, and regulatory decision making. Drug Intell Clin Pharm 22:336–344
Okrent D (1987) The safety goals of the U.S. nuclear regulatory commission. Science 236:296–300
Petak WJ, Atkisson AA (1982) Natural hazard risk assessment and public policy. Springer, Berlin Heidelberg New York Tokyo
Pfund P (1982) Recht und Risiko. Tagung Nov 22/23, Zürich-Oerlikon, Referat 12. Schweiz. Vereinigung für Atomenergie, Bern
Renn O (1989) Risk communication at the community level: European lessons from the Seveso Directive. J Air Waste Manage Assoc 39(10):1301–1308
Ricci PF, Molton LS (1981) Risk and benefit in environmental law. Science 214 Dec 4:1096–1100
Richard BW (1987) Drug regulation in the United States and the United Kingdom: the Depo-Provera story. Ann Intern Med 106(6):886–891
Ris CH, Preuss PW, EPA (1989) Risk assessment and risk management: an institutional process. Adv Mod Environ Toxicol 15:1–21
Rodricks JV, Taylor MR (1989) Comparison of risk management in USA regulatory agencies. J Hazard Materials 21(3):239–254
Roth DH, Wyzga RE, Hammerstrom T (1984) The use of risk assessment in developing health-based regulations. ASTM Spex Techn Publ 845:46–65

Sauer F (1989) EEC regulatory initiatives on drug information. In: Bogaert M, Vander Stichele R, Kaufman JM, Lefebvre R (eds) Patient package inserts as a source of drug information. Excerpta Medica, Amsterdam
Scheuplein RJ (1987) Risk assessment and food safety: a scientist's and regulator's view. Food Drug Cosmet Law J 42:237–250
Schroeder CH (1986) Rights against risks. Columbia Law Rev 86:495–562
Shulman SR (1989) Public health and the law: the broader message of accutane. Am J Public Health 79(11):1566
Silverglade BA (1983) The risks of risk assessment and risk-benefit analysis. Food Drug Cosm Law J 38:318–324
Smith MV (1984) Use of risk assessment in regulatory decision making. Food Technol Oct:114–118
Spivey RN, Lasagna L, Trimble AG (1987) New indication for already-approved drugs: time trends for the new drug application review phase. Clin Pharmacol Ther 41(4):368–370
Taylor MR (1984) The role of law in risk management. Fundam Appl Toxicol 4:408–417
Travis CC, Richter SA et al. (1987) Risk and regulation. Chem Tech Aug:478–483
Tunkel V (1989) Drug trials: who takes the risk? Lancet 2 (8663):609–611
van Andel FG (1985) On regulating perceived risk. Effective Health Care 2(6):231–237
Walker SR (ed) (1989) International medicines regulations – a forward look to 1992: executive summary, CMR workshop Ciba Foundation and internat. symposium Royal College of Physicians, London Sept 1988. Centre for Medicines Research, Carshalton, Surrey UK
Walker VR (1988) Quantitative risk assessments as evidence in civil litigation. Risk Anal 8(4):605–614
Young FE (1987) Risk assessment: the convergence of science and the law. Regul Toxicol Pharmacol 7:179–184

# 56. RAD-AR Bibliography

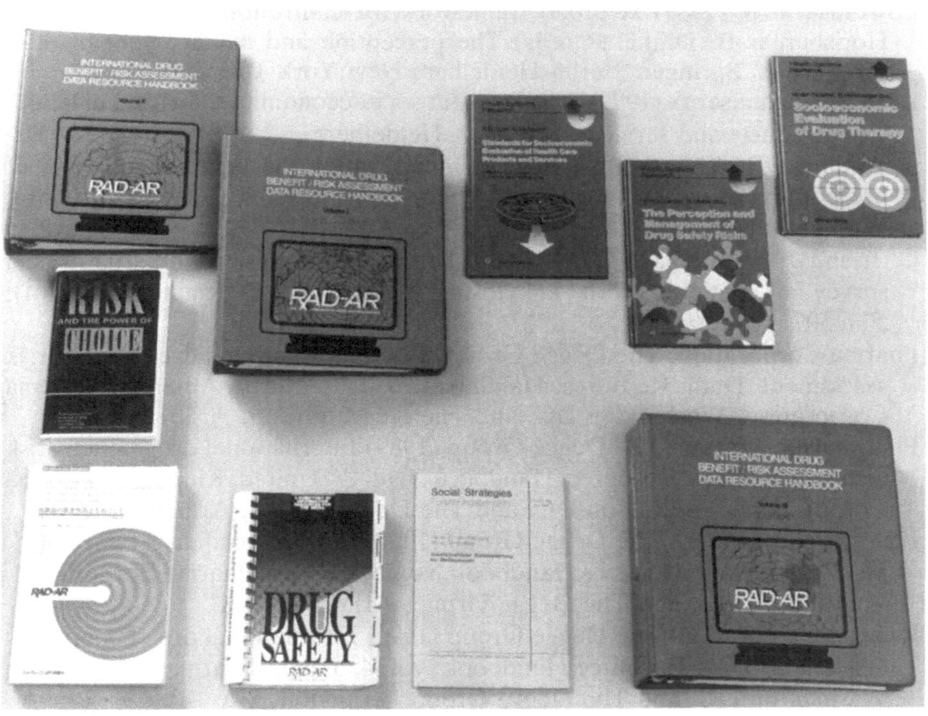


RAD-AR proceedings, reports and sponsored publications

Anderson GM, Spitzer WO, Weinstein MC, Wang E, Blackburn JL, Bergman U (1990) Benefits, risks, and costs of prescription drugs: a scientific basis for evaluation policy options. Clin Pharmacol Ther 48(2): 111–119

Burley D, Inman WHW (eds) (1988) Therapeutic risk: perception, measurement, management. Wiley & Sons, New York

Burley D, Silverstone T (eds) (1988) Medicines and road traffic safety. CNS Publishers, London

Ciba-Geigy (Japan) (1988) Report on public awareness survey on medical care and drugs (summarized edition). Ciba-Geigy Ltd, Japan

Ciba-Geigy (Japan) (1988) Report on physician's survey on drugs and ADR. Ciba-Geigy Ltd, Japan

Hammond K, Victor D (1988) Annotated bibliography for risk perception and risk communication. Center for research on judgment and policy, University of Colorado at Boulder

Horisberger B, Dinkel R (eds) (1989) The perception and management of drug safety risks. Springer, Berlin Heidelberg New York Tokyo

Hubbard S (1989) RAD-AR: an innovative drug safety initiative. Swiss Pharma 11 (5a): 13–16

Lappe H, Slovic P, Kraus NN, Letzel H, Malmfors T (1990) Risk perception and communication of prescription drugs. In: Gow HBF, Otway H (eds) Communicating with the public about major accident hazards. Elsevier, London: 510–527

Lowrance WW (1989) A broad framework for confronting health risks. In: Horisberger B, Dinkel R (eds) The perception and management of drug safety risks. Springer, Berlin Heidelberg New York Tokyo: 9–18

Luce B, Elixhauser A (1990) Standards for socio-economic evaluation of health care products and services. Springer, Heidelberg

McCallum DB, Yenney SL (1989) Communicating the benefits and risks of prescription drugs. Inst for Health Policy Analysis, Georgetown University, Washington DC

O'Brien BJ, Elswood J, Calin A (1990) Perception of prescription drug risks: a survey of patients with ankylosing spondylitis. J Rheumatol 17(4): 503–507

Pharma Corporation, The Degge Group (1988) International drug benefit/risk assessment Data Resource Handbook, vol. 1: North America. Pharma Corporation, Washington DC, and The Degge Group, Arlington, VA

Pharma Corporation, The Degge Group (1989) International drug benefit/risk assessment Data Resource Handbook, vol. 2: United Kingdom. Pharma Corporation, Washington DC, and The Degge Group, Arlington, VA

Pharma Corporation, The Degge Group (1990) International drug benefit/risk assessment Data Resource Handbook, vol. 3: Europe. Pharma Corporation, Washington DC, and The Degge Group, Arlington, VA

Pharma Corporation, The Degge Group (1990) International drug benefit/risk assessment Data Resource Handbook, vol. 4: Japan. Pharma Corporation, Washington DC, and The Degge Group, Arlington, VA

Shimizu N, Tanaka Y, Jones J, Taylor D (eds) (1990) Improving drug safety: the assessment, management, and communication of the therapeutic benefits and risks of pharmaceutical products. The official proceedings of the RAD-AR symposium 1989. Pharma International, Tokyo, Japan

Slovic P (1989) The perception and management of therapeutic risk. CMR Annual lecture, June 1989. Centre for Medicines Research, Carshalton, Surrey, UK

Slovic P, Kraus NN, Lappe H, Major (M) (1989) Risk perception of prescription drugs: report on a survey in Canada. Decision Research, Eugene, Oregon, USA, unpublished manuscript

Slovic P, Kraus NN, Lappe H, Letzel H, Malmfors T (1989) Risk perception of prescription drugs: report of a survey in Sweden. Pharmaceut Med 4: 43–65

The RAD-AR Center (1989) A RAD-AR conference sponsored by the Centre for Pharmaceutical Medicine, Stratford-upon-Avon, England, October 1988. Executive summary, The RAD-AR Center, Basle, Switzerland

The RAD-AR Center (1989) A meeting of the International Working Group on Risk/Benefit Perception and Communication, Washington DC, USA, June 1989. Executive summary, The RAD-AR Center, Basle, Switzerland

The RAD-AR Center (1989) A "decision-conferencing" meeting at the London School of Economics, London, England, March 1989. Executive summary, The RAD-AR Center, Basle, Switzerland

The RAD-AR Center (1989) A meeting of the International Pharmacoepidemiology Working Group, Georgetown University, Washington DC, USA, March 1989. Executive summary, The RAD-AR Center, Basle, Switzerland

The RAD-AR Center (1989) RAD-AR International Foundation. Consultation meeting of interested parties. Tufts European Center, Talloires, France August 1989. Executive summary, The RAD-AR Center, Basle, Switzerland

The RAD-AR Center (1989) RAD-AR Bibliography. The RAD-AR Center, Basle, Switzerland

The RAD-AR Center (1989) RAD-AR Report, No 1, 2, 3. The RAD-AR Center, Basle, Switzerland

The RAD-AR Center (1990) RAD-AR Report, No 4, 5. The RAD-AR Center, Basle, Switzerland

The RAD-AR Center (1990) Drug Safety: a directory of information resources for the media. The RAD-AR Center, Basle, Switzerland

The RAD-AR Center (1990) Risk and the power of choice. Video. The RAD-AR Center, Basle, Switzerland

The RAD-AR Center (1990) Bibliography – "Improving drug safety: a joint responsibility", Wolfsberg Conference, Switzerland, April 1990. The RAD-AR Center, Basle, Switzerland

The RAD-AR Council Japan (1989) The RAD-AR Council, Japan, Tokyo, Japan, May 1989. Executive summary, The RAD-AR Council Japan, Tokyo, Japan

The RAD-AR Council Japan (1989) RAD-AR Expert Committee Reports. Executive summaries in English, The RAD-AR Council Japan, Tokyo, Japan

van Eimeren W, Horisberger B (eds) (1988) Socioeconomic evaluation of drug therapy. Springer, Berlin Heidelberg New York Tokyo

von Wartburg WP (1988) Identification, assessment, and management of drug risks. April 25, Switzerland

von Wartburg WP (1989) Overview of the drug safety issue and Ciba-Geigy's response: RAD-AR. In: Horisberger B, Dinkel R (eds) The perception and management of drug safety risks. Springer, Berlin Heidelberg New York Tokyo von Wartburg WP, Versteegen U (1990) Gesellschaftliche Risikobewertung bei Medikamenten – die RAD-AR Initiative. In: Leisinger KM, Trappe P (eds) Social strategies, Forschungsberichte 4(1). In press

Walker SR (ed) (1989) International medicines regulations – a forward look to 1992: executive summary, CMR workshop Ciba Foundation and international symposium, Royal College of Physicians, London, September 1988. Centre for Medicines Research, Carshalton, Surrey, UK

# 57. Curriculum Vitae of Authors and Editors

ARNOLD, RICHARD B.
Ph. D.
Executive Vice President, International Federation of Pharmaceutical Manufacturers Associations (IFPMA), Geneva, Switzerland
1977–1984 Director of the Association of the British Pharmaceutical Industry (ABPI)

ARNTSON, PAUL
Prof. Ph. D.
Professor and Chairman, Communication Studies, Northwestern University, Evanston, ILL, USA; Faculty Associate, Center for Urban Affairs and Policy Research

Ph. D., Communication Arts and Educational Psychology, University of Wisconsin, USA
Educational consultant, Medical Education Department, Northwestern Medical School, and Oxford Regional Commitee for Postgraduate Education in General Practice

BANKOWSKI, ZBIGNIEW
Prof. Dr. med.
Secretary-General, Council for International Organizations of Medical Sciences (CIOMS), Geneva, Switzerland

M. D. and Ph. D., Lublin, Poland
Teaching and research positions in experimental pathology at Lublin, Lodz, Warsaw, Paris and Tunis
1965–1972 Coordinator of research and training programs, World Health Organization, Geneva
Since 1975 Secretary-General of CIOMS, responsible for management and coordination of CIOMS/WHO programs on bioethics, international nomenclature of diseases and drug development and use
Editor of CIOMS round table conference proceedings

BRÄUTIGAM, HANS HARALD
Prof. Dr. med.
Medical Editor, *Die Zeit*, Hamburg, FRG

1955 Board certified obstetrics and gynecology
1961 Dept. obstetrics and gynecology, Kansas City Medical School, USA

1962 Chairman Dept. obstetrics and gynecology, Marienkrankenhaus, Teaching Hospital, University of Hamburg
1966 Lecturer in obstetrics and gynecology, University of Hamburg

## Bruppacher, Rudolf

M. D., Ph. D.
Head of Pharmacoepidemiology, Ciba-Geigy Ltd., Basle, Switzerland; Associate Professor, University of Basel

M.D., University of Zurich, Switzerland
1969 M. P. H., Harvard University, USA
1972 Ph. D., Public Health, Tulane University, USA
1979–1986 Director, Swiss National Research Program on Efficiency in Health Care
1982–1986 President, Swiss Health League Conference

## Carpenter, Peter F.

President, ALZA Development Corporation, Palo Alto, CA USA; Advisor on Organizational Values and Missions, Institute of Medicine, Affymax, NV, Palo Alto, CA and Ciba-Geigy Ltd., Basle, Switzerland

1962 A.B., Chemistry, Harvard University, USA
1965 M.B.A., University of Chicago, USA
1973–1976 Assistant Vice President for Medical Affairs, Stanford University, Stanford, CA, USA
1975–1976 Executive Director, Stanford University Medical Center, Stanford University, Stanford, CA, USA
1976–1989 Alza Corporation, Palo Alto, CA, USA
Director, American Foundation for AIDS Research; member of the Executive Committee, California AIDS Leadership Committee

## Dinkel, Rolf

Dr. rer. pol
Managing Director, HealthEcon Ltd., Basle, Switzerland

M. B. A., Ph. D., Economics, University of Würzburg
1969–1972 Director, Dept. Organization and Planning, Glanzstoff Ltd., FRG
1973–1981 Managing Consultant, Prognos Ltd., Basel, Switzerland

## Domeischel, Jack R.

Vice President, International Public Affairs, Searle, Chicago, ILL, USA

1976 B. S., Public Health Education, State University of New York at Stony Brook, NY, USA
1985 M. A., Public Health Administration, Long Island University, Greenvale, NY, USA

## Faich, Gerald A.

M. D., M. P. H
Director, Office of Epidemiology and Biostatistics, Center for Drug Evaluation and Research, Food and Drug Administration, Rockville, MD, USA

B. Sci. (Mathematics) and M. D., University of Wisconsin
M. P. H., Harvard University
Fellow – American Colleges of Epidemiology, Physicians, Preventive Medicine (FACE, FACP, FACPM)

## Follath, Ferenc

Prof. Dr. med.
Head of Clinical Pharmacology Division, Kantonsspital, Basel, Switzerland

M. D., University of Basel, Switzerland
Postgraduate training, Hammersmith Hospital, London
Research in cardiovascular pharmacotherapy, antibiotics

## Fülgraff, Georges M.

Prof. Dr. med.
Scientific Counselor and member of several committees in the European Community and FRG

Studies in Law, Economy, Psychology and Medicine
1959 M. D., University of Munich, FRG
1972 Professor of Pharmacology and Toxicology, University of Frankfurt/Main, FRG
1974 President of the Federal Health Office (BGA), Berlin
1980 State-Secretary of the Federal Ministry of Youth, Family Affairs and Health, Bonn, FRG

## Gordon, Arnold J.

Ph. D.
Executive Director, Scientific Affairs and Safety Assurance, Pfizer International Inc., New York, NY, USA

1960 B. S., Chemical Engineering, Northeastern University, USA
1962 M. S., Organic Chemistry, New York University, USA
1964 Ph. D., Chemistry, New York University, USA
1964–1966 Captain, U.S. Army Chemical Corps
1966–1971 Assistant Professor, Chemistry Dept., Catholic University of America, Washington, DC, USA
1971–1974 Associate Director/Group Director, Scientific Affairs, Pfizer Pharmaceuticals, New York, NY, USA

## Gorovitz, Samuel

Prof.
Dean, College of Arts and Sciences and Professor of Philosophy, Syracuse University, Syracuse, NY, USA

Author of several publications, including *Drawing the Line: Life, Death, and Ethical Choices in an American Hospital*, Oxford University Press, 1990

## Haas, Joanna F.

M. D.
Director, Corporate Drug Safety, Boehringer Ingelheim GmbH, Germany

B. A., M. D., Boston University School of Medicine, Boston, MA, USA
M. Sc., Epidemiology, Columbia University School of Public Health
Fellow of the American College of Physicians; Fellow of the American College of Preventive Medicine

## Horisberger, Bruno

Dr. med.
Director of Interdisciplinary Research Centre for Public Health, St. Gallen, Switzerland

1952 graduated, University Zurich
1957–1959 Research Fellow in Occupational Physiology, Swiss Federal Institute of Technology
1959–1960 Research Fellow, Chronic Disease Research Institute, Buffalo, NY, USA
1963–1979 Surgery and Head of Surgical Intensive Care Unit, Cantonal Hospital, St. Gallen
1971 Founder and Director, Interdisciplinary Research Centre for Public Health
1980 Chief Medical Officer, Canton of St. Gallen
Member of the editorial board of the *International Journal of Health Sciences* and co-editor of the book series on Health Systems Research by Springer-Verlag

## Jones, Judith Karen

M. D., Ph. D.
President, The Degge Group, Ltd., Arlington, VA, USA; Medical Director, Health Information Designs, Arlington VA, USA

1962 B. A., Baylor University, Waco, TX, USA
1966 M. D., Baylor College of Medicine, Houston, TX, USA
1973 Ph. D., University of California, San Francisco, CA, USA
1974–1978 Chief, Division of Clinical Pharmacology, Presbyterian Hospital, San Francisco, CA; Assistant Clinical Professor, University of California, San Francisco, CA, USA
1978–1985 Special Assistant to Director/Director, Center for Drugs and Biologics, U.S. Food and Drug Administration, Rockville, MD
Since 1985 Associate, Clinical Prof., Geriatrics/Medicine, Georgetown University, School of Medicine, Washington, DC

## Koide, Goro

Commentator, NHK (Japan Broadcasting Corporation), Tokyo, Japan

Degree in Radioecology, University of Tokyo, Japan
Producer/director of television series, including *The Universe Within: Human Body*
Author of various publications, including *The Brain* and *Energy Strategy*

## Kreutz, Gottfried

Prof. Dr. med.
Head, Department Arzneimittelverkehr, Institute for Drugs, Federal Health Office (BGA), Berlin

1967–1973 Studies in Medicine, Free University, Berlin; University of Sheffield, UK
1973–1974 Medical internship
1975–1979 Studies in chemistry, Technical University, Berlin
1982 Dr. med.
Postgraduate studies in internal medicine, pharmacology and toxicology

## Leisinger, Klaus M.

Prof. Ph. D.
Deputy Director, Ciba-Geigy Ltd., Basel, Switzerland

Ph. D., Economics and Social Sciences, University of Basel, Switzerland
Professor for Development Policy, University of Basel, Switzerland
Former manager of Ciba-Geigy Pharmaceuticals in Sub-Saharan Africa
Member of the Business and Industry Advisory Committee, Organization for Economic Cooperation and Development (OECD), the Advisory Committee for International Development Cooperation, Swiss Federal Council, and the Expert Group, Swiss National Research Fund
Consultant to the United Nations
Author of a series of books and articles on development policy and business ethics

## Lewandowski, Guenter

Head of Pharma Policy Department, Pharmaceutical Division, Ciba-Geigy Ltd., Basle, Switzerland

Studies in Law (West Berlin, FRG, and Lausanne Switzerland); former Vice-President of the Federal Health Office (BGA), FRG

## Lowrance, William W.

Ph. D.
Senior Fellow and Director, Life Sciences and Public Policy Program, The Rockefeller University, New York, NY, USA

1965 A. B., Chemistry and Biology, University of North Carolina, Chapel Hill, NC, USA
1970 Ph. D., Organic and Biological Chemistry, Rockefeller University, New York, NY, USA
Author of the books *Of Acceptable Risk: Science and the Determination of Safety, Modern Science and Human Values* and *Confronting Health Risks*

## Luce, Bryan R.

M. B. A., Ph. D.
Director, Medical Technology Assessment Program, Battelle Human Research Center, Washington, DC, USA

## Maccoby, Nathan

Janet M. Peck Professor of International Communication, Emeritus, Stanford University, USA; Associate Director, Stanford Center for Research in Desease Prevention

1950 Ph. D., Psychology, University of Michigan, USA
Fellow, Academy of Behavioral Medicine, American Psychological Association, and International Communication Association

## Mann, Ronald D.

M. D.
Medical Services Secretary, Royal Society of Medicine, London, UK

1952 M. B., B. S., Westminster Hospital, London, UK
1969 M. D., University of London
Author of several publications, including *Risk and Consent to Risk in Medicine* (1989) and *Oral Contraceptives and Breast Cancer* (1990)

## MORRIS, LOUIS A.

Ph. D.
Acting Director, Division of Drug Advertising and Labeling, Food and Drug Administration, Rockville, MD, USA

Scholar-in-Residence, Center for Marketing Policy Research, American University, Washington, DC, USA
Ph. D., Psychology, Tulane University, New Orleans, LA, USA
Author of 75 articles and the recent book, *Communicating Therapeutic Risks*

## NAKAGAWA, HISAO

Director, Office of ADR Information, Pharmaceuticals and Chemicals Safety Division, Ministry of Health and Welfare, Tokyo, Japan

1971–1976 Department of Chemical Synthesis, National Institute of Hygienic Sciences; Pharmaceutical Affairs Bureau, Ministry of Health and Welfare, Tokyo, Japan
1976–1979 Chemical Specialist, Office for the Safety of Household Products, Environmental Health Bureau, Ministry of Health and Welfare, Tokyo, Japan
1979–1982 Deputy Director, Biological Products Division, Pharmaceutical Affairs Bureau, Ministry of Health and Welfare, Tokyo, Japan
1983–1988 Chemical Specialist, Department of Environmental Health, Environment Agency
1988–1989 Deputy Director, Inspection and Guidance Division, Pharmaceutical Affairs Bureau, Ministry of Health and Welfare, Tokyo, Japan

## PFANNER, JEAN

Dr. jur.
Director, Intercantonal Office for the Control of Medicines (IOCM), Berne, Switzerland

1959 Law degree, University of Berne, Switzerland
1959–1960 Postgraduate studies in London and Salzburg
Several positions in the private sector and with Swiss cantonal authorities
Former Director of the Schweizerische Genossenschaft für Getreide und Futtermittel (GGF)

## SIMON PETER

Director General, Head of Pharmaceutical Division, Hoffmann-La Roche Ltd., Basle, Switzerland

Master of Business Administration, University of Basel, Switzerland
1973 General Manager, Ogden Filter Company, Los Angeles, CA, USA
1977 General Manager South Africa and Marketing Director Europe, Africa and Middle East, Schering Plough Corporation, USA
1985 Regional Manager Europe and North America, Pharma Division, Hoffmann-La Roche, then Pharma Marketing Director

## Spitzer, Walter O.

Prof., M. D.
Professor and Chairman, Department of Epidemiology and Biostatistics, Strathcona Professor of Preventive Medicine, and Professor of Medicine, McGill University, Montreal, Canada

1962 M. D., University of Toronto, Canada
1966 M. H. A., University of Michigan, USA
1970 M. P. H., Epidemiology and Public Health, Yale University, USA Editor of *Journal of Clinical Epidemiology* and founder of *Clinical and Investigative Medicine*

## Stearns, Beverly Peterson

Freelance writer and editor, Basle, Switzerland

1967 B. A., Journalism, University of Washington, Seattle, WA, USA
Experience as a journalist with The Associated Press, Canadian Press and, currently, with AP-Dow Jones, Zurich

## Strandberg, Kjell

M. D., Ph. D.
Director, Dept. of Drugs, National Board of Health and Welfare, Uppsala, Sweden

1967 M. D.
1971 Ph. D., Pharmacology
1971–1974 Lecturer in Clinical Pharmacology
1974–1976 Resident in Pulmonary Medicine
1977–1982 Professor of Pharmacotherapeutics, National Board of Health and Welfare, Dept. of Drugs
1977–1984 Head of the Division of Clinical Pharmacology, University Hospital, Uppsala, Sweden
Since 1984 Director, WHO Collaborating Centre for International Drug Monitoring, Uppsala, Sweden
Chairman, EFTA Expert Group on Pharmaceutical

## Takeuchi, Tetsuo

Manager, Medical Information Dept., Yamanouchi Pharmaceutical Co., Ltd., Tokyo, Japan

Bachelor of Pharmacology, Toyama University
Since 1955 with Yamanouchi Pharmaceutical Co., Ltd.

## Tanaka, Yasumasa

Prof., Ph. D.
Professor of Social Psychology and Communication, Department of Political Science, Gakushuin University, Tokyo, Japan
B. A., Political Science, Gakushuin University, Tokyo, Japan
M. A., Political Science, University of Illinois, USA
Ph. D., Communication, University of Illinois, USA
Litt. D., Psychology
President, Japan Election Studies Association; member of the Board of Directors, Japan

Political Science Association, Japan Atomic Energy Forum, and Japan Nuclear Safety Research Association
Author of nine books in Japanese, and 200 articles and papers in Japanese and English

## Taylor, David

Ph. D.
Manager of Corporate Communications and Projects, Ciba-Geigy (Japan) Ltd., Takarazuka, Japan

1969 B. A., Philosophy, Rutgers University, NJ, USA
1974 Ph. D., Political Philosophy, Rutgers University, NJ, USA
1981–1985 Director of Public Policy for Pharma Division, Ciba-Geigy, Summit, NJ, USA
1986–1989 Head of Pharma Policies and Issues Group, Pharma Policy and Economics Department, Ciba-Geigy Ltd., Basle, Switzerland
1989–1990 Deputy Head of the Pharma Policy and Public Affairs Department, Pharma Division, Ciba-Geigy (Japan) Ltd., Takarazuka, Japan

## Tolo, Kenneth W.

Prof. Ph. D.
Vice Provost, University of Texas, Austin, and Professor, Lyndon B. Johnson School of Public Affairs, University of Texas, Austin, TX, USA

1962 B. A., Mathematics, Concordia College, Moorhead, MN, USA
1968 Ph. D., Mathematics, University of Nebraska, USA
1972 M. A., Public Affairs, University of Minnesota, USA
Author or editor of various public policy publications

## Vander Stichele, Robert H.

M. D.
General Practitioner, City of Gent, Belgium

Coordinating officer of the Belgian PPI Evaluation Research Project, Heymans Institute of Pharmacology, State University of Gent, Belgium; Secretary of the Flemish General Practice Research Institute

## Von Wartburg, Walter P.

Prof. Dr. jur.
Member of the Pharma Management Committee, Ciba-Geigy Ltd., Basle, Switzerland

1963 Doctorate, Faculty of Law, University of Basel, Switzerland
1965–1966 Legal and economic studies at Princeton University, USA, and Harvard Law School, USA, Master of Law degree
Professor of Public Health Policy, Graduate School of Economics, Business and Public Administration, St. Gallen, Switzerland

## Walker, Stuart R.

Prof. Ph. D.
Director of the Centre for Medicines Research, Carshalton, Surrey, England; Honorary Professor of the Welsh School of Pharmacy, Cardiff, Wales

Current research includes assessment of new medicines, improving methodology for assessing quality of life in the determination of the benefits of medicines and evaluation of post-marketing surveillance schemes
Author of six books and over 100 research papers

## WHITEHORN, KATHARINE, E.

Columnist and Associate Editor, *The Observer*, London, UK; Vice-President, The Patients' Association; Vice-President, Open Section, Royal Society of Medicine

M. A., Newnham College, Cambridge
Director, Nationwide Anglia Building Society
Publication of various books, including *View from a Column*, and *How to Survive in Hospital*

## WIHOLM, BENGT-ERIK

M. D., Ph. D.
Associate Professor, Head, Pharmacoepidemiology Section, Division of Pharmacoepidemiology and Information, Medical Products Agency, Uppsala, Sweden; secretary of the Adverse Drug Reactions Advisory Committee

Associate Professor of Clinical Pharmacology, Department of Clinical Pharmacology, The Karolinska Institute, Huddinge University Hospital, Sweden

## YOUNG, ERNLE, W. D.

Ph. D.
Co-Director, Stanford University Center for Biomedical Ethics

Clinical Professor of Medicine and Pediatrics (Ethics), Stanford University, CA, USA
B. A. and M. A., Systematic Theology, Rhodes University, Grahamstown, South Africa
Ph. D., Theological Ethics, Southern Methodist University, Dallas, TX, USA
Chaplain to the Stanford Medical Center
Associate Dean, Stanford Memorial Church
Author, *Alpha and Omega: Ethics at the Frontiers of Life and Death* and co-author of *A Time to Be Born, A Time to Die: Ethics and Conflicts in an Intensive Care Nursery*

# 58. International Life Sciences Institute

The International Life Sciences Institute (ILSI) is a nonprofit public foundation which was established in 1978 to advance the sciences of nutrition, toxicology, and risk assessment. The membership includes more than 160 food, pharmaceutical, and chemical companies worldwide, which pool their resources to resolve health and safety problems. Through sponsoring research, conferences, publication, and educational programs, ILSI brings together scientists from government, academia, and industry to work on health and safety issues.

ILSI is headquartered in Washington, DC, has branches in Australia, Europe, Japan, and North America and is expanding to Brazil, Mexico, and Malaysia. The branches enable members to respond to local issues by working with governments and scientists immediately involved while also utilizing ILSI's global network of scientists and resources.

In 1988, the World Health Organization (WHO) officially recognized ILSI as a nongovernmental organization, a designation which allows it to work officially with WHO on nutrition, food safety, and risk assessment issues. An ILSI scientist is located at the WHO offices in Geneva to better collaborate with scientists there.

ILSI supports programs to resolve long-term basic scientific issues, as well as programs to address issues of regional and more immediate concern. For example, it has established the Risk Science Institute to improve the scientific basis for risk assessment and the Research Foundation to support basic research and educational activities in nutrition and toxicology. In 1989, it set up the Health and Environmental Sciences Institute to address safety issues in an area which includes pharmaceutical, chemical, petrochemical, and automobile industries. The founding members and current Board of Members of the Health an Environmental Sciences Institute include 14 companies.

ILSI Europe, established in 1986 with headquarters in Brussels, has 47 member companies and working groups on nutrition, toxicology, packaging materials, microbiology, and food technology. This group prepares short monographs on a number of scientific subjects and also shares information with its members about regulatory developments in Europe.

The Board of Trustees of ILSI is the principal policy-making body and consists of an equal number of private sector and public trustees. The private sector trustees are representatives of ILSI's member companies; the public trustees come from universities, research organizations and foundations. This leadership and ILSI's structure as a member-driven organization with international branches and scientific institutes, have encouraged an exchange of ideas by experts on a variety of issues, regardless of scientific backgrounds and locations. ILSI itself does not maintain a permanent research staff or laboratory facilities. Instead, it sponsors scientific studies at major universities and research centers and thus retains flexibility to respond to the latest advances or emerging public health issues.

ILSI has recognized the area of risk perception, communication, and research as one which has consistently received little serious attention, and it has undertaken to change this situation. The Risk Science Institute focuses on one project in the area of risk communication or risk perception each year at some academic setting in the United States. Like other ILSI committees and programs, the Risk Science Institute works with various government agencies. RSI has a cooperative agreement with the United States Environmental Protection Agency to sponsor workshops and conferences on scientific issues of critical importance for health risk assessment. In addition, RSI was the sponsor of the National Academy of Science publication, "Improving Risk Communication." One of the recommendations of this document was to develop a consumers' guide to risk and risk communication, to articulate key terms, concepts and trade-offs in risk communication for the lay audience, and to make audiences better able to discern misleading and incomplete information. A working group is now following through on efforts to write such a guide.

It is the view of ILSI that major challenges of the 1990s will lie in the areas of risk assessment, risk perception and risk communication. Through its Risk Sciences Institute and its Health and Enviromental Sciences Institute, ILSI will continue to focus in on various facets of risk with an aim to advance the understanding of science for the benefit and good health of all countries.

# 59. International Medical Benefit/Risk Foundation – RAD-AR

By the close of the Wolfsberg dialogue conference, many participants had expressed a wish to see the kind of projects generated under the RAD-AR umbrella translated into a broader, more formal structure of an international body. Since April, a great deal of research has been carried out into the kind of organization that would answer current and future needs with regard to medical benefit/risk assessment.

Now a foundation is being set up as a fully independent, nonprofit organization, whose governance, funding and work will be open to a wide audience of interested and committed parties. The foundation will be headquartered in Geneva, in order to take advantage of the city's neutrality and accessibility.

A number of major multinational corporations have made a firm commitment to membership in the RAD-AR Consortium, and quite a few more firms are expected to join. Professor William W. Lowrance of The Rockefeller University in New York is serving as the Acting Executive Director of the foundation. The foundation will be officially established and launched in early 1991.

The International Medical Benefit/Risk Foundation – RAD-AR will strive to enhance public health by facilitating judicious benefit/risk assessment and application of pharmaceutical products and other medical technologies by health-care providers and consumers.

More than any particular techniques or procedures, the foundation is devoted to fostering an approach, an outlook, an attitude encouraging a "culture of informed weighing" of medical benefits against risks. As its name indicates, the foundation's potential scope may include a wide range of medical benefit/risk issues, such as those surrounding over-the-counter preparations, diagnostic procedures, vaccines, biotechnological innovations, and therapeutic choices in general. Initially it is likely to focus on pharmaceutical questions.

**The foundation will pursue its purpose by:**

- Helping advance the state-of-the-art of relevant scientific methods, decision-making approaches, and communication techniques;

- Supporting development of capabilities for gathering, evaluating, and disseminating needed scientific information, such as statistical analyses of medical benefits and risks of drugs in actual use (pharmacoepidemiology);
- Addressing the perception and ethical evaluation of medical options by the health-care professions and institutions, manufacturers, and the public;
- Fostering fuller professional and public understanding and adoption of benefit/risk approaches to making health-care decisions;
- Assisting in the resolution of controversies that arise in connection with pharmaceutical and other medical approaches; and
- Generally serving as a major resource and coordination center for addressing medical benefit/risk problems.

To achieve its ends, the foundation will sponsor and coordinate social and economic research, develop case studies of controversies and decisions, establish networks, convene workshops and conferences, pursue educational and training activities, provide forums, and nurture the development of organizations having related interests. The foundation will sponsor and fund other bodies in conducting some projects, and will conduct some projects itself. Wherever feasible, the foundation will work in collaboration with other organizations that are involved in addressing these problems.

The foundation will actively coordinate with existing national RAD-AR councils and working groups, seeking ways to work synergistically. Also it will help establish councils in additional nations.

Various other committees and affiliations will be established wherever desirable. The foundation offers to work cooperatively with regulatory agencies, and with such bodies as the World Health Organization and the Commission of the European Community. Similarly, it intends to work with patient/consumer representatives and other organizations concerned with health care. The foundation invites approaches from all interested parties.

# 60. Subject Index

MIX
Papier aus verantwortungsvollen Quellen
Paper from responsible sources
FSC® C105338

If you have any concerns about our products,
you can contact us on
**ProductSafety@springernature.com**

In case Publisher is established outside the EU,
the EU authorized representative is:
**Springer Nature Customer Service Center GmbH**
**Europaplatz 3, 69115 Heidelberg, Germany**

Printed by Libri Plureos GmbH
in Hamburg, Germany